It's Not Just Growing Pains

It's Not Just Growing Pains

A Guide to Childhood Muscle, Bone, and Joint Pain, Rheumatic Diseases, and the Latest Treatments

THOMAS J. A. LEHMAN, MD, FAAP, FACR

OXFORD
UNIVERSITY PRESS
2004

OXFORD
UNIVERSITY PRESS

Oxford New York
Auckland Bangkok Buenos Aires Cape Town Chennai
Dar es Salaam Delhi Hong Kong Istanbul Karachi Kolkata
Kuala Lumpur Madrid Melbourne Mexico City Mumbai Nairobi
São Paulo Shanghai Taipei Tokyo Toronto

Published by Oxford University Press, Inc.
198 Madison Avenue, New York, New York 10016
www.oup.com

Library of Congress Cataloging-in-Publication Data
Lehman, Thomas J. A.
It's not just growing pains : a guide to childhood muscle, bone, and joint pain, rheumatic diseases, and the latest treatments / Thomas J. A. Lehman.
p. cm.
Includes bibliographical references and index.
ISBN 0-19-515728-1
1. Pediatric rheumatology. 2. Rheumatism in children. I. Title.
RJ482.R48 L448 2004
618.92'723—dc21
2003010938
Rev.

1 3 5 7 9 8 6 4 2
Printed in the United States of America
on acid-free paper

This book is truly dedicated to the many children around the world with muscle, bone, or joint pain or arthritis—and to their families and the physicians and other professionals who care for them. It is intended to help them by helping parents and professionals to be sure these children are being properly diagnosed and treated.

On a more personal note, I would like to dedicate this book to the memory of five physicians who greatly inspired me but are no longer with us:

Dr. Harry O. Zamkin, a pediatrician who loved his patients;

Dr. Virgil Hanson, a pediatric rheumatologist who taught me that pediatric rheumatology was not learned from textbooks—it is learned by listening and carefully evaluating the children you treat, every time you see them;

Dr. Barbara Ansell, a pediatric rheumatologist who taught me that an "atypical case of A" was most likely a "typical case of B" that I had not thought of, and so much more;

Dr. Arthur D. Schwabe, a gastroenterologist who taught me to never stop asking questions of the children, their families, and myself until all the answers fit together and made sense;

Dr. John Decker, for many years the "Dean" of rheumatology at the National Institutes of Health in Bethesda who inspired so many by his quiet confidence combined with a willingness to endorse any idea that seemed sensible, no matter that it had "never been done before";

and last, to **Dr. Jack Klippel** (who is very much still with us!), for continuing to say, "If not you, who? It's your idea—do it."

Contents

PART II: THE RHEUMATIC DISEASES AND RELATED CONDITIONS

PART III: LIVING WITH A CHILD WHO HAS A CHRONIC CONDITION

Introduction

This is not a textbook. It is a guidebook. Like a traveler's guidebook it will help you find your way in unfamiliar territory. This book provides both the information an intelligent parent of a child with muscle, bone, or joint pain or arthritis needs to make sure his or her child is getting the best care and the information a health professional, unfamiliar with pediatric rheumatology, needs to guide them. My goal is to help you understand what is happening to your child (or the child you care for) and why.

For parents, this book will serve as a guide to help understand the many causes of muscle, bone, and joint pain, to help understand their doctors' decisions, and to help understand what to expect for their child in the future. This book will give parents the information necessary to ask meaningful questions and properly evaluate the alternative choices available for their child's care.

For physicians, this book is designed to help in the recognition and care of children who need to be referred to a specialist. Often parents will seek help from their primary physician or other health professionals because they have questions about the specialist's recommendations. This book provides the information needed to explain these recommendations and help parents understand their choices. It also provides the information necessary to allow health care professionals to ask the specialist meaningful questions.

This is not a textbook of pediatric rheumatology or pediatric orthopedics. It is a guide to the chronic rheumatic and orthopedic conditions of childhood. Like every guidebook, it does not cover everything. I have emphasized the more common conditions and the more important problems. Not everyone will agree with all that I have written—just as traveler's guidebooks may disagree on which are the best restaurants and hotels in a given city. If you are looking for long lists of detailed references, put this book down. The phone book will tell you every restaurant, every hotel, and every museum in the city with complete objectivity. A guidebook will not list them all but will tell you which ones the authors believe you should choose. This book will provide you with the insights I have gained from over twenty-five years of experience in caring for children with muscle, bone, and joint pain and rheumatic diseases.

In this day and age, millions of dollars are spent annually on research into causes of disease and newer medications, but few of the children I see do poorly because doctors lack the necessary tools to treat them. The majority of children with rheumatic disease do well. Most who do poorly do so because too much time elapsed before they came to proper medical attention or because their parents and caregivers had too little understanding of the many treatments available and the importance of proper treatment.

I am writing this book for an audience of both parents and professionals in the hope that it will speed the proper diagnosis and referral of many children with unrecognized or improperly treated problems. The parents will find words that are sometimes unfamiliar, and the professionals definitions for which they have no need. My apologies to all of you. There is a glossary at the end of the text.

Much of the information in this book is not in textbooks, and in many cases it has not been rigorously proven. This is the type of information for which you go out of your way to find an experienced specialist. Any physician can go to the library and read the chapter in the textbooks. Often when parents discuss treatment options with their physicians, reference will be made to "controlled clinical trials." It is important to understand that there are far too few children with rheumatic disease for large-scale controlled trials of any but the simplest questions.

The absence of controlled trials is upsetting to both parents and the many physicians in the field. However, it is impossible to fill an auditorium with children with rheumatic disease and agree that everyone on the left gets treatment A and everyone on the right gets treatment B. Even without worrying about funding, we don't have enough children with most of these diseases *whose disease is similar enough in severity* for proper comparison. The most important questions regarding which treatment gives the best long-term results require five or ten years of follow-up. We can't wait that long to start treating your child.

When physicians, trained in the field, cannot all agree on the right answers, how are parents going to make the proper choices? This book reflects my experience. My goal is to give you the benefit of that experience to help you get the best outcome for your child. The care of children with muscle, bone, and joint pain and arthritis is still more an art than a science. As in cooking, the best results depend far more on experience, careful monitoring, and minor adjustments than on strict adherence to the written recipe. Not every physician will share my opinions. Not every physician is willing to go beyond the "proven" in reaching for the best possible outcome. The final decisions will always be yours.

A note on the case histories:
I have included many illustrative stories throughout the text. The names, ages, and other identifying details have been changed to protect patient confidentiality, but the examples are all real ones from my experience.

How to Use This Book

The purpose of this book is to guide families and their health care providers through the process of determining and responding to whatever is causing the children they care for to have muscle, bone, or joint pain or arthritis. *Everyone reading this book will have different needs and a different background.* I have tried to make the writing clear and the science easily understood, with as little medical jargon as possible. However, I've been caring for children with these problems for over twenty-five years. What seems obvious to me may not be to you. *If a word confuses you, look in the glossary at the back.*

If a section confuses you, take this book with you to the doctor's office and ask the doctor or nurse to take a minute and explain it. But don't surprise a busy physician with a request that takes extra time. If you want your child more carefully evaluated or need time to ask extra questions, call ahead and ask the physician's office to schedule a long appointment. You want your physician to be relaxed and to take time with you and your child.

If you are the parent of a child who has been given a diagnosis, you should begin by reading about that diagnosis to see whether it describes your child. For parents who know their child's diagnosis, this book has useful chapters on medications, the meaning of laboratory test results, family issues, getting the best care for your child, and reconstructive surgery. You will find a lot of information that will allow you to make informed choices and get the best possible results for your child.

If you are the parent of a child who does not have a diagnosis, or the diagnosis does not seem correct to you, you should begin with Chapter 2,

"Figuring Out What's Wrong." It is my goal to help you think about what the correct answer might be. Then you should approach your physician and discuss your thoughts. It is to be hoped that he or she will be happy to discuss the situation with you, to help you to understand why the diagnosis is correct, or to rethink the diagnosis with you. Don't be afraid to call your physician's office and ask for a long appointment, as discussed above.

This book will help you to understand why physicians ask the questions they ask, and perhaps what questions they should have asked, but didn't. *Don't be afraid to volunteer information that the physician didn't ask for.* Make sure your child is getting the time and attention needed. If you are dissatisfied after discussing your child's care with your physician, see Chapter 27, "Getting the Best Results for Your Child."

If you are a health care professional who is not a pediatric rheumatologist, this book will give you the information you need to evaluate children with musculoskeletal pain before you refer them. This book will help primary care physicians to know what tests to do and to decide whether and to which specialist to refer the child. This book will also help nurses, primary care physicians, and other health care providers to evaluate the advice their patients are being given. *Specialists need your help in explaining to families what they are doing to take care of the children and why.* If the situation doesn't make sense to you, call the specialist yourself. If you don't get the answers you need to make things clear to the family, there's a problem. Knowing when to recommend that your patient seek an additional opinion is one of the most important services you can provide. No specialist should ever be afraid of listening to a different viewpoint.

If you have questions, get answers. Do not sit still and do nothing. Many of the answers can be found in this book. If you don't find the answers to all your questions here, this book will give you the information you need so that you can ask the right questions of the specialist and evaluate the answers you receive with confidence.

Part I

MY CHILD COMPLAINS OF PAIN

1

Growing Pains?

Little Jennifer S. was fourteen months old when her mother noticed that she did not want to put her left foot firmly on the floor when she was taken out of her crib one morning. She did not seem to walk right for a few minutes, but an hour later she seemed fine. It did not happen again until a couple of weeks later. After six weeks, Jennifer's mother noticed that it was happening more frequently. She mentioned this to the pediatrician when Jennifer was in for her immunizations one afternoon. The pediatrician wiggled Jennifer's leg around, watched her walk a few feet, and reassured Jennifer's mother that she was fine. When Mrs. S. called the pediatrician a month later to discuss bringing her in, she was told it was probably just "growing pains." By the time Jennifer was seen in the pediatric rheumatology clinic at the age of two years, the left knee was markedly swollen, she could not straighten her left leg out all the way, and the muscles of her left leg were much weaker than the right side. Jennifer had obvious arthritis. Reassured by what the pediatrician had told her, her mother had continued to believe Jennifer just had growing pains until Jennifer screamed when the nurse tried to straighten her leg at her two-year-old checkup.

Things you need to know

- Growing pains never occur during the daytime.
- No matter how severe the pain at night, children with growing pains are always fine the next morning.
- Any child with pain on waking up in the morning or during the day requires a full medical evaluation.

Whenever a child limps or complains that an arm or leg hurts, our first thought is that he or she must have injured it. Even if a child is old enough to deny an injury, we often assume that the child just does not remember. The family is likely to seek medical advice only if the pain is very severe or persists for more than a day or two. Even when the pain or limp continues beyond a few days, parents and many physicians often dismiss the problem as growing pains. Children do have growing pains; in fact they are fairly common. But unfortunately, many children with serious problems are misdiagnosed with growing pains for weeks or even months. Children with arthritis are often first noticed because they walk abnormally when they wake up in the morning, but since "they get better in a few minutes," no one is concerned.

Growing pains typically occur in young children between the ages of three and eight years. The child will wake up suddenly from a deep sleep complaining that his or her legs hurt. Parents become aware of the problem because the child is crying in bed. Most often the episode occurs a few hours after the child has gone to sleep, but it can occur in the middle of the night. Typically, the child will point to the front or back of the knee, or the muscles just above the knee. The pain will usually disappear with ten or fifteen minutes of gentle massage and be completely gone in the morning. The pain is almost always in a large joint such as the knee, not a finger or toe. Sometimes the pains will wake the child up two or three nights in a row, but more often they occur episodically over a period of weeks or months. Growing pains often occur after days of extra activity. They may disappear for months or a year only to start up again during another period of rapid growth.

The key finding in evaluating a child for growing pains is that the child is absolutely fine when he or she wakes up in the morning. There is no pain, limp, or any other abnormality. If any pain is still present when the child wakes up in the morning or any pain occurs while the child is awake, this must not be dismissed as growing pains. Such pains are not always due to a serious condition, but they are not growing pains.

For a child with typical growing pains, a trip to the doctor is not usually necessary. If a child has absolutely classic pains and is always fine in the morning, the family can usually treat the child with gentle reassurance. However, if the pains are persistent or unusually severe, a medical examination is warranted. Any child with pain during the day should be medically evaluated.

If blood tests or X rays are done at the time of medical evaluation, a child with growing pains should have absolutely normal results. Bone scans, magnetic resonance images (MRIs), and other special tests are not necessary for a child with growing pains. But they may be necessary to exclude other causes of pain in children who have atypical findings or pain during the day.

There are a variety of explanations for growing pains, and doctors are not in complete agreement regarding which explanation is correct. The best explanation is that growing pains are the result of tendons and muscles being stretched as the bones of the legs become longer. There is evidence that the body produces more growth hormone at night, and some doctors believe the body is actually growing faster at night, leading to the pain. A more likely explanation is related to the gate control theory of pain. This is easy to explain. As you read these words you will suddenly become aware of feeling the shoes on your feet (if you're wearing shoes). A minute ago you probably were not aware of the feeling. The nerves in your feet that feel the pressure from your shoes did not suddenly turn on. They were always sending their message to your brain. However, the center in your brain that receives information from all the different nerves in your body filters this information and decides what to make you aware of and what you can ignore.

During the day when children are active, any message to the brain from tendons and muscles being stretched by growth is lost in all the other things going on. But when a child is falling asleep at night and there are no distractions, the pain impulses from stretching the muscles and tendons may be passed on to the higher brain centers, causing the child to wake up. As a result, growing pains occur most often during periods of rapid growth and after days of extra physical activity (when they may be joined by muscle complaints).

Growing pains can be disturbing to both parents and children, particularly when they occur several days in a row. Most often gentle massage and reassurance are enough to help the child get back to sleep. Children with more severe pain usually will respond to a dose of acetaminophen or ibuprofen just as you would treat them for a headache during the day. If they wake up with pain several nights in a row, it may be helpful to give them a dose of medication at bedtime. This will decrease the perception of pain and may prevent the child from waking up. After two or three nights without episodes, the medication should be stopped.

Growing pains will go away. They may come back when the child goes through another period of rapid growth, but they never stay. While inconvenient, they are not of any long-term significance. They do not interfere with proper growth or development. But remember, growing pains never occur during the day. If the child is complaining of pain during the day, a more complete investigation should be done.

If the pains persist despite medication or return as soon as the medication is stopped, a full medical evaluation should be done. The first step is to be sure that the cause is just growing pains. Surprisingly, growing pains tend to run in families. If one of your children is having a lot of growing pains, ask your parents and your spouse's parents. It's likely one of you also had a lot of growing pains.

2

Figuring Out What's Wrong

Before medical school I had to take all the required classes in college. Many of the classes required for medical school satisfied the requirements for majoring in zoology in college. I enjoy the outdoors and was happy to sign up for field zoology as one of the required courses. Armed with guidebooks, we walked around the local hills in small groups with an instructor looking for and identifying birds. Sometimes the instructor would hear a noise or see a bird vaguely in the distance and tell us what it was. Frequently, it was too far away to see the identifying characteristics noted in the guidebook, but when we got closer we would see that he was correct in his identification. Other times one of us would become very excited and announce that we had just seen a bird we had never seen before and we were sure it was, for example, a Mexican jay. The instructor would just shake his head. No matter how sure we were that it matched the picture in the book, he would point out that we were not in (or even close to) Mexico and that a common bird in our area looked a little bit like the Mexican jay. A few minutes' investigation would invariably prove that he was right and we were wrong. He had been teaching this course in the same hills for many years. Each different bird had a typical behavior, a typical place it was likely to be seen, and a typical time of year it was likely to be there. These things were not in our guidebooks, but the instructor knew them from experience. With years of experience it was easy for him to recognize birds from much further away than we could and to know when we could not have seen what we thought we saw. He knew that there were rare exceptions, but they were always unlikely.

Things you need to know

- Just like the birds above, diseases have characteristic behaviors.
- There is a typical age when they occur.
- There are typical complaints from the parents and child.
- There are things that the diseases typically do not do that should make you question the diagnosis.
- A complete history involves listening to your complaints and asking many questions that you will think cannot possibly have anything to do with your child's problems.
- Always give your child a chance to talk—even young children can explain more about what's happening to their bodies than you think. Many have symptoms of which you may not be aware.
- A complete physical examination involves looking at your entire child, not just the part that you know hurts.

When evaluating a child with muscle, bone, or joint pain it is important to understand that each of the conditions that may be responsible has a typical set of problems it causes (symptoms), a typical age group where it occurs, and other typical findings that make it easy for an experienced physician to diagnose—just as it was easy for my instructor to recognize the birds in a familiar park. At the same time, if a child does not have the typical problems or is not the typical age, it's much less likely that the suspected condition is the proper explanation. This is why your physician should always start the evaluation by asking you questions about the problem. As you read through this book you will see that I have clearly indicated the typical presentation for each of the conditions a child might have.

TAKING AND GIVING A HISTORY

As a parent evaluating your own child, ask yourself these questions and think about the answers. Your physician will want to know the answers to help arrive at an appropriate diagnosis. In addition, knowing the answers to these questions, and what diseases they suggest, will help you in determining whether the physician's diagnosis makes sense to you. If it does not, discuss what you have noticed with your physician. If the physician is not interested in your child's history, something's wrong.

The first thing you should have in mind when you go to the doctor's office is your *chief complaint*. What is it that you want the doctor to fix? Do not tell the doctor things other doctors have told you. Tell the doctor what the problem is as clearly as you can. For example, "My left knee hurts." Or sometimes the problem is more general: "I ache all over and I feel very weak." If your child is old enough to explain, let him (or her) answer the questions in the doctor's office. You may have to help out, but you'd be shocked to realize how often parents are surprised by meaningful findings their child tells the doctor of which the parents were not aware. For teenagers it is very important to let them explain their own problems. You may have to help out, but let them go first.

The key pieces of information for the physician often can be summarized in just a few words.

- He or she needs to know the quality of the problem: Is it a sharp pain or a dull ache?
- He or she needs to know the exact location of the problem. Some problems cause the front of the knee to hurt; some the side. Sometimes the pain is above the knee; sometimes it's below. Each suggests a different diagnosis.
- How long has the pain been going on, and how did it start?
- Is it getting better over time, or worse?
- What lessens the pain, what makes it worse?

These sound like simple questions, but for an experienced physician they can rapidly lead to the diagnosis. Imagine, if you will, that a fourteen-year-old boy is brought to the doctor because his knee hurts. "Most of the time I'm fine, but when I put my foot down and turn to the left, I get a sudden sharp pain on the side of my knee. After five or ten minutes the pain gets better, but then it happens again if I put my foot down and turn left again." (This story clearly suggests a mechanical problem in the knee and probably a torn meniscus.) If the same fourteen-year-old boy says, "My knee hurts all the time," we have much less information. "It hurts when I walk on it," does not tell us very much. We need to know if it is stiff when he wakes up in the morning or hurts only with activity. Sometimes the children and parents are not sure. An experienced physician will ask the same question several different ways. "Are you stiff when you wake up in the morning? Do you have trouble getting out of the car after a long car ride? Do you have trouble getting out of your seat in the movie theater after a long movie? Suppose you and I are walking in a shopping center, how far can you walk without stopping? If we stop and sit, does your knee immediately get better or does it take five or ten minutes to get better? If we get up to go again after your knee has improved, does it start to hurt immediately and get worse? Does it seem stiff, but then get better after a few steps? Is it fine until we've been walking for ten or fifteen minutes again?" The answers to these questions will help an experienced physician to determine the correct diagnosis.

Mechanical problems often hurt after a period of use. They get better with rest. Then they start to hurt after a period of use again. Arthritis may begin to hurt after a period of use and then get better with rest, as well. However, children with arthritis will be stiff when they get up to walk again but improve after a few steps (see Part II). That's not what happens with injuries. Sometimes children and families are quite sure of the answers, sometimes not. You have to ask the same type of question several different times and consider each answer. The child with arthritis will often describe trouble with long car rides or sitting in a movie theater. Children with injuries are much less likely to do so.

Sometimes you need to go in a different direction. A child with chondromalacia patella (a mechanical irritation of the knee; see Chapter 5) may be brought to the physician's office with the same chief complaint of knee pain. There is no suggestion of stiffness, but it hurts when he or she walks long distances. If you ask whether it hurts more going up- or downstairs, children with chondromalacia patella characteristically complain of more pain going downstairs. In contrast, children with unrecognized dermatomyositis might also be complaining of leg or knee pains (see Chapter 16). They will have much more trouble going upstairs. Children with these different diseases might be the same age and the same sex. They both might complain of leg pains and point to their knees, but these are very different conditions with different causes and different treatments. Knowing that one child has more trouble going upstairs and the other more trouble going downstairs helps to guide the evaluation and eliminate unnecessary tests.

Another important question is how the pain began. If the child says, "My knee hurt immediately after I was tackled from the left crossing the forty yard line with the football," the list of possible causes (differential diagnosis) is very different from the child who cannot explain how the pain began. At the same time, you need to be very careful about histories of trauma. In small children and even in teenagers I have often seen swollen fingers or toes with the explanation, "We did not see anything, but we assumed she must have jammed it." Someone in the family should remember if a child has injured a finger or toe badly enough for it to be markedly swollen. Children who exhibit an unexplained "sausage digit" often have psoriasis-associated arthritis (see Chapter 9). I also see lots of children with spondyloarthropathies who complain of repeatedly spraining their ankles or wrists. They cannot really tell you when they sprained it; it just happens "all the time." These are not sprains at all. It's a type of arthritis that commonly causes tendons to be inflamed, mimicking a sprain.

Typically, children with injuries know exactly what happened. But children with arthritis or other diseases cannot tell you exactly how or when it started. They just assume they must have twisted it or otherwise somehow injured the joint. Parents of children with pauciarticular onset arthritis are rarely able to tell you when it began. This is a subtle arthritis that most often sneaks up on people. If the parents can tell me the child was fine until Tuesday, I know the diagnosis is not pauciarticular onset arthritis. Many other diseases also begin gradually and the parents and children cannot really tell you when they began.

Children with a history of injury

Most children with a definite history of injury have an orthopedic problem. These problems are usually easily diagnosed by the appropriate history, physical examination, X rays, or MRIs. If the problem was that straightforward, you probably would not be reading this book. Sometimes there is a definite history of injury that leads everyone in the wrong direction. A child may be brought to the emergency room limping because he or she fell a few days earlier and is not getting better. The X-ray evaluation may show arthritis or a bone infection, not an injury. In this situation, it used to be taught that the child probably fell because of the infection or arthritis and that the fall brought attention to the problem. However, we now know that an initial injury can alter the dynamics of the bone and joint, making the child more vulnerable to the onset of an infection or arthritis.

Often when I'm evaluating a child with pain that started on a certain day, I ask about what happened in the days or weeks "just before that." In the section on infection-associated arthritis in Chapter 9 you will read about types of arthritis that often begin ten to fourteen days after an episode of sore throat or flu. Another situation in which the history is important is making a diagnosis of palm frond synovitis. This type of arthritis is the result of a palm frond breaking off inside the child's knee at the time of a fall. The fall usually took place six or eight weeks before the child developed symptoms. The family has no reason to think their trip to Florida in February has anything to do with the child's knee pain in April. As a result, they will not think to mention it unless the physician asks about travel. There are many similar situations. As the parents, you cannot always rely on the physician to remember to ask you about travel, unusual pets, or other findings that might be important. Tell the physician anything you think might be important.

I was once working as a general pediatrician in the farm country of California. A mother called me and asked whether I had any experience with malaria. Knowing that malaria does not occur in California, I asked, "Why?" She explained that she and her family had been living in a malarial region of Southeast Asia until two months previously. She was working there as a teacher. She and her family had returned to California, but now one of her own children was "showing the same symptoms the children in my classes in Southeast Asia showed when they had malaria. I must have stopped the medicine we were taking to prevent malaria too soon." This was easy. But imagine how long it would have taken for a physician to suspect malaria and do the right tests if the parent had simply brought the child to the doctor and said, "He has a fever and looks sick."

Physicians do not know all about the lives of the children they are taking care of. Parents do not know what is important to the physician and what is not. The key to the best possible care is an open exchange of information. Often at the very end of a long history, one parent will say, "I do not know if this is important, but . . ." Surprisingly often, that may be the key piece of information that leads us to an accurate diagnosis. To get this information, physicians will ask families a lot of questions that seem unrelated and unimportant. I ask all families these questions, because I have no way of knowing, in advance, when the answers will make a difference.

- Is the child growing well?
- Has there been any fever or rash?
- Has the child had frequent infections?
- Has there been any recent travel?

General questions that will help me to get a feel for your child's health include questions about whether they have been growing well and gaining weight as expected. Children with chronic problems or severe problems often have been losing weight. Have they been having fevers or night sweats? These types of problems often suggest a long-standing problem and perhaps a more severe one. Has the child had a lot of infections? Children with frequent ear or upper respiratory infections may have immunoglobulin A (IgA) deficiency or other immune deficiencies that are associated with an increased frequency of arthritis and other rheumatic diseases (see Chapter 9). All these questions may seem a silly waste of time if your answer is no, but they are very important when the answer is yes.

Medications

It is important to tell the physician all of the medications your child is taking, including vitamins, herbal supplements, and medications you are obtaining without a prescription. ("I gave Johnny one of Grandma's pills that she had left over from when she had a cold" can turn out to be the explanation for the entire problem. It was an allergic reaction to Grandma's medicine.) The physician needs to know what has been done to treat the problem in the past. He also needs to know what other medical problems the child is being treated for and how. Furthermore, the physician needs to be sure the child is not on a medication that may be causing the problem, including one that has recently been stopped. In addition, it is important for the physician to be sure that the child is not taking a medication that will interact with the medications the physician wants to prescribe. *If your child is allergic to medicines, know which ones they are when you go to your appointment.* Do not leave the office with your doctor "guessing" the child is not allergic to the one being prescribed today.

Past medical history

This is another long set of questions that doctors ask and families frequently wonder about. The physician needs to know whether the child has other illnesses that may be related to the joint pains or the treatment. You should try to give him or her as much information as possible. A child might be ten or eleven years old, but the strange problem he or she is having may be the result of something that happened in the neonatal intensive care unit shortly after birth. The physician cannot even begin to suspect that if he does not know that the child was in the neonatal intensive care unit. If your physician forgets to ask, you might just remind him.

> Not long ago a child was sent to me because of blood in the urine and joint pains. The referring physician was worried about lupus. After I'd gotten all the relevant information from the mother and was asking about past medical problems, she told me the child had frequently been treated for an infected parotid gland. Then I asked the child whether he had trouble making tears or eating certain foods. When I got the right answers, I knew to evaluate him for Sjogren's syndrome. Despite several years of the child's being treated for various symptoms, the correct diagnosis had not been previously considered because no one obtained the pieces of information necessary to see how everything fit together to suggest this diagnosis.

Family history

This is one of the most important parts of evaluating children with chronic disease. Many diseases have a tendency to run in families. Often I request extra tests for a disease that I would not initially have suspected because there is a strong family history of the disease. I have discovered children with inflammatory bowel disease (IBD) long before they were having abdominal symptoms because I requested the appropriate tests when I realized that they had joint pains and a family history of bowel disease. Celiac disease, rheumatic fever, psoriatic arthritis, spondyloarthropathies, and many other diseases tend to run in families.

> One of the clues to the genetic nature of diseases such as arthritis, psoriasis, diabetes, and thyroid disease comes from genetic studies. If you were to randomly pick 100,000 people on the street, all of these diseases would have the reported low frequency found in the normal

population (e.g., 15 cases per 100,000 people). However, if you select 100,000 relatives of people with one of these diseases, that disease and all of the other diseases in this group would occur far more often than expected (e.g., 75 cases per 100,000 people). From a parent's point of view, this is like knowing that a bunch of kids tend to hang out together. If Frankie and Johnnie and Pete are close friends, you should look around for Pete when you see Frankie and Johnnie. He will not always be there, but you should be looking.

Social history

Many people think social history consists simply of asking where a child goes to school, what grade he is in, and what he wants to be when they grow up. But it also includes asking about smoking or ethanol and other drug use in teenagers. It means that I know whether a child lives at home or in a boarding school. Does the child come home to mom or a babysitter or go to an after-school club? All these pieces of information may provide the answer to the problem. It's easy to consider psittacosis (pigeon fancier's disease) if you know that a child raises birds as a hobby or helps someone who does. But you have to ask about hobbies to know the answer.

Review of systems

The review of systems is your doctor's last try to find out anything you forgot to mention. Is the child allergic to any drugs? Does the child have any bleeding problems? Are there any problems with the hair, eyes, or ears? I ask about everything from the top of the head to the bottom of the feet. Not the physician, the child, nor the family knows for sure whether the answer to the problem is going to become obvious from these questions. Often it does not, but no one knows until one asks.

THE COMPLETE PHYSICAL EXAMINATION

Sam was a fourteen-year-old boy brought to my office by his mother because his ankle hurt. Sam was a good athlete and loved to play baseball and basketball. Over the last year he had suffered from repeated ankle sprains. He'd been evaluated by several orthopedists and sports medicine doctors and given a diagnosis of tendonitis. When his complaints did not go away despite casting and physical therapy, he was referred to me for a "chronic pain syndrome." Sam's ankle had been X-rayed, and CAT (computer axial tomography) scanned, and an MRI had been done. Sam and his family were very frustrated. He could not play and the doctors seemed to be implying he did not want to get better. After taking the history from Sam and his family, I sat down next to him and begin to examine his fingers and wrists. Sam immediately complained, "It's my ankle that hurts, not my hands." A moment later he jumped when I flexed his wrist fully. Careful examination revealed that Sam had inflammation in many tendons and obvious limitation of motion in his back and hips. After completing my examination I told Sam and his family he had mild arthritis and prescribed medication. They were dubious at first, but two weeks later Sam was back at basketball without problems. The key was in examining all of Sam's joints, not focusing only on the one he complained about. Even Sam had not realized he had other problems. A complete examination of "all of Sam" was the key to the proper diagnosis.

There are several key aspects to a physician's physical examination of a child. If you have a child with an obvious injury to an arm or leg, then you want the physician to examine carefully that arm or leg. However, if your child is having recurrent problems with injuries or has complaints without an obvious explanation, you want to be sure the child is examined completely. Physicians who are used to dealing with injuries often forget this.

Margie was the twelve-year-old daughter of a doctor. She had not been feeling well for several weeks. One morning she woke up with severe pain in her left knee. The pediatrician could not find anything wrong with the knee and sent her to an orthopedist. The X rays were normal and the orthopedist was stumped. When I saw Margie the next day, she was tense and anxious. Lying on the examination table, she was holding her knee bent and complaining of pain. I sat down next to her and had her relax as best she could, then carefully moved her knee. It was easy to move and not swollen. However, when I squeezed her thigh above the knee, she was tender when I compressed the bone. Then I put my hand on her abdomen and immediately noticed an enlarged, hard spleen. Margie had leukemia. Since she was complaining about her knee pain, her leg had been carefully evaluated, but no one had done blood work or examined the rest of her. When I did, the diagnosis was immediately evident.

The key to getting a proper diagnosis is a careful and complete physical examination. The physicians caring for your child need to know to look everywhere for the answer, not just where the child points. There are far too many specific findings that an experienced physician will look for to list them all here. As a parent you cannot know all the things to look for, but you can know whether the doctor evaluated your child completely or "just looked at what hurt." Diagnosing illness is like solving puzzles. You'll never do a good job if you do not collect all the clues.

> George was a sixteen-year-old boy whose family moved to the Southwest because he had severe problems with his fingers getting numb in the cold. He had been diagnosed with Raynaud's phenomenon (see Chapter 14) and given medicine. Moving to the Southwest had mostly corrected the Raynaud's, but he was having ankle pain. When George walked in to be examined, he had noticeable round red spots on his face and hands. He had seen a dermatologist who told him he had telangiectasia. This is a common finding and nothing to be worried about. In talking to George I also learned that he had seen a gastroenterologist because food sometimes got stuck going down. He had been told that his esophagus was weak. When I examined him, his fingers were long and thing and there were little sores on the fingertips. Careful examination also revealed dilated blood vessels in his nail folds (you need a magnifying glass to see this—see Fig. 21, page 199). George also had a lump on his left elbow. An orthopedist had seen this and told him it was calcium buildup, "probably from an old injury." CREST syndrome is a variant of scleroderma (see Chapter 15). The key findings are calcinosis (the bump on his arm), Raynaud's, esophageal problems (the difficulty swallowing certain foods), sclerodactyly (long thin fingers), and telangiectasia (the red spots on his face and hands). Different physicians had seen George for each of the findings, and when asked he knew about all of them. But no one had put them all together to make the proper diagnosis.

When examining a child with pain in the muscles, bone, or joints, there are several important steps. The first is to determine carefully where the pain is.

- Is the pain in the joint (where the bones come together)?
- Is the pain just above or below the joint?
- Is the pain in the middle of the arm or leg—far away from a joint?
- Is the child in pain without being touched, or does it hurt only if you squeeze?

- Is this the only joint that hurts or do other joints hurt if I squeeze them?
- Is the area that hurts hot or warm to the touch?
- Is it red? Is it obviously swollen?
- Does the child have other findings (a rash, bumps, etc.)?

If you are worried about a joint, can the child bend it without pain? Can they bend it all the way? Normal children under age ten can put their heels on their buttocks without difficulty. Young children should also be able to bend their hips so that their heels can reach their abdomen. Often I see children who were told they were normal because they could do everything a forty-year-old can do. Children should be much more flexible than forty-year-olds.

No physician knows everything. If you go in for an ear infection, it is highly unlikely the physician will check your child's knees. As a parent you cannot be expected to do a careful examination yourself, but you can be expected to notice whether the physician did a careful examination of your child. If your child's problems aren't getting better, you want to be sure he or she has been properly evaluated.

LABORATORY TESTS AND OTHER EVALUATIONS

Proper diagnostic testing may include blood tests, radiographs (X rays), bone scans, MRI, ultrasound (sonograms), and even biopsies of affected joints and tissues. Chapter 24 is an extensive discussion of the laboratory and diagnostic tests commonly used in the evaluation and monitoring of children with muscle, bone, or joint pain or arthritis. It is important to remember that diagnostic tests are not a substitute for knowledge and judgment. I often have children referred to me with thousands of dollars of wasted tests and the wrong diagnosis. The key to proper diagnosis and treatment is a careful history and a thorough physical examination as discussed above. After those have been done, appropriate diagnostic tests can help to pinpoint the cause of the problem and aid in planning treatment.

Simply performing a large battery of poorly thought-out tests not only wastes time and money, but also exposes the patient to unwarranted risks associated with both the testing procedures and the pursuit of false leads. I am often asked to evaluate children who had a positive blood test that suggested a rheumatic disease when no one can tell me why the test was done. The child never had any of the symptoms associated with the disease the test suggests, but somehow it was ordered and now no one knows what to do with the result.

Proper evaluation consists of taking a careful history and doing a complete physical exam. In the hands of an experienced physician, this is often sufficient to establish the diagnosis. Further testing should be ordered only to confirm the diagnosis and assure that there is nothing else wrong. Only if physicians are having difficulty finding the cause of a child's problems is a much more extensive evaluation warranted (see Chapter 4).

I have seen several children who complained to their parents of knee pain. When their physicians noted that the knee appeared swollen and there was no history of injury, the children were sent for MRIs. The MRIs were interpreted as showing "synovial tissue proliferation" and the children were operated on for possible tumors. A careful history and physical examination made it clear that they had typical juvenile arthritis. In many cases it was obvious the problem was not a tumor because there were other swollen and tender joints when a full examination was done. Thousands of dollars were wasted and the children were put through unnecessary hospitalizations and operations. Even the initial MRI that suggested a "possible tumor" would not have been needed if the child had been carefully examined.

Even when appropriate tests are done, it is important to be sure they are properly interpreted. A ten-year-old boy was sent to me because of hip pain. The child was having severe pain, but could walk. The family brought an X ray of the hip that had been interpreted by the radiologist and showed "no hip damage." A bone scan of the hip was also done that showed "no abnormal uptake in the hip," that is, no damage. When I examined the child, it was clear that his pain was not in the hip, but adjacent to it. The X ray and the bone scan brought to me by the family were indeed negative for hip damage, but both showed a fracture of the pubic ramus (a bone near the hip). Looking at just the hip, the doctors had overlooked the fracture nearby. The child pointed right to the location of the fracture when he was asked where it hurt.

3

Common Causes of Pain

KNEE PAIN

When evaluating a child with knee pain, it is important to separate mechanical problems from problems resulting from infections or inflammation. Most knee pain is initially thought to be the result of an injury. If we do not remember having seen a fall, we assume the child must have twisted it. If your child is complaining of knee pain, here is a list of questions to which you should know the answers before you go to the doctor's office.

- Did the pain begin immediately after an injury? Or did you notice the child was in pain and then have to "remember" the injury?
- Does the knee hurt all the time?
    - Does it hurt only in the middle of the night?
    - Does it hurt only when the child is out running on the soccer field?
    - Does it hurt only in the evening?
- Can the child play, but then has to come off the field?
    - If the child comes off the field, is he or she better in five minutes and back in the game?
    - Or is the child out for the rest of the day?
- When the child wakes up the next morning, does he or she feel better? Or worse?

- Is the knee stiff the next morning? Does it loosen up in the morning after the child gets up and gets going?
- Has the knee ever been swollen?
- Are any other joints ever stiff or swollen?
- Has there been any fever?
- Has there been any recent diarrhea or viral illness?

The answers to these questions will suggest a variety of different explanations for the pain. Knowing the answers in advance should help your doctor to pinpoint the problem quickly.

Children with mechanical problems typically hurt with activity. Stop the activity and the pain goes away. Resume the activity and the pain comes back. If there is a fracture or an infection the pain is there all the time. If there is a torn ligament or meniscus, the pain may be intermittent. It will come on with activities and clear more slowly. The following is a list of conditions that commonly cause knee pain in children.

Mechanical conditions
Osgood-Schlatter disease
Osteoid osteoma
Blount's disease
"Growing pains"
Meniscal injuries
Torn ligaments
Overuse syndromes (see Chapter 5, on sports injuries, for a discussion of these problems)
  Iliotibial band
  Chondromalacia patella
  Osteochondritis dissicans
Other orthopedic conditions

Common infections
Staphylococcal infections
Tuberculosis
Lyme disease

Rheumatic diseases
Juvenile arthritis
Spondyloarthropathies (enthesitis-associated arthritis)
Systemic lupus erythematosus
Dermatomyositis (weakness in the thighs may be described as "knee pain")
Psoriatic arthritis

Miscellaneous conditions
Pigmented villonodular synovitis
Plant thorn synovitis

Metabolic diseases
Hemophilia
Sickle-cell anemia

Pain after a fall

If a child is in severe pain after a fall, he or she should immediately be taken to the physician for appropriate evaluation. In these cases X rays are usually done. Most often fractures are immediately obvious on the X ray. However, some fractures may be very small and will be seen only on a follow-up X ray. This is because the bone will form a large callous as part of the healing response. This is easily seen on the follow-up X ray, even though the original small fracture was not evident on the first X ray. Sometimes children with pain who do not have an obvious fracture are presumed to have a growth plate injury that is hard to see on the X ray. The growth plate is the junction between the shaft and the end of the bone where rapid growth is occurring (see the Glossary). If a fracture is seen or suspected, the child will be put in a cast for an appropriate period. Following cast removal, the child should recover quickly. Repeated injuries in which the fractures are hard to see should be regarded with suspicion. Many children with arthritis are originally incorrectly diagnosed with "small fractures."

If the X rays are negative, the child is often diagnosed with a sprain. If there is no obvious swelling, such children are often treated with an Ace wrap and crutches. These children need careful medical follow-up. Often it all goes away quickly and there is no need for concern. However, injuries to the supporting ligaments of the knee or the menisci will require further attention. These injuries are most often associated with swelling. If a physician removes the fluid from (aspirates) the knee, it will often be bloody. Careful orthopedic evaluation is mandatory, as bloody synovial fluid suggests a significant injury. Children with hemophilia may have recurrent bleeding in their knees. A rare type of synovial disease called pigmented villonodular synovitis (see the Glossary) is also associated with bleeding into the knee joint.

If a child continues to have knee pain after the initial treatment, a repeat, thorough examination should be done. Repeat X rays of the knees may be needed. It is also important to be sure the hips have been carefully evaluated. Some children with problems in their hips complain about pain in their knees. Everyone is fooled because the knees are normal. The most common example of this is a child with a slipped capital femoral epiphysis of the hip (SCFE) (see the next section in this chapter on common causes of hip pain). The child should also have blood work that includes a complete blood count, a metabolic profile, and muscle enzymes.

Continuing knee pain during the day should not be dismissed as growing pains or Osgood-Schlatter disease without thorough evaluation. Some children with muscle disease will initially complain of knee pain (in fact, it is probably thigh pain). There are also children with infections or tumors of the bones and joints and children with arthritis who are first brought to the doctor because of pain after falling. Most of these conditions are evident on MRI, if the appropriate area is examined.

Pain that comes and goes

Pain that comes and goes may have many different explanations. If the pain comes and goes with changing levels of activity, it may have a mechanical explanation. On the other hand, pain that comes and goes with changing barometric pressure (rapid rising or falling air pressure as when a storm is coming) may be the beginnings of arthritis or the result of an old injury or a chronic infection. Pain that is much worse with activity but disappears when the activity stops suggests a mechanical problem.

Pain that begins with activity but does not disappear when the activity is stopped and often results in stiffness the next morning suggests arthritis. Physicians are often fooled when examining children because they believe that arthritis in childhood must be associated with either a positive test for rheumatoid factor or an elevated sedimentation rate. Neither is required for a child to have arthritis (see Chapter 7). Children who have stiffness when they wake up in the morning or difficulty getting out of the car after a long ride or out of their seat after a long movie need to be carefully evaluated for arthritis. Small children may have obviously swollen knees and difficulty walking when they first wake up, but never seem to be in pain. Again, this is often a sign of arthritis.

A key distinction in children with knee pain is to be sure the pain is in the knee joint and not in the shaft of the bone (the femur is the bone above the knee and the tibia the main bone below it). At the beginning, children with tumors or infections in the bone may complain of intermittent pain. Most often these conditions are diagnosed by X ray or bone scan (see Chapter 24). Typically, these children have pain in the bone itself rather than the joint. The child will say only that the knee hurts, but this distinction can be made easily if the child is carefully examined. Children with growing pains may have intermittent complaints of pain in and around the knee. Normal test results and the occurrence of pain only at night help to differentiate them from more serious conditions (see Chapter 1).

Proper evaluation

The key elements in evaluating a child with knee pain are the presence or absence of stiffness and the description of the pain. X rays are important if the pain seems to be coming from the bone. If the joint is swollen, then withdrawing fluid from the knee may provide useful answers. Discovering bacteria in the fluid will indicate an infection, while a large amount of blood suggests an injury (see synovial fluid analysis in Chapter 24).

If the knee appears to be absolutely normal, it is important to examine the child and make sure the pain is not coming from the shaft of the bone or even the hip. Blood tests may be helpful in detecting an infection or arthritis. A bone scan can also help. MRIs can be very useful in diagnosing injuries to the soft tissues around the knee. See Chapter 24 for a more complete discussion of these tests.

Specific conditions

Osgood-Schlatter disease. This condition is the result of inflammation of the attachment (insertion) of the patellar tendon (which transmits all of the force from the muscles in the thigh to forward motion of the lower leg) where it attaches to the lower leg (anterior tibial tubercle).

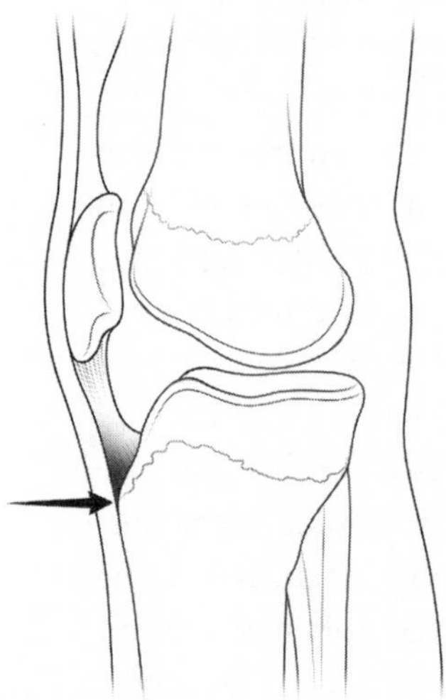

FIG 1. *Inflammation of the tendon insertion in Osgood-Schlatter's disease producing pain just below the knee. The arrow indicates the anterior tibial tubercle.*

In children who are developing rapidly (nine- to fifteen-year-old age group), the muscles often strengthen more rapidly than the bones. Lots of running and kicking, such as while playing sports, leads to repeated pulling on the tendon where it attaches to the bone. With repeated pulling, children develop inflammation at the tendon insertion. As a result, the anterior tibial tubercle (bump just below the knee) becomes swollen and tender (Fig. 1).

The pain in Osgood-Schlatter disease is brought on by activity and relieved by rest. It is never associated with stiffness or swelling of the knee itself—just the bump below the knee. It does not cause pain when children wake up in the morning and it does not wake children up from sleep. The key to diagnosing Osgood-Schlatter disease is to realize that the pain is not in the knee (although that is how the children usually describe it). On careful examination, the knee is entirely normal. The pain is reproduced by pressing on the anterior tibial tubercle (the prominent bump just below the knee). Most often the tenderness is present on both sides, but it may be only the dominant side (e.g., the right if the child is right-handed). The key to resolving this situation is to enforce relative rest so the inflamed tendon and bone can heal and the bone can become stronger so that it can withstand the pulling by the muscles.

Osteoid osteoma. Osteoid osteomas are benign tumors of the bone, much like knots in wood. Often they never cause difficulty. However, in some children they cause pain. Most often the pain occurs in the middle of the night and is sufficiently severe to wake the child. They occur in boys more often than girls and frequently become symptomatic during the teenage years. They are most common in the region of the hip (see below), but may occur either above or below the knee. Osteoid osteomas around the knee are usually easily diagnosed on routine X rays. The pain from an osteoid osteoma is usually easily relieved by acetaminophen or ibuprofen. All children in whom there is any consideration that the lesion may be a serious bone tumor and all children whose pain is not easily relieved by these medications require careful evaluation by an orthopedist with extensive experience in these lesions.

Plant thorn synovitis. Plant thorn synovitis is an arthritis that occurs in children who have fallen on a palm frond or similar piece of sharp plant material and a part of the plant has broken off inside the knee. The typical story is a four- to six-year-old child who is brought to the doctor with a single swollen knee. The knee is usually red and hot with no history of injury. The family doctor sends the child to an orthopedist, who removes fluid from the knee. The fluid looks infected. The orthopedist sends the child to the hospital for intravenous antibiotic therapy. When the cultures of the knee fluid fail to reveal any bacteria and the knee fails to improve after four or five days of antibiotic therapy, it may be thought that this is Lyme disease that is not responding to the antibiotics. When the knee still does not get better after changing antibiotics, a diagnosis of juvenile arthritis is considered.

The key to recognizing plant thorn synovitis is in taking a proper travel history. Usually the child has traveled to someplace warm (e.g., Florida, the Caribbean, Southern California) several weeks before the problem started. These are typically children who are just old enough to get out of sight and fall down. They have a small cut on the knee that heals quickly. No one remembers this cut when the knee is hot and swollen weeks later.

It is important to recognize plant thorn synovitis because it will not respond to antibiotics or nonsteroidal anti-inflammatory drugs (NSAIDs; see Chapter 22). Proper treatment requires a synovectomy (cleaning out all of the inflamed tissue lining the knee). When this is done, the diagnosis of plant thorn synovitis can be confirmed by looking at the tissue under polarized light. This will show starch granules from the plant material that broke off inside the knee.

Orthopedic conditions

Blount's disease. Blount's disease refers to bowing of the legs (genu varum). There are two major groups of children with Blount's disease. Young children may develop Blount's disease without any apparent explanation. There is a sudden shift in growth of the tibia (the lower leg bone) so that the inner edge does not grow as well as the outer edge. With progressive growth of the outer edge the legs are forced to bow. In small children, this is most often painless and it affects both sides.

In teenagers, Blount's disease is associated with obesity. In these children, it is suspected that the excessive weight puts too much stress on the inner side of the lower leg bone (medial side of the tibia) and the growth plate is damaged. Under these circumstances, one side may be affected without the other. Blount's disease in teenagers may be associated with progressive pain. At first the pain may be intermittent and relieved by acetaminophen or other pain relievers, but over time it may steadily worsen. If it is left untreated, the pain will continue and the damage to the joint may result in the premature development of mechanical arthritis. An orthopedic surgeon should monitor children of all ages with Blount's disease. Bracing and surgical intervention are sometimes necessary.

Overuse syndromes

Chondromalacia patella, osteochondritis dissicans, and iliotibial bands. These are all mechanical conditions that primarily result from excessive wear and tear on the knee and surrounding tissues. Because these diagnoses are frequently given to explain pain with athletic activities, I have chosen to discuss these conditions in detail in Chapter 5, on injuries.

Infections

There are two types of infection that must be considered in a child with joint pain. Septic arthritis is an infection in the joint itself. Osteomyelitis is an infection in the bone. In the region of the knee, osteomyelitis is more common than septic arthritis. Often osteomyelitis occurs near the ends of the bones and produces pain in the joint near the infected bone. The pain of osteomyelitis may wax and wane, but the child is never free of pain. In children with osteomyelitis, the pain usually gets steadily worse over a few days at most. These children often have fevers and look ill, but occasionally the child looks well and is only limping. If the infection has been present for a period of time, it should be easy to see on X rays. However, during the first few days after an infection begins, the X ray may not show changes. Bone scans and MRIs will demonstrate infections in the bone even at the earliest stages when pain is present.

One problem that requires attention is the possibility of a "sympathetic effusion." In this situation, there may be an infection or a tumor (even leukemia) in the bone. At the same time the child will complain of pain and have an obviously swollen knee. Aspiration of the knee will show fluid that suggests arthritis and not an infection. The key to suspecting this situation is that these children are in more pain than would be expected. In addition, careful examination will indicate that they are very tender in the shaft of the bone, not just in the joint itself.

Bone cysts

Unicameral bone cysts are large cystic malformations of the bone that may occur in the femur or the humerus (shoulder bone). They usually are entirely asymptomatic unless there is a fracture, in which case the child should be cared for by an experienced orthopedist. Fractures that occur will have to be treated appropriately. Following healing of the fracture, the orthopedist may choose to treat the lesion by direct injections of corticosteroids or curettage. Aneurismal bone cysts differ in having a significant blood vessel component in the cyst. They tend to grow more rapidly than unicameral bone cysts and are more likely to be discovered because they are causing pain. Like unicameral bone cysts, they are easily discovered by routine X ray and should immediately be referred to an experienced orthopedist.

Bone tumors

While many bone tumors are benign, some are malignant and life-threatening. The key to recognizing bone tumors is appropriate evaluation of the child with pain. Like tumors elsewhere, bone tumors begin very small and grow relatively slowly. Often they are easily visible on routine X ray by the time they are producing pain. Children with pain during the day should never be dismissed as simply having "growing pains" without further evaluation (see Chapter 1). It is true that growing pains and tumors may both wake up children during the night. However, the child with growing pains is fine during the day, while the child with a tumor will most often have pain during the day if carefully examined.

A full discussion of the types of bone tumors and their treatment is far beyond the scope of this book. If you desire further information on this subject you should contact your local office of the American College of Orthopedic Surgeons or a similar organization.

HIP PAIN

Hip pain is a particularly disturbing finding in children. Most often, children with hip pain walk with a very abnormal gait. If the pain is sudden and severe, the child may not be able to walk at all. A child who is suddenly unable to walk after trauma or a fall needs immediate medical evaluation to exclude fractures and other orthopedic injuries. A child who, without warning, wakes up in the morning with hip pain and has difficulty walking may be suffering from a variety of conditions. If the pain does not disappear after a few minutes, the child should be brought for immediate medical attention to exclude the possibility of an infection. All children with hip pain should receive a careful and thorough medical evaluation, including children with pain that disappears after a few minutes but keeps coming back.

The box lists the common causes of hip pain in childhood, along with the ages at which they occur.

Small children (under age 10)
Toxic synovitis
Observation hip
Bacterial infection
Legg-Calve-Perthes disease
Tumors
Osteoid osteoma
Sickle-cell anemia

Teenagers
Slipped capital femoral epiphysis
Sports injuries
Stress fractures
Apophysitis
Labrial tears
Meralgia paresthetica
Osteoid osteoma
Tumors
Iliotibial band syndrome
Spondyloarthropathies

Often pain in the hip is in fact pain in various parts of the pelvis. With excessive physical activity it is common to develop pain at muscle insertions around the pelvis. These are often referred to as pointers. Children with chronic hip injuries typically report pain with certain movements and activities. The pain is relieved by rest. The hip is a deep-seated joint, and injuries such as ligamentous tears are infrequent in childhood.

Chronic and recurrent hip pain in younger children may be the result of Legg-Calve-Perthes disease, arthritis, an infection, or tumor in the bone (see below). In older children, slipped capital femoral epiphysis (SCFE; described below) and spondyloarthropathies (enthesitis-associated arthritis; see Chapter 9) are more common. These conditions often begin with vague complaints of hip pain that become progressively worse over time. Children with all of these conditions may initially describe knee or thigh pain. None of these conditions is difficult to diagnose if the child is properly evaluated with X rays, blood tests, and, if necessary, a bone scan or MRI.

Specific conditions

Toxic synovitis. Toxic synovitis is an inflammation of the hip that typically occurs in children in the four- to six-year-old age group. Although it often occurs in children with evidence of a viral respiratory infection, its cause is unknown. Children with toxic synovitis have a very characteristic story. Most often the child went to bed well or with "a slight sniffle" the night before. In the morning the child has severe hip pain and is unable to walk. Because the symptoms are so dramatic, the children are immediately brought to the doctor. Often there is a low-grade fever and blood tests may show an elevated white blood cell (WBC) count and slight elevation of the erythrocyte sedimentation rate (ESR). The immediate concern is to exclude a bacterial infection of the hip. Frequently, these children are referred to an orthopedist who may aspirate the hip to look for bacterial infection. Bacterial infections of the hip rapidly worsen over a period of hours. In contrast, I have often seen children with toxic synovitis who are already improving by the time they reach my office. If the physician is in doubt, aspiration of the hip, hospitalization, and antibiotic therapy are appropriate, until the possibility of an infection has been excluded.

Once the diagnosis of toxic synovitis has been made, children may be treated with NSAIDs and rest. They usually recover completely within a few days. However, careful examination may reveal residual irritability of the hip for several weeks. The prognosis for these children is very good. It has long been thought that the incidence of Legg-Calve-Perthes disease (LCP; see below) in children who have recovered from toxic synovitis is higher than in the general population. However, more recent reports suggest that the two conditions are unrelated.

Children with "recurrent" toxic synovitis should be regarded with suspicion. Some have Legg-Calve-Perthes disease that has not been recognized. In other children, recurrent episodes of synovitis in the hip may be the first manifestation of what will ultimately become an obvious spondyloarthropathy. Any child with recurrent toxic synovitis should have a thorough evaluation by a pediatric rheumatologist, if possible. True toxic synovitis is not a recurrent condition and the correct explanation for the recurrent hip pain should be vigorously sought.

Legg-Calve-Perthes disease. LCP results from softening of the head of the femur (the long bone of the leg), which gradually becomes distorted and may flatten or crumble (see Fig. 2). It is thought that this results from problems with the blood supply to the head of the femur. These problems may be the result of an injury or congenital abnormality. One report has suggested that LCP occurs far more frequently in the children of parents who smoke. However, problems with the blood supply cannot be the whole answer, since LCP occurs four times more often in boys than in girls.

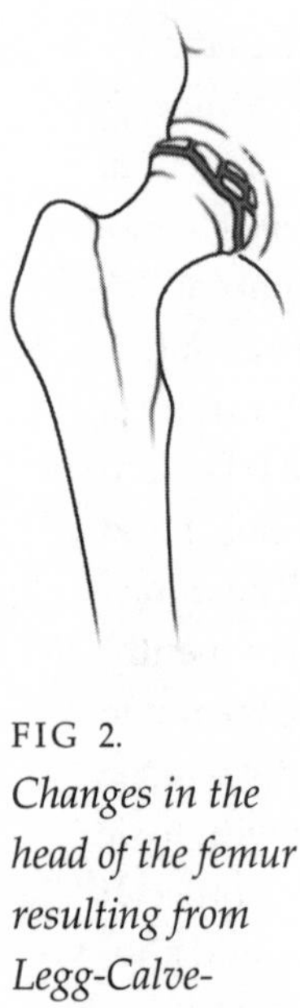

FIG 2. *Changes in the head of the femur resulting from Legg-Calve-Perthes disease.*

LCP usually begins in young children (four to six years of age most commonly), who are usually noticed to be limping before there is any complaint of pain. Over time, the limp becomes more noticeable and the child may begin to complain of pain. At the earliest stages an MRI may be required to diagnose LCP. However, if the symptoms have been present for more than several weeks, it should be possible to make the diagnosis with a regular X ray of the hip. This will show flattening of the head of the femur. Most cases of LCP involve only one hip, but in a few children both hips are involved. Premature birth and problems during the newborn period increase the risk of LCP, as does a family history of the disease.

Children diagnosed with LCP should be under the care of an orthopedist. Treatment often consists initially of traction followed by casting. Once the cast is removed, physical therapy is important to restore strength and range of motion. The purpose of the traction and casting is to keep the femur properly seated in the hip while decreasing the pressure on the femoral head. Often this allows the bone to reestablish its blood supply and begin to repair itself. The precise details of your child's treatment will depend on the age of your child and the degree of damage to the bone at the time the problem is discovered. You should discuss the treatment in detail with your orthopedist.

Children with bilateral LCP should be thoroughly evaluated. In some instances, this is a sign of an underlying condition such as hyperthyroidism or sickle-cell disease. In others, the deformed head of the femur may be the result of more widespread conditions, such as multiple epiphyseal dysplasia or spondyloepipheseal dysplasia tarda. These conditions are recognized by the presence of abnormal epiphyses in multiple joints when a skeletal survey is done. (The epiphyses are the ends of the bone that insert into the joints; see the Glossary. A skeletal survey is a complete set of X rays to show all the bones and joints.) These are orthopedic conditions that are beyond the scope of this book.

The long-term prognosis for children with LCP who are diagnosed early is good. If the disease has been present for a long time, the bone may already have begun healing itself by the time the disease is recognized. In many children, this healing is adequate and things go well. However, in some children, there may be permanent damage to the bone. There is also concern that children with residual damage from LCP may have persisting mechanical problems that will cause them to have mechanical arthritis of the hip, leading to problems when they become adults.

Sickle-cell anemia. Sickle-cell anemia may cause pain in the bones because of blood vessels being blocked by the abnormally shaped blood cells. This may occur in the blood vessels that supply the hip and result in damage to the hip bone (femur). When it does, it looks exactly like—and essentially is—LCP. In children with severe sickle-cell anemia, other bones may be damaged and there may be widespread joint problems. Usually a child with these problems will have been recognized to have sickle-cell disease long before the bone problems begin.

Infections. There are two basic types of infections that must be considered in children with hip pain. **Septic arthritis** is an infection in the joint itself. There are foreign organisms growing in the space between the bones. Osteomyelitis is an infection in the bone. In the hip, septic arthritis is more common than osteomyelitis. **Hemophilus influenzae** was the most common bacterial infection of the hip for many years. Now most children are vaccinated against this infection (with the HIB vaccine) and it has become rare. Staphylococcal and streptococcal infections of the hip do still occur. It is also possible to have a tuberculosis infection in the hip. At present, Lyme may be the most common cause of infectious arthritis involving the hip for people living in endemic areas of the United States (see Chapter 10, on Lyme disease).

Most infections in the hip are sudden in onset and associated with rapidly worsening symptoms of pain, fever, and difficulty in walking. A child with these symptoms should be seen by a physician as soon as possible. Tuberculosis may cause slowly worsening symptoms of hip pain. A child with an acutely painful hip should be seen by an orthopedist. Although there may be some confusion with toxic synovitis, children with toxic synovitis are usually rapidly improving without treatment. If there is serious consideration that the joint may be infected, it should be aspirated for appropriate studies, including bacterial cultures. Chronic hip pain associated with stiffness is more likely to be the result of enthesitis-associated arthritis involving the hip (see Chapter 9), but the possibility of an infection should always be given careful consideration.

Osteomyelitis is an infection in the bone. Often osteomyelitis occurs near the ends of the bones and produces pain in the joint near the infection. The pain of osteomyelitis may wax and wane, but the child is never free of pain and the pain usually gets steadily worse over a period of a few days. Children with osteomyelitis often have fevers and are ill appearing, but occasionally the child looks well and is only limping. If the infection has been present for more than a few days, it should be easy to detect on X rays. However, during the first few days after an infection begins, the X ray may not show changes. Bone scans and MRIs will demonstrate infections in the bone at the earliest stages when pain is present.

Pain in the lower abdomen near the hip may be a cause of confusion. When dealing with younger children, it can be difficult to know exactly where the pain is coming from. Children with severe lower abdominal pain may walk with an abnormal gait, suggesting arthritis or an infected hip. As a result, occasionally I have seen children brought for evaluation of hip pain and limp who turned out to have an abscess resulting from an appendix that had ruptured. This possibility should always be considered in children with pain in the right side of the pelvis without an obvious explanation. It can be easily detected by appropriate CAT scan or ultrasound examination of the hip and abdomen.

Osteoid osteoma. Osteoid osteomas are benign tumors of the bone, much like knots in wood. Often they never cause difficulty. However, in some children they cause pain. Most often the pain is low-grade but constant. It typically is worse in the middle of the night and often is sufficiently severe to wake the child. Careful evaluation is required because malignant bone tumors can also cause chronic bone pain that may awaken a child at night. The pain from an osteoid osteoma is usually easily relieved by acetaminophen or ibuprofen. All children in whom there is any consideration that the lesion may be a serious bone tumor, as well as all children whose pain is not easily relieved, require careful evaluation by an orthopedist with extensive experience in these lesions.

Osteoid osteomas occur more often in boys than girls. Most frequently, they become symptomatic during the teenage years. However, they may cause pain and become troublesome earlier. They are most common in the region of the hip but may also occur around the knee. Osteoid osteomas in the region of the hip are easily diagnosed on routine X rays or bone scans. In most cases, no therapy is necessary once the diagnosis has been established. However, in some children the pain is more severe. Surgical removal of the lesion is possible in most of the troublesome cases.

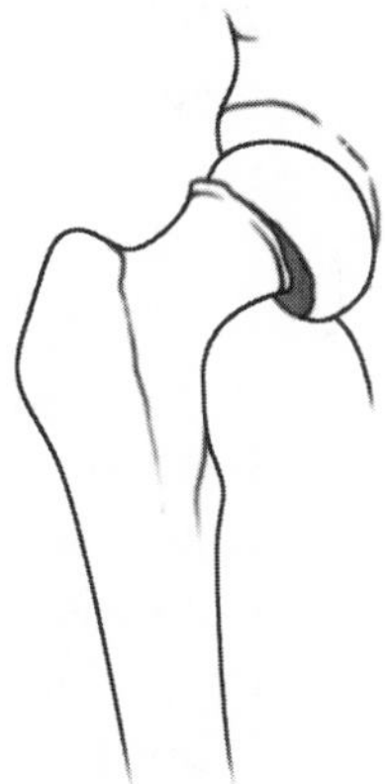

FIG 3. *This is the characteristic appearance of a slipped capital femoral epiphysis. The epiphysis is the rounded portion of the bone in the hip joint. It has literally slipped off the end of the long bone (femur). Compare this with Fig. 2, where the epiphysis has crumbled but remains in the proper position.*

Slipped capital femoral epiphysis. Slipped capital femoral epiphysis (SCFE) is an injury to the growth plate of the femur (the long bone of the leg) that results in the growing end of the bone slipping off from the shaft (see Fig. 3). This injury occurs most often in boys between the ages of ten and fifteen years but may occur in girls and occasionally in older children. It occurs more often in African Americans and in children who are overweight. The most dramatic cases of SCFE occur as an injury with sudden slipping of the epiphysis. This produces acute hip pain and inability to walk. These children are promptly taken to the physician, where X rays confirm the diagnosis. The X rays should include both standard views and "frog leg" views in which the child is instructed to bend the knees and spread them apart. SCFE may be missed on standard views of the hips, but the "slippage" is usually obvious on the "frog leg" views.

Some children develop SCFE on a more gradual basis. No one is sure why this happens. These children will have progressive onset of pain and stiffness in the involved hip. Because deep pain may be difficult to localize, the child may describe the pain as coming from the groin, the thigh, or the knee instead of the hip. Children with a chronic slip usually have an obvious limp. The changes in the bone may force the hip on the affected side to rotate outward. The abnormal alignment of the bones that results triggers muscle spasm. This muscle spasm causes children with chronic SCFE to report stiffness with rest and increased pain with activity, symptoms that suggest arthritis. The chronic slip should be evident on X ray. In uncertain or difficult cases, an MRI may be useful to confirm the diagnosis.

SCFE may occur in children with hypothyroidism and other growth problems. In about one-third of children, the disease is bilateral. The slip on the opposite side may be present when the first SCFE is noted or may occur later. SCFE is treated by orthopedists. They will put a pin in the bone to hold the epiphysis in place while the bone heals. If detected and treated early, children with SCFE usually do well. Chronic SCFE that is not promptly treated may result in damage to the head of the hip bone (femur). This can result in a permanent limp, difference in the length of the two legs, and early onset of arthritis due to mechanical damage.

Iliotibial band syndrome. Iliotibial band syndrome may produce pain at the hip or knee. When it produces pain at the hip, children typically complain of a snapping sensation with certain movements. Often this is associated with trochanteric bursitis (see Fig. 4), which may be the result of excessive activity. Iliotibial band syndrome may also occur in children with a spondyloarthropathy (see Chapter 9). Iliotibial band syndrome itself is a benign condition that does not normally require therapy. However, if the snapping is associated with a sensation of pain, further evaluation is warranted.

Trochanteric bursitis. The greater trochanter is the large bump that sticks out on the side of the hip bone (femur) where it turns toward the knee. Because this protrusion is just under the skin at the side of the hip, it is protected by a bursa. The bursa is a small sac of fluid that allows easy movement of the tissues over the bone (see Fig. 4). With excessive running or other activities, this bursa may become inflamed. Typically, this is a problem of teenagers or adults and not younger children. The classic complaint is pain along the side of the leg that can be reproduced by pressure over the greater trochanter. The pain often is described as

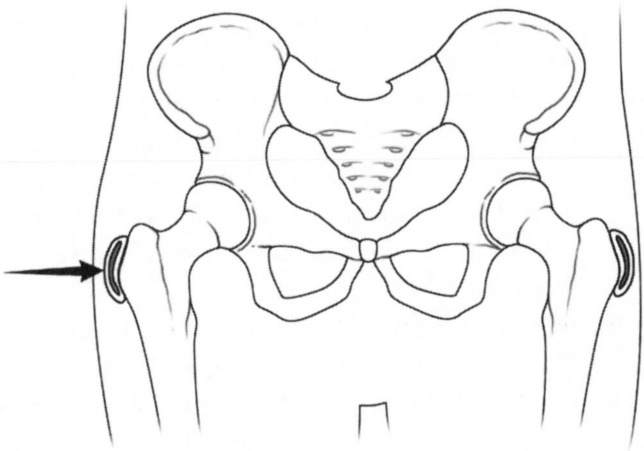

FIG 4. *Trochanteric bursitis results from irritation in the fluid-filled sacks (bursas) that are located just under the skin and over the greater trochanter.*

moving both up and down the side of the leg. Trochanteric bursitis is treated with ice, stretching exercises, and in more severe cases, nonsteroidal anti-inflammatory drugs (NSAIDs). In rare cases, children require injection of steroids into the bursa for relief.

Congenital hip dislocation. Congenital hip dislocation results from improper formation of the sockets into which the heads of the hip bones insert on the pelvis (improper development of the acetabulum, which covers the femoral head). This condition should be diagnosed in early childhood. Often it is first suspected when the pediatrician notices a "hip click" in the nursery. This is a sensation of clicking when the hip is moved in what is called the Ortolani maneuver. In most children, the hip click will go away after a period of observation and perhaps "double diapering." However, if it persists, the pediatrician should pay careful attention and orthopedic evaluation is needed.

Children with congenital hip dislocation walk with a waddling gait that is obvious to a trained observer but may be overlooked by parents. If the hip dislocation is present on only one side, it may be suspected when the parents or physician notice that the line under the curve of the buttock is not in the same position on both sides (asymmetric gluteal folds). The children will have decreased range of motion of the hips, if carefully examined, and abnormal X rays. However, because the condition has always been there, the children may never have complained of pain.

Congenital hip dislocation is easily diagnosed if appropriate X rays are done. It is treated by orthopedists. Cases detected in early life can often be managed without surgery. However, in severe cases surgical correction is necessary. If it is not detected and corrected, the hips may become severely damaged because of mechanical damage leading to degenerative arthritis. It is important that any child who walks with a waddling gait be appropriately evaluated and not simply dismissed because "she's always walked like that."

Arthritis involving the hip joint. The hip joint is rarely the first joint involved in children with juvenile arthritis (Chapter 7), but it may become involved over time. In contrast, the hip is commonly the first joint involved in children with spondyloarthropathies (Chapter 9). These children often begin with complaints of stiffness in the hip or lower back when they wake up in the morning. Over time, they develop symptoms in other joints. However, they often have to be asked and examined carefully for evidence of pain or limitation in the back, wrists, knees, or ankles, as they will not associate the complaints in other joints with their hip pain. This often results in a delay in proper treatment while they are investigated for the cause of their repeated injuries (see Chapter 9 for more detail). Since spondyloarthropathies rarely begin in children before the age of ten, younger children with hip pain must be carefully evaluated to exclude other causes.

Mechanical arthritis may occur in children who have had damage to the bones of the hip resulting from SCFE, congenital hip dislocation, or previous infection. These conditions and the mechanical cause of the arthritis are often evident on routine X rays. If the routine X rays do not provide an explanation for the pain, an MRI may be necessary to exclude less common causes of hip pain.

Muscle and systemic diseases. Some children with muscle or systemic diseases will experience significant pain in the muscles in the front of the thigh. This pain may be mistakenly reported as coming from the hip or the knee (and in fact, hip and knee problems may cause pain in the same muscles). Whenever a child is complaining of chronic pain and disability without obvious findings in the bones or joints, a careful evaluation for muscle or systemic diseases should be performed. Over the years I have seen children with hypothyroidism, hyperthyroidism, dermatomyositis, leukemia, lymphoma, and rhabdomyosarcoma who were referred with "hip" problems. Proper evaluation for these conditions includes blood tests with muscle enzymes, thyroid function studies, a complete blood count, and appropriate MRIs and X rays.

Bone cysts and bone tumors. Unicameral bone cysts are large cystic malformations of the bone that may occur in the femur or the humerus (shoulder bone). They usually do not produce any symptoms unless there is a fracture. Like bone cysts near the knee, they should be cared for by an experienced orthopedist. The common bone tumors of childhood are briefly discussed in the section above on knee pain. They should be considered in the evaluation of children who initially have pain in the hip, as well.

BACK PAIN

In this age of increasingly large book bags and backpacks, backache is becoming an increasingly common complaint among adolescents. A friend's daughter carefully loaded up her book bag for her first day in seventh grade, sat down on a bench, and promptly went over backward with the weight. Despite the muscle strains associated with heavy book bags and other activities, it is fortunate that serious back problems remain uncommon. As is true for other regions of the body, the key to assisting the physician in properly diagnosing the cause of your child's back pain is the information you provide. When you take your child to be evaluated, you should be prepared to tell the physician the answers to the following questions.

- When the pain began, did it come on suddenly following an injury or fall? Or slowly over a period of days without an injury?
- Does the pain wake the child up at night?
- Is the pain associated with stiffness and worse when the child first gets up in the morning? Or does the pain begin only with activities?
- Is the pain relieved by rest? Or does the child stiffen up if he or she sits for a long period?
- What position or activity makes the pain better? What position or activity makes the pain worse?
- Is the pain confined to a single location or does it move up and down the back?
- Does the pain extend down into one leg or out into one shoulder?

The answers to all of these questions are important in providing a clear understanding of the cause of your child's pain. Common causes of back pain are listed in the box.

Common causes of back pain in childhood

- Scheuermann's disease
- Spondylolisthesis
- Spondylolysis
- Disc disease
- Spondyloarthropathies
- Scoliosis
- Benign tumors
- Infections
- Disciitis
- Osteoid osteomas

Serious back injuries are typically associated with severe trauma, such as accidents, falls, and sports activities. Trauma and serious injuries will not be covered here. True backaches not associated with injuries are rare in childhood. Structural abnormalities are the most common cause. Back pain due to structural abnormalities is extremely unusual before the age of ten years. Any young child complaining of back pain requires careful evaluation. Infections and tumors are serious causes of back pain that may be present in this age group. These problems must not be ignored. In older children, scoliosis and spondylolisthesis are the most common structural abnormalities that cause back pain. Usually they begin without symptoms, but over time compensatory changes occur that often cause mechanical pain. Scoliosis and spondylolisthesis rarely come to medical attention before the age of ten years.

Scoliosis is an abnormal curvature of the spine with rotation of the vertebrae. This curvature often results in one shoulder appearing higher than the other or the hips appearing uneven. Since the curvature occurs with growth, it is rare for scoliosis to become evident before the age of ten years. Once detected, it should be carefully evaluated and followed. Many children have only mild curvatures and require no treatment, but others have progressive disease requiring bracing and, less frequently, surgery. Scoliosis is usually painless and detected only on examination (see Fig. 5). Pain suggests that the scoliosis has been present for a prolonged period with secondary mechanical problems.

Children are routinely screened for scoliosis at school, but the expertise and thoroughness of the examiners varies widely. Most scoliosis is idiopathic (unexplained). In rare cases, scoliosis may be the result of tumors, infections, or damage to the spinal cord. These cases may appear at an earlier age than idiopathic scoliosis and be more severe. Any child whose spine appears crooked should have a careful orthopedic evaluation.

It is easy to examine a child for scoliosis. Have the child stand in front of you with both feet together and the heels lined up with each other. Then have the child bend forward to touch the toes. Two findings suggest a scoliosis. The most common finding is a "rib hump," which means that the ribs on one side stick up higher than the ribs on the other (Fig. 5). In some children, there is a prominent low back (lumbar) component that is easily felt by putting your hand on the lower part of the back. If one side of the back is lower than the other, further evaluation by an orthopedist is necessary.

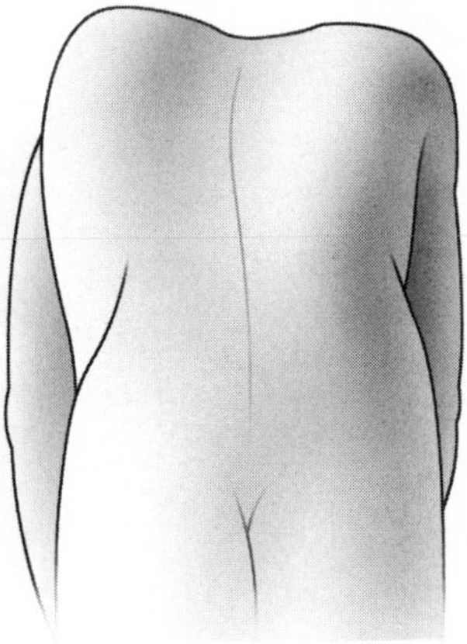

FIG 5. *A positive scoliosis screen with the ribs on the left side appearing higher than the right when the child bends over. The shoulders may also appear uneven when the child is standing up, but this is more difficult to notice.*

Spondylolisthesis is an anterior slippage of one vertebra over another. Most often this occurs at the junction of the lumbar and sacral spine (L5 S1 level). Some cases may be due to a congenital weakness, while other cases may be due to poor healing after an injury. Either cause results in weakness of the bone bridges (posterior elements) that hold the spine in place (see Fig. 12 below). Spondylolisthesis results when this weakness allows one bone segment to slide forward over another. Although mild degrees of spondylolisthesis may be asymptomatic, more severe involvement characteristically leads to low back pain that may radiate down the back of the thighs. Most children with this condition can be followed conservatively, but some require orthopedic intervention. Because the symptoms can worsen over time, all children with chronic back pain should be followed by an experienced orthopedist.

Kyphosis is an excessive curvature of the spine in which the spine is bent forward. Looking at the child from behind you will not see a curvature, but if you look at the child from the side when he or she is bending over, you will see that the upper part of the back angles forward sharply instead of the normal C shape (see Fig. 6). This abnormal forward curvature may be the result of abnormalities in the bone resulting from fractures or infections. However, most often it occurs without explanation. In severe cases the child may appear to have a hunchback.

Some children have a **postural kyphosis**. This is usually a mild increase in the forward bend of the spine, leading to the appearance that

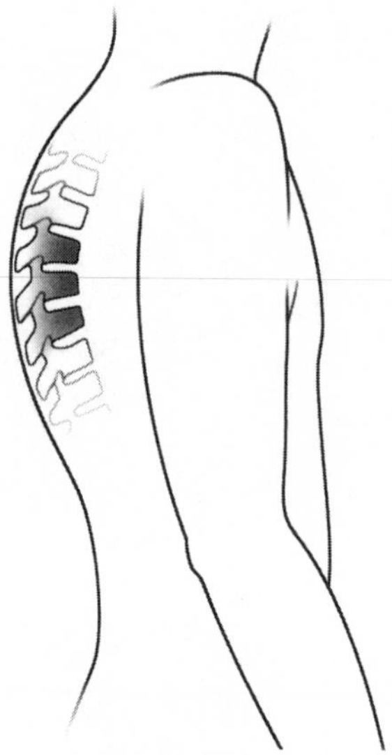

FIG 6. *Appearance of the spine with wedge-shaped vertebrae in a child with kyphosis due to Scheuermann's disease.*

they are always slumping over. These children often have no abnormal findings on X ray. These children can lie face down with their backs perfectly flat. Children with more significant abnormalities usually have changes in the bones. As a result, they cannot lie perfectly flat on their stomachs. These children all need to be investigated by an orthopedist with appropriate X rays to find out why they have kyphosis. For children without significant abnormality, a program of exercises is often adequate.

Scheuermann's disease is a common cause of kyphosis in teenagers. It is thought to result from abnormalities in the growth of the bones of the back (vertebrae), which results in the front being compressed relative to the back (see Fig. 6). The diagnosis is easily made when the abnormal bone structure is seen on appropriate X rays. Children with this condition may need to wear a brace to relieve their pain and prevent worsening of their condition. More severe or worsening cases may require orthopedic surgery.

Kyphosis may also be the result of damage to the bones of the spine by an infection, tumor, or poor bone formation. These conditions are all rare. Children with conditions that are known to damage the spine should be carefully monitored. Parents of children with poor bone formation or children who are taking medications that can damage the bones need to be reminded that their children should be watched carefully for spine problems. If a child has been diagnosed with an infection or a tumor in or around the spine, the family should be aware of the need to monitor the spine as the child grows.

There are a variety of infections that may damage the spine. Fortunately, none of them is common in childhood. Staphylococcal bacteria are common causes of infections that may affect the bones of the spine. Tuberculosis can also affect the bones of the spine. In the old literature, tuberculosis that affects the spine is called **Potts' disease**. Bacterial infections of the spine are usually very painful. They are easily diagnosed by either X rays or bone scans (Chapter 24). Despite many claims to the contrary, back pain in children is not a result of Lyme disease. The last child I saw with "back pain from chronic Lyme" had cancer that had gone undetected and untreated through six months of chiropractic and antibiotic treatment.

Disciitis is a confusing cause of back pain in younger children. Typically, it affects children under the age of ten. These children may have initial symptoms of a cold or flu-like illness. They then develop severe back pain, but in this age group they may not be able to describe it. *The key to recognizing this illness in very young children is that they suddenly refuse to sit up or walk.* The etiology of disciitis remains unclear. In some cases, a bacteria such as staphylococcus is identified and the infection is treated with antibiotics. In many cases, no causative bacteria is identified. This illness is usually diagnosed on the basis of the typical clinical picture with a bone scan and MRI or X rays to be sure that no other problem is present.

Osteoid osteomas are a cause of chronic low-grade bone pain that may occur in many different locations. While many osteoid osteomas never cause sufficient discomfort to attract attention, some are very problematic. Osteoid osteomas in the spine typically come to parents' attention when a child complains of chronic back pain that comes and goes without explanation. Larger osteoid osteomas are easily seen on X rays. Smaller lesions may be found on bone scans. A typical child with an osteoid osteoma reports a sense of deep aching pain, often worse at night. The pain is usually relieved by NSAIDs but continues to recur until the osteoid osteoma is removed. Untreated painful osteoid osteomas may cause major problems because the pain causes muscle spasms.

Herniated discs are a common complaint among adults and a frequent explanation for back pain that starts in adulthood. Disc herniation is usually the result of an excessive stress put on the spine with the resultant rupture of the cushioning material in one of the intervertebral discs. This condition is quite rare in children because they have more flexible bones and are less likely to be doing the work-related heavy lifting that often causes disc problems. Although an MRI of the spine is very accurate at identifying disc problems, finding minor disc problems on the MRI is not a reliable explanation for back pain. Many individuals who deny ever having back pain have minor disc herniation on an MRI. Although it is not impossible for a teenager to have a damaged disc, parents should be extremely skeptical about this diagnosis as the cause of back pain. Gradual onset of back pain with stiffness on awakening is more likely to be associated with a spondyloarthropathy or other illness.

Low back pain and morning stiffness are commonly due to spondyloarthropathies in teenagers. However, adolescents rarely come to the doctor complaining of low back pain when they wake up in the morning. Since the onset is very gradual, most accept this stiffness as normal. The key to suspecting a spondyloarthropathy as the cause of an adolescent's back pain lies in carefully examining the teenager and finding evidence of arthritis or tendon insertion pain (enthesitis) elsewhere. A strong family history of back pain also should suggest this diagnosis even though the other family members with back pain will all have "good excuses" for why their backs hurt. A key indication is that children with spondyloarthropathies almost never have the ability to bend over and touch their toes. See Chapter 9 for a full discussion of spondyloarthropathy.

NECK PAIN

Neck pain in children is rare. Most often it is due to muscle irritation involving the muscles that hold the head and shoulders in the proper position. Muscle irritation that the child describes as neck pain may be the result of an improperly carried backpack, especially if a heavy backpack is slung over just one shoulder. Carrying an excessive weight on one side places unnecessary strain on the back, the shoulder itself, and the neck muscles.

Before you go to the physician's office with your child's complaints of neck pain, think about the answers to the questions at the beginning of the section on back pain. Since the neck is simply the top portion of the back, the same questions need to be asked about complaints here. Several additional questions should also be asked.

- Is the child having headaches? Do they occur at the same time as the neck pain?
- Is the child having jaw pain? (Spasm in the muscles around the jaw may be reported as neck pain.)
- Is the child having problems seeing?
- What type of pillow does the child use?

Muscular irritation

Wryneck is a condition in which the child holds the head to one side because of problems with the sternocleidomastoid muscle. This muscle

Common causes of neck pain in childhood

Muscular irritation

- Wryneck
- Sprains and strains (e.g., whiplash)
- Severe sore throat
- Jaw pain
- Uncorrected visual problems causing the child to hold the head tilted

Bone problems

- Congenital abnormalities
- Osteoid osteoma
- Herniated disc (rare without known injury)
- Infection
- Spondyloarthropathies (enthesitis-associated arthritis)
- Juvenile arthritis

at the front of the neck is sometimes injured at birth and becomes shortened as a result of the injury. Children with this problem do not usually report pain, since it has been present since birth. However, they may develop neck pain as their muscles try to compensate, if the problem is not corrected as they get older. Wryneck in older children is due to muscle irritation (see below).

Sprains and strains are the most common cause of neck pain in children. The muscles of the neck must simultaneously support the head and protect the spinal cord while allowing maximum flexibility for looking up, down, and to both sides. This combination of strength and flexibility can be accomplished only using several overlapping sets of muscles. Injury to any one of these muscles will be reported as neck pain. If the pain is severe, there may be muscle spasm, forcing the child to hold the head tilted to one side for comfort. Pain due to irritation of the sternocleidomastoid muscle radiates into the front of the chest. In contrast, pain due to irritation of the trapezius muscle radiates down into the middle of the back and out toward the shoulder on the affected side.

Older children may injure the sternocleidomastoid muscle or the trapezius muscle, causing pain and a tilted head position. They also may suffer an overuse injury when they carry a heavy backpack on just one side. Constant contraction of the muscles necessary to keep the head level when the shoulders are slanted by a heavy load will fatigue the muscles, leading to spasm. The child may go to bed the night before without complaint but wake up stiff and sore, unable to straighten his or her neck out. The muscles of the neck may also become inflamed by severe sore throat, resulting from infections in the tonsils and infections or other causes of irritation elsewhere in the nose and throat. Similar problems may result from irritation of the jaw, producing spasm of the muscles where the neck and jaw meet. Any child in whom this is a persistent problem without explanation should be evaluated by an ear, nose, and throat specialist (otolaryngologist).

There are congenital bone problems that affect the neck, such as the **Klippel-Feil syndrome**. These are easily diagnosed on X ray. Other bone problems such as **osteoid osteoma** may occur in the neck with findings identical to when they occur lower in the back. **Herniated discs** and **infections** may also occur in the neck as elsewhere. *It is important to recognize that these problems may initially be reported as headaches and not recognized to be coming from the neck.*

Spondyloarthropathies predominantly affect the low back. However, there are children with neck pain due to irritation of the muscle insertions. In most, but not all cases, they will have previously been recognized to have involvement of multiple joints. Certain forms of juvenile arthritis commonly lead to problems with the bones in the neck. These children have limited neck motion (often they cannot look up or down or turn their heads from side to side without moving their backs). In some cases, this loss of motion is associated with pain, but more often it occurs gradually and the patient is not immediately aware of the problem.

Any child with prolonged, severe, or unexplained neck pain should be thoroughly investigated with a complete physical examination. If the problem is persistent and the answer has not been found, consideration should be given to evaluation by a neurologist, an ear, nose, and throat specialist, a neurosurgeon or orthopedist who deals with neck problems, and a rheumatologist.

FOOT, ANKLE, HEEL, AND TOE PAIN

It takes a moment to realize that when a child says, "My feet hurt," he or she could be referring to their heels, their toes, their ankles, or anywhere in the middle of the foot. Each area of the foot has a different set of common problems and solutions. Often parents initially assume foot pain in childhood is the result of shoes that do not fit properly. It is only when the pain continues despite a new pair of shoes that medical care is sought.

When you go to the physician because your child is complaining of foot pain, you need to be able to tell the physician whether the pain is in the toes, the ball of the foot (the area just behind the toes), the middle of the foot, the heel, or the ankle. You can both ask the child to point and examine the child's foot yourself to see whether any part of the foot is red, swollen, or tender. As with most other complaints of muscle, bone, and joint pain in childhood, the physician's first response is likely to be: "Maybe he or she banged or sprained it." If the pain has been present for more than a few days, you should insist that a more thorough evaluation be done.

There are some very knowledgeable podiatrists, but children should be thoroughly evaluated by an orthopedist and, if appropriate, a rheumatologist before being referred to a podiatrist. Do not forget that heel pain is a common early manifestation of a spondyloarthropathy. Putting cushions in the shoes may alleviate the heel pain, but it will do nothing to correct the associated problems in children with arthritis. X rays will exclude major fractures, but beware of the diagnosis of hairline fractures or growth plate fractures. These are real conditions, but they are also often convenient explanations when the child hurts and nothing is evident on the X rays. The information you give the physician and the care with which the child is examined are the keys to finding the correct diagnosis. Common conditions causing pain in the toe, heel, and mid-foot are listed in the boxes below.

Toe pain

In young children, toe pain is often a source of confusion because small children cannot reliably tell you what happened. When a child points to one toe and says it hurts, we all start by thinking that it was banged, got stepped on, or is being pinched in the shoe. Real trauma to the toe is usually obvious. A fractured toe is not subtle. The toe is very painful and there is often bleeding under the skin so that a large area of the toe appears bruised. Whenever this occurs, the foot should be X-rayed to make sure nothing is broken. With the exception of fractures, minor trauma to the toe should be better in a day or two.

Common causes of toe pain

- Trauma
- "Tennis toe"
- Ingrown toenails
- Dactylitis with arthritis
- Freiberg's infarct

When the toe has been injured, there is often discoloration under the toenail. If there is no discoloration and the pain persists, you should look carefully to see whether the toe is red or swollen. Compare it to the same toe on the other foot. If it is very red and swollen, it may be infected. This should be evaluated by a physician immediately. Any child with red marks spreading up the foot that are warm and tender should be assumed to have a serious infection. If one toe looks bigger than the one on the other side, but the child is not complaining, squeeze it gently. Often the toe is tender and the child will pull the foot away. If that happens, gently take the foot in your hand and squeeze just behind where the toe attaches to the foot. If that is also tender it suggests arthritis. Certain forms of arthritis commonly start with tender swelling involving the entire toe that is often mistaken by physicians for an infection or tumor.

Tennis toe is pain due to bleeding under the toenail. It is most commonly an injury in older children but may occur in younger children whose shoes are too small. It is the result of the toes forcibly colliding with the front of the shoe during activities. The acute pain can be relieved by allowing the blood to escape from under the toenail which releases the pressure (this can be done by a physician). It is important to recognize that it is an indication of improper foot wear and that the shoes should be changed.

Ingrown toenails may result from a variety of conditions. Although a number of possible explanations have been put forward, the most common cause of ingrown toenails in children is that the nails were cut too short. This results in the nail growing under the skin in front of it. Most often, ingrown toenails can be treated with warm soaks and local antibiotic creams. But this can be an extremely painful condition and may be associated with serious infections. Severe cases may require antibiotics and surgical removal of the offending toenail. Prevention is important. Do not cut your child's toenails too short.

In older children, toe pain may be due to a variety of injuries. **Freiberg's infarct** is a degeneration of the end of the metatarsal bone. The metatarsals are the long bones in the foot that extend to the base of the toes. Freiberg's infarct most often occurs in girls and usually at the base of the second toe. It is easily diagnosed if the appropriate X rays are taken. It is treated with casting and use of an orthotic device to relieve the pressure placed on that portion of the foot. This condition may occur in other toes, but rarely if ever involves the small toe.

Children complaining of pain at the base of the toes should be carefully examined for problems in other joints. A number of children have come to me after being treated with casting and orthotics for months. The orthopedists were considering surgery. However, the children were not getting better because the toe pain was due to arthritis. This was not obvious from examining the toe, but when the whole child was examined, there was obvious arthritis in other joints. The toes got better when the arthritis was treated.

Heel pain

Direct trauma to the heel is rare. It may occur if the foot is stepped on or if something falls on it. These injuries are obvious. Injuries to the heel may also occur with landing wrong after jumping, but again the injury is immediately evident. Chronic heel pain associated with activities may be thought to be **Sever's disease**. This is a common condition of pre-teenagers that is associated with increased physical activity. In this condition, the bone of the heel is often tender to pressure and the heel cords may be tight. Some physicians will make this diagnosis based on X rays showing irregularity and increased density of a portion of the bone behind the heel bone (sclerosis of the calcaneal apophysis). This is incorrect, as identical changes are commonly found on X rays of children without foot pain. *Sever's disease is not associated with pain in the tendons above or below the heel. Heel pain accompanied by pain in these tendons is often a sign of a spondyloarthropathy* (Chapter 9).

Common causes of heel pain
Trauma
Sever's disease
Plantar fasciitis
Achilles tendonitis
Spondyloarthropathies

Children may develop recurrent injuries and irritations of the tendons in the foot. In small children, these are thought to be cysts, sprains, and strains. In older children, they are often thought to be recurrent athletic injuries. Isolated **plantar fasciitis** (pain at the bottom of the heel where the tendons from the front of the foot attach) and **Achilles tendonitis** (pain at the back of the heel where the tendons coming down from the calf muscles attach) occur as overuse injuries in runners and other athletes. Since these findings may also be part of a spondyloarthropathy, the key to proper diagnosis is a careful history and physical examination. Often a child with recurrent ankle sprains turns out to have back stiffness and hip limitation, too, all of which are indicative of a spondyloarthropathy. Once the entire history has been obtained and a careful examination done, it is clear that the ankle sprains are part of a larger diagnostic picture.

Mid-foot pain

A number of different conditions may cause pain in the middle of the foot. Again, acute injuries are obvious and easily recognized with appropriate X rays. Chronic pain in the middle of the foot is often the result of a variety of bony abnormalities. The most common of these is **flat feet**. Painless flat feet are most often a variation of normal and require no treatment. However, if a child with flat feet has foot pain, it requires evaluation. Often no significant abnormality is found and the pain is relieved with the use of an orthotic.

Common causes of mid-foot pain

- Flat feet
  - Tarsal coalition
  - Accessory tarsal navicular
- Bunions
- Kohler's disease
- Pes cavus
- Arthritis of the subtalar joint

Some children have a "rigid" flat foot. This is easy to recognize because it is difficult to move the different parts of the child's foot in relation to each other. (You should be able to simply hold the child's foot in your hand and turn the front part in different directions, while holding the heel steady [see Fig. 7]. If the child has normal feet, this is easy to do and causes no pain.) In children with a "rigid" flat foot, it is necessary to determine whether the rigidity is being caused by **tarsal coalition** or another correctible abnormality. Every child with a rigid flat foot should be evaluated by an orthopedist.

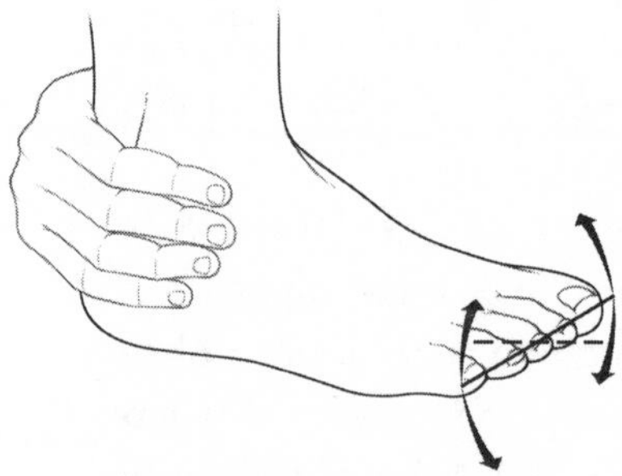

FIG 7. *Twisting the front of the foot while holding the heel steady. This is how to evaluate for the possibility of a "rigid" flat foot. The front of the foot should twist easily.*

Tarsal coalition refers to the formation of fibrous bands between two or more of the bones in the middle of the foot (the tarsals). These fibrous bands restrict motion and thus reduce the flexibility of the foot itself. This fibrous banding is thought to be present at birth, but becomes symptomatic only over time. It can be diagnosed with routine X rays or CAT scans. Casting may provide relief, but surgery is necessary for more difficult cases.

An **accessory tarsal navicular bone** is an extra little piece of bone that forms at the base of the navicular bone in the mid-foot. The extra bone is easily seen on X ray. This extra piece of bone sticks out on the inside of the foot and may be painful and tender where it rubs against the inside of the shoe. Many people have these and never realize it. If there is pain where the shoe rubs against the inside of the foot, stretching the shoe or wearing wider shoes often will eliminate the problem. Rare cases may require surgery.

Bunions are commonly thought of as a disease of adults. However, they may occur in teenagers, girls more often than boys. With activity these bunions may cause pain. Treatment usually centers on finding properly fitting shoes and other conservative measures. Surgery is generally unnecessary.

Kohler's disease is an irregularity of the navicular bone located in the middle of the foot, behind the metatarsal of the big toe. A typical patient with Kohler's disease is a child under the age of ten who complains of pain when walking and tenderness when the bone is pressed. Kohler's disease usually resolves without treatment. Severe or persistent cases of Kohler's disease are often treated by casting. This can be diagnosed by appropriate X rays or a CAT scan.

Pes cavus refers to the condition in which the arch of the foot is unusually high. Children with this condition often complain of foot pain when running or with other activities. This is not a common condition. Usually both feet are affected equally. If only one side is affected, there is often a neurologic problem. Even when both sides are affected, there may be an underlying neuromuscular condition. All children with pes cavus should be carefully examined by an orthopedic specialist. Surgery to correct the deformity may be necessary.

Arthritis involving the subtalar joint may occur as a complication of many different forms of childhood arthritis. (The talus is the major bone in the foot where it connects to the leg at the ankle joint. The subtalar joint is located in the middle of the foot, where this bone connects to the bones of the front of the foot.) Because the subtalar joint is responsible for twisting movements of the foot, children with arthritis of the subtalar joint experience pain and difficulty walking on uneven surfaces. Subtalar joint involvement is just one part of a much larger picture in children with arthritis. Careful and complete examination of the child makes it easy to recognize that the subtalar arthritis is not an isolated finding. This arthritis is easily diagnosed by careful examination of the foot. It may be treated with NSAIDs or local injection. Some children with persistent pain benefit from the use of orthotics that prevent motion in the subtalar joint by holding the foot in a rigid position inside the shoe.

Diffuse foot pain is infrequent. One of the most common causes is **reflex sympathetic dystrophy** that may begin after an injury to the foot. Children with reflex sympathetic dystrophy often experience color changes in the foot accompanied by profound hypersensitivity. Many of these children cannot put on a shoe or even a sock. This is a complex condition requiring specialized treatment. See Chapter 20 for more details regarding reflex sympathetic dystrophy.

ELBOW, SHOULDER, WRIST, AND FINGER PAIN

Pain in the fingers, wrists, elbows, and shoulders is common in older adults. But in young children, complaints are infrequent. Most complaints of pain in children under the age of ten are associated with minor injuries. Over the age of ten, overuse with athletic competition becomes more of an issue.

Elbow pain

"Nursemaid's elbow" is one of the more common causes of distress in young children. Parents usually notice that a young child (two to three years is the peak age group) is holding the arm bent and not using it. It is most often the left arm, but either may be involved. Typically, the injury occurs when a parent or sibling who is anxious to get going tugs hard on the arm. It might happen with crossing the street, arguing over whether or not it is time to leave the playground, or any other time the child is leaning away from you while you are pulling him or her toward you by the arm. It can also happen if you pick the child up by the arm (this should be avoided). The excessive stress on the elbow causes the bones to shift out of position, or dislocate. As a result, the child has pain and cannot straighten the arm.

Commonly, the dislocated "nursemaid's elbow" will snap back into place by itself, but if not, an experienced physician can usually snap the elbow back into place by holding the elbow steady and rotating the thumb toward the middle of the body. The bones often shift back into place with a pronounced clunk. A physician should evaluate children complaining of continuing elbow pain because there may be an associated fracture or other problems requiring correction. Elbow fractures are not always easily seen on X rays. Although isolated episodes of "nursemaid's elbow" happen to almost everyone, parents should be careful in handling their children. Repeated or prolonged dislocations of the elbow may lead to permanent damage. The most common causes of hand, wrist, elbow, and shoulder pain are listed in the box.

Trips and falls are the major cause of pain in the hand or wrist. Serious fractures are unusual without major trauma, but **green stick** or **buckle fractures** may occur. In these situations a child falls on an outstretched arm and immediately experiences pain. The arm may seem okay, but if it remains very tender at a specific point, the child should be taken for X rays. In these fractures, one side of the bone breaks, but the break does not go all the way through. These should be cared for by an orthopedist, as improper treatment could result in unbalanced growth of the bone causing the arm to curve. All fractures require immediate orthopedic care.

Common causes of pain in the elbow, shoulder, hand, and wrist

- Elbow
  - Nursemaid's elbow
  - Green stick or buckle fractures
  - Little Leaguer's elbow
  - Osteochondritis dissicans
  - Tennis or golfer's elbow
- Shoulder
  - Little Leaguer's shoulder
  - Rotator cuff injuries
- Wrist and fingers
  - Trauma
    - Mallet finger
    - Boutonniere deformity
    - Navicular fractures
  - Dactylitis

Chronic elbow pain in childhood is most often the result of overuse. The bones and ligaments of young children lack the strength to endure the repeated stress associated with throwing hard and other sports-related activities. While the number of innings pitched during games is strictly limited in organized Little League baseball, many parents fail to recognize that too many hard pitches in practice can also cause damage. *Parents concerned about their child's possible future career in professional sports must recognize that excessive hard practice at an early age will most likely result in injuries that make a professional career impossible.* Symptoms of "**Little Leaguer's elbow**" include pain or swelling along the inner aspect of the elbow and difficulty straightening the arm fully. Although X rays may be normal, children with these complaints should be forced to rest and not be allowed to throw until the symptoms have entirely disappeared. Continuing to throw despite elbow pain most likely will lead to long-term disability.

Older children in throwing sports such as football and baseball may develop **osteochondritis dissicans** of the elbow. In this condition, a small fragment of the end of the upper arm bone (humerus) may drop off the end of the bone. It is the result of repeated stress on the bone from overuse. This can be extremely painful. If the fragment falls into the joint space, it may block normal motion of the joint and cause locking. This can be detected by X ray or MRI. If the fragment is blocking normal motion, surgical removal may be necessary.

Tennis elbow is a degenerative change at the insertion of the muscle that is used to flex the wrist for activities such as backhanding a tennis shot. This muscle (the extensor carpi radialis brevis) is anchored to the arm just below the elbow. Excessive jerking of the muscle with strong contractions causes pain and irritation where it attaches to the bone. This is rarely seen in young children but may occur in adolescents who are overusing the arm. **Golfer's elbow** is a similar injury occurring on the inside of the elbow with excessive tugging on a different group of muscles. As with all such overuse injuries, these problems are best treated with rest and modification of the activity to prevent further injury.

Juvenile arthritis infrequently begins in the elbow joint without findings of pain, swelling, or limitation of motion elsewhere. However, any child who exhibits swelling of the elbow and difficulty straightening the arm fully should be carefully evaluated for other explanations. Children with arthritis beginning in the elbow may be labeled as having pauciarticular onset arthritis, but such children most often go on to have more widespread joint disease over time (see Chapter 7).

Shoulder pain

Fractures in the area of the shoulder are usually the obvious result of direct trauma. All require orthopedic intervention. The most common chronic conditions producing pain in the shoulder are overuse injuries associated with sports. "**Little Leaguer's shoulder**" is an inflammation of the growth plate in the shoulder. It results in pain when the shoulder is pressed and, in more severe cases, weakness. Advanced cases are easily diagnosed on X ray, but any child experiencing pain should be restricted from further throwing and other stressful shoulder activities until the pain has resolved. Excessive use of the shoulder can occur with tennis, gymnastics, swimming, baseball, basketball, football, and many other sports. As with overuse injuries in other joints, continuing the activity despite pain is more likely to produce chronic disability than an athlete of superior ability.

The great range of movement possible at the shoulder is due to the fact that unlike the hip, the shoulder is not limited by a deep bone socket. As a result, the shoulder is much more dependent on strong ligaments to maintain proper alignment. Young athletes with relatively loose ligaments are therefore uniquely susceptible to recurrent shoulder injury and dislocation. Any child with recurrent shoulder dislocations without obvious explanation should be carefully evaluated for ligamentous laxity and associated conditions (see Chapter 18).

Rotator cuff injuries are typically the result of irritation of the muscles in the rotator cuff being compressed between the upper bone of the arm (humerus) and the scapula (the bone that attaches the arm to the body; see Fig. 8). This compression is thought to result from imbalances in the strength of the muscles and ligaments that normally keep the bones properly aligned. Most often the children report pain with throwing and other overhand activities. Children with these problems should be carefully evaluated, rested, and begun on a careful program of rehabilitation. Allowed to rest and rehabilitate appropriately, most children can resume full activity. X rays are rarely helpful in this condition. MRI may be warranted if the problems persist. Surgical intervention is infrequently necessary.

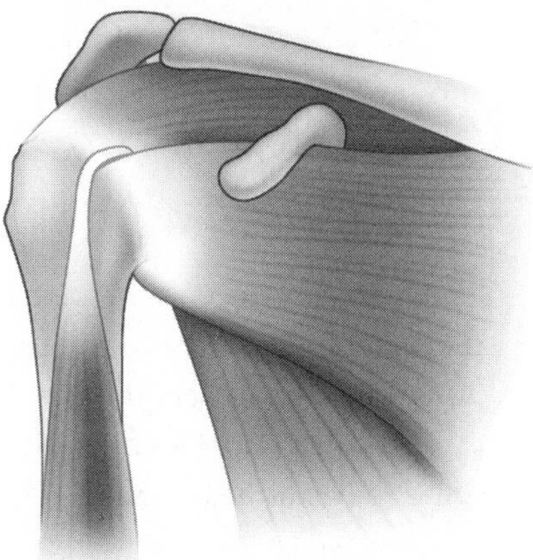

FIG 8. *The muscles of the shoulder and the rotator cuff. Injuries often result from the muscles enlarging with athletic activity to the point where they are irritated as they pass between the bones.*

Children with chronic shoulder pain and repeated injuries should be carefully evaluated for the presence of underlying conditions. Some adolescents with chronic shoulder problems have underlying conditions such as spondyloarthropathies or ligamentous laxity, which require further investigation and specialized treatment (see Chapters 9 and 18).

Hand, wrist, and finger pain

Finger injuries are extremely common in children of all ages. Obvious fractures are easily recognized and quickly diagnosed by appropriate X-ray examination. Children with persistent finger injuries require careful evaluation. Children with blunt trauma to the ends of the fingers may suffer damage to the tendons resulting in mallet finger or boutonniere deformity. A mallet finger is one in which the tip of the finger is pointed downward. It cannot be brought up because of damage to the tendon. Whenever a child suffers a blunt injury to the end of the finger, parents should check that the child can move all of the individual parts of the finger appropriately. If a tendon is ruptured, with the result that the child cannot move the tip of the finger up or down, the injury should be corrected surgically. **Boutonniere deformity** results from trauma to the finger tendons as they pass over the middle knuckle of the finger. As a result, the damaged tendon may slip down while the tip of the finger is pulled up (see Fig. 9). These are common sports-related injuries. However, boutonniere deformity may also be the result of arthritis.

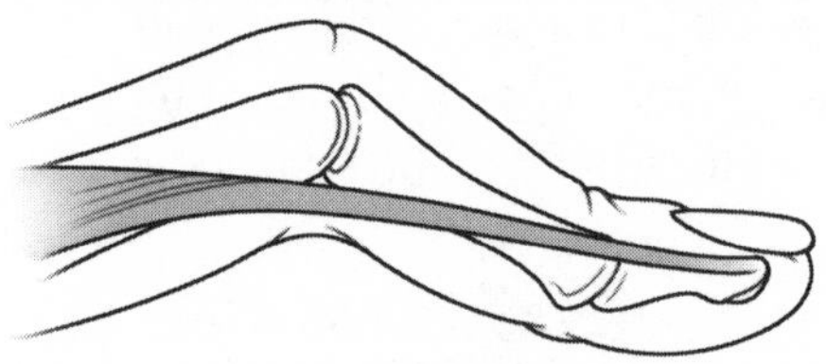

FIG 9. *Boutonniere deformity resulting from tendon slippage.*

Young children with swollen fingers or toes without explanation are often thought to have banged or stubbed them. But if the pain or swelling persists, the child should be carefully examined for evidence of arthritis. Persistent swollen fingers (**dactylitis**, or a sausage digit) may be the first manifestation of serious arthritis. Unfortunately, relatively few physicians are aware of this association (see Chapter 9).

Wrist injuries are common in normal athletic activity. Younger children rarely experience wrist fractures, but they commonly occur in adolescents engaged in vigorous sports activities. As with other parts of the body, most fractures are immediately apparent and easily diagnosed with appropriate X rays. One exception is fractures of the scaphoid bone. This bone is located at the center of the wrist. Fractures usually occur when a child falls hard on the outstretched hand. Although the child may complain of pain in the wrist, there is often no obvious problem. However, the pain will persist and the wrist will be tender if it is moved in the direction of the thumb or pressure is applied to the space at the base of the thumb (see Fig. 10). Fractures of the scaphoid often are not seen on

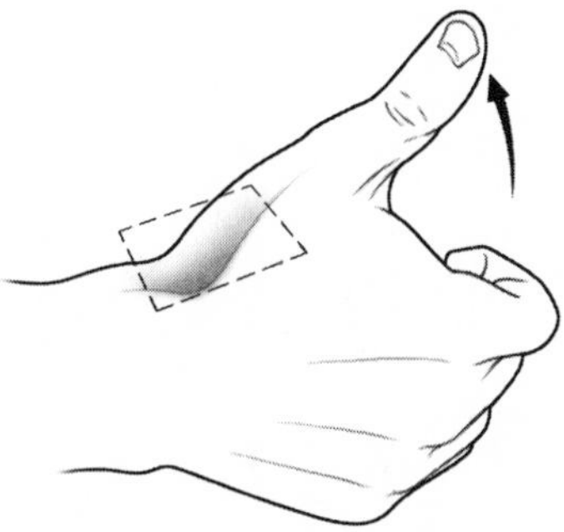

FIG 10. *Pain in the "anatomic snuff box," the base of the thumb, is an important finding suggesting a fracture of the scaphoid bone in the wrist.*

regular X rays unless special views are taken. Children with persistent wrist pain after a fall should be evaluated by an orthopedist.

Tendon irritation, sprains, and strains are uncommon in children under the age of ten except as the result of trauma. In older children, overuse injuries are common, especially with tennis and gymnastics. Children experiencing wrist pain in association with sports activities should be allowed to rest and recuperate to avoid worsening the inflammation.

Several forms of arthritis commonly begin in the wrist. Although long-standing arthritis is obvious on X rays, the key to recognizing arthritis early lies in a careful examination. Most children with arthritis have several joints involved that will be noted on careful examination of the whole child. Children with a chronic injury usually have only one involved joint.

4

The Child Who Hurts All Over

Children who are not doing well or complain of constant pain are a source of great concern for both parents and physicians. Some parents are concerned that their child is not able to keep up with the other children when playing. Others are concerned about repeated athletic injuries, wondering why their child has so many sprains and strains. Still other parents are concerned that the child seems withdrawn, irritable, or has lost interest in activities. There are many possible explanations when a child is not doing well. They range from serious illnesses to problems adjusting at home or in school.

Most physicians who care for adolescents are aware that a dramatic change in behavior without obvious findings on examination might be a sign of drug use or depression, but it may also be the first indication of rheumatic or other serious diseases. Inability to keep up with other children may simply be an indication that the child in question is not athletic, but it can also be the first sign of many serious illnesses, including muscle weakness from dermatomyositis or arthritis due to any of its many causes. Repeated athletic injuries and recurrent tendonitis may be due to poor stretching techniques, but they may also be the first signs of a spondyloarthropathy that can be easily treated.

Because there are so many possible causes, children without an obvious explanation for their complaints often become a source of frustration. This frustration can be minimized if everyone agrees to take a systematic approach. *Parents who are concerned that their child is not doing well should make a scheduled appointment with their physician for a full physical examination. It is best if the parents inform the physician's office at the time the appointment is made that this is not an appointment for a routine physical examination. You want your physician to be taking time and thinking about the problem.* You want your physician to know in advance that you are worried. This will not happen if you just happen to mention that your child seems out of sorts during a visit for a sore throat or a routine vaccination. Those are scheduled short appointments. Most likely, you are catching the physician both off guard and in a hurry. *You are far more likely to get the time and consideration your child deserves if your physician knows why you are coming and is thinking about the problem in advance.*

One of the greatest difficulties for families and physicians is that some children with widespread complaints do not look ill. A routine physical examination of the heart, lungs, and abdomen will not reveal muscle pain, weakness, or tender joints. Physicians unfamiliar with rheumatic diseases are unlikely to carefully evaluate the child for joint pain or weakness. As a parent, you must express your concerns. If necessary, you may need to insist on blood tests, X rays, or a specialist referral. For very young children, the physician is able to rely on a standard evaluation of the child who is "failing to thrive." Every pediatrician is trained to do this standard evaluation for babies and small children who are not growing as expected. Unfortunately, pediatricians are not trained to do a standard examination on older children who are not doing well. As a rheumatologist, I have developed my own standardized list of tests to evaluate these children (see box on the following page).

It is not practical to recommend that a physician do all of these tests on every child who does not feel well. Most children who I evaluate with these complaints have previously seen a number of physicians or have been complaining for a long period of time. I do all tests in the first portion of the list on every child I evaluate who is reported to not be "doing well." I reserve the amylase and lipase for children with complaints of abdominal pain, the IgG, IgA, and IgM for children with complaints of frequent infections, and the HLA B27 for children with joint pains. The clotting studies are reserved for children with easy bruising or bleeding, heavy menses, or chest pain.

The majority of children with a significant illness of the musculoskeletal system have specific findings on physical examination or abnormalities on at least some of these laboratory tests. Sometimes the abnormalities will seem only minor, but they must be viewed as part of a pattern of findings that may indicate the diagnosis. In isolation, *normal values on these laboratory tests are not enough to eliminate a significant medical condition.* There

Tests for the evaluation of children who are just not doing well

PPD (skin test for tuberculosis)

Complete blood count (CBC)

Erythrocyte sedimentation rate (ESR)

T3, T4, TSH anti-thyroid antibodies, anti-thyroid peroxidase (thyroid function studies)

IgA tissue transglutaminase (anti-endomyseal antibodies, associated with celiac disease)

Creatinine phosphokinase, a muscle enzyme (CPK)

Aldolase (another muscle enzyme)

Complete metabolic profile (this is a broad panel of general tests, including liver and kidney function)

Glucose, calcium, albumin, and total protein

Electrolytes including sodium, potassium, CO_2 (carbon dioxide, bicarbonate), and chloride

Kidney tests including blood urea nitrogen (BUN) and creatinine

Liver tests including alkaline phosphatase (ALP), alanine amino transferase (ALT, also called SGPT), aspartate amino transferase, (AST, also called SGOT), lactic acid dehydrogenase (LDH), and bilirubin

Urine analysis (UA)

Serologic markers including antinuclear antibody (ANA), rheumatoid factor (RF), and Lyme titer

Amylase and lipase if there is abdominal pain, dry eyes, or dry mouth

Total immunoglobulin levels including IgG, IgA, IgM

Clotting studies prothrombin time (PT) and partial thromboplastin time (PTT)

HLA B27

Note: I do not routinely screen for drug use in my rheumatology practice. However, in the setting of a general pediatric practice this may be necessary. Testing for HIV and other sexually transmitted diseases may also be needed in the appropriate situations.

are a number of children with spondyloarthropathies and other conditions who do not have any laboratory abnormalities. Nonetheless these children can be easily diagnosed by careful physical examination. Sometimes children have vague complaints during the earliest stages of a disease, even before obvious abnormalities occur. It may not be possible to make a definite diagnosis in these children and they may not require treatment. However, it is one thing to know your physician is taking your concerns seriously and will follow up on the problem, and another to simply be told, "There's nothing wrong with your child."

Family history may be the key.

I recently saw a five-year-old boy whose mother was concerned that he was recurrently waking up at night complaining of pain in his knees. At first the story sounded like a typical case of growing pains. However, as I continued to take the history, the mother described episodes of pain in the back and ankles that occurred during the day as well. The pains were usually short-lived (minutes to hours). A careful evaluation had been done by the referring physician, including an MRI of the spine because of concerns for a possible tumor. All of the laboratory tests and X rays were entirely normal. But the pains had been occurring for a period of months.

When I completed the history and physical examination of the child, there were only two key points. On examination the child was certainly "normal," but he was not limber. He had some tightness in his hips and at his ankles. However, it was not enough to be termed "abnormal." In addition, when taking the family history, I learned that the father had significant ulcerative colitis. This form of inflammatory bowel disease (IBD) is associated with arthritis (see Chapter 9) and the arthritis may precede the abdominal manifestations. I did not tell the mother that the child had arthritis. Nor did I tell her that the child had inflammatory bowel disease. What I did tell her was (1) that her child's complaints were not "normal," (2) that there was a possibility that the child's complaints were an early indication of inflammatory bowel disease, and (3) that no treatment was necessary at present, but routine follow up was important so that we could monitor for the possible development of IBD or increased symptoms that did require therapy.

I do not know whether this child will ever develop IBD. I do know that he is at increased risk, just based on the family history. Knowing that there was a possible explanation for the child's complaints and that he would be followed gave this mother reassurance that she had not gotten from being told, "Everything is normal." Someone might want to argue that I have unnecessarily made this mother worried about her child developing IBD. However, she already was concerned

Diseases that hurt all over
Fibromyalgia
Lupus (SLE)
MCTD
Scleroderma
Dermatomyositis
Spondyloarthropathies
Leukemia
Lymphoma
Neuroblastoma
Tuberculosis
Epstein-Barr virus (infectious mononucleosis)
Parvovirus B19 infections
Lyme disease
HIV and other sexually transmitted diseases

and knew IBD could be inherited. What she did not know was that it could produce joint pains. Knowing she was being listened to and carefully followed did not make her more worried. It made her more comfortable that her child was being watched carefully and would be treated appropriately if more problems developed.

The key to the diagnosis of diseases that hurt all over (see box) is a careful history, an appropriate physical examination, and appropriate diagnostic testing.

LABORATORY FINDINGS

There are two key elements that must be considered when evaluating the laboratory results of a child who is "failing to thrive." *The first is that entirely normal tests do not assure the absence of disease.* Many children with chronic diseases begin to lose their energy and feel unwell long before their routine laboratory results become abnormal. It is important to make sure that all of the appropriate tests have been done. *The second key element is to remember that things change over time.* On a number of occasions I have evaluated children who have been followed for months with unexplained chronic complaints. Many blood tests were done when the child was first brought to a physician, and all were normal. However, when the tests were repeated four to six months later, this was no longer the case. In the search for an explanation for a chronically ill child, it is important to reevaluate everything periodically.

Often the earliest abnormalities include a mild elevation of the ESR, a mild anemia, or mild hypoalbuminemia (see Chapter 24). Each of these findings is nonspecific, but an increasing number or gradual worsening of these nonspecific findings should alert the physician.

Many children with normal laboratory testing, but continued complaints, are labeled as having fibromyalgia or a similar condition. However, the physician must take responsibility for thoroughly excluding other significant illness before ascribing a child's complaints to a chronic illness or psychological problems. This is especially true if the child has any abnormal laboratory findings including an ANA, elevated ESR, or anemia. Careful evaluation of such children often includes a bone scan and a gallium scan, which may reveal the presence of infections, tumors, or other causes of inflammation. Tests such as MRI or ultrasound may be helpful in further evaluation of an area that has been identified as abnormal, but the bone scan and gallium scan have the advantage of evaluating the entire body in order to determine where more precise evaluation may be helpful (see Chapter 24).

WHEN NOTHING IS FOUND

Families and physicians become frustrated when, despite an entirely normal diagnostic evaluation, a child continues to complain of feeling unwell and is unable to continue his or her normal daily activities. Often the physician-family relationship becomes adversarial. The family *knows* there is something wrong with the child, but the physician *knows* he or she cannot find anything wrong. *It is vital for everyone involved to recognize that they are on the same side.* Often in this situation physicians will recommend a psychological evaluation. Parents often interpret this as a suggestion that they or their child are crazy. However, both the physician and family are doing everything possible to get at the root of the problem and restore the child to good health.

To get the best possible outcome, it is important for both the physician and the family to realize that, while psychological illness may cause chronic complaints of pain, chronic pain may also cause psychological illness. Both issues need to be addressed. The child who is unable to attend school needs psychological support, whether or not the cause is "physical." At the same time, referral of the child to a psychologist should not stop the ongoing medical evaluation of the child. *I often explain to families that in medicine we have the luxury of being able to go in two directions at once.* It is easy to ask for a psychological evaluation and an MRI on the same day. Sometimes parents ask me how I can justify doing both. The answer is that it is always justified to do everything possible to find the cause of a child's complaints. Looking in only one direction at a time may not be in the child's best interest.

If a child is able to attend school and carry out essential activities, it may be necessary to continue to monitor and to repeat periodically the diagnostic evaluation while awaiting the outcome of psychological intervention. For some families, this situation becomes unbearable. There is no single correct piece of advice. *The family must have complete confidence in the physician. If for any reason the family does not, a second opinion should be sought. Every reasonable physician has the child's best interest at heart. If another physician has a useful suggestion, everyone benefits. If the relationship between the physician and family has foundered and the family can establish a better relationship with a new physician, again everyone is better off.*

I often evaluate children who have seen many physicians. Sometimes these children have significant problems that have been overlooked or misinterpreted by other physicians. As a specialist, I am able to diagnose and treat a number of unusual conditions that other physicians might not recognize. Sometimes children have a slowly evolving disease that was not evident initially but becomes more obvious over time. However, some of the families I evaluate are simply "looking for the answer they want to hear." *Unfortunately, there are no adequate guidelines that can be written in a book that will distinguish the child with normal laboratory tests who has an unrecognized illness from the child with a disturbed psychosocial situation. Nor are the two mutually exclusive.* Both parents and physicians must rely on their own experience and judgment in deciding when to go further and when to stop. Neither will always be correct.

5

Sports Injuries

THINGS YOU NEED TO KNOW

Sports injuries are the most common causes of muscle, bone, and joint pains in childhood. Most are minor injuries related to trauma, easily recognized because the pain started right after falling, running into another child on the field, twisting an ankle, and so on. Often these are minor muscle and tendon injuries (bangs, scrapes, and sprains) that resolve over a few hours or days at most. Pain that is severe or persists requires medical attention.

Any child who needs to be carried off the field or brought home because of an injury should have a prompt and thorough medical evaluation. Acute sports injuries are not the focus of this book. However, the child who is repeatedly injured or in pain every time he or she participates needs to be carefully evaluated to find out why.

Children with chronic or recurrent "sports injuries" are often ignored because they seem to get better with rest. This is a mistake. Children with chronic and recurrent injuries may be suffering from overuse syndromes, unrecognized arthritis, or a variety of other medical conditions. Many of the children with spondyloarthropathies have been misdiagnosed as having chronic sports injuries by physicians who are unfamiliar with childhood arthritis (see Chapter 9).

The common athletic statement, "No pain, no gain," is incorrect. While it is true that muscle pain with activity may be associated with building stronger muscles, *bone and joint pain is never associated with gain*. Continued activity on bones or joints that hurt is causing injury and may be causing permanent damage.

Athletic coaches and trainers are not physicians. Their primary goal is athletic achievement. Many of the conditions described below are the result of overuse of the bones and joints or imbalance between rapidly increasing muscle strength and more slowly strengthening bone strength. Some trainers, sports physicians, and orthopedists feel these conditions should be treated with icing and taping. They commonly recommend that sports be continued unless "the athlete is unwilling or unable to tolerate the symptoms." This is a shortsighted approach. There are many adults complaining of chronic joint pains in their thirties and forties that they ascribe to high school and college athletics. Are this season's sports worth a lifetime of pain that could have been avoided by simply resting and letting the bones mature?

> I often evaluate children who have significant athletic ability and chronic pain. One of these was a young girl who was training for the Olympics. Tania had grown up in Eastern Europe, and because of her talent she had been selected to come to the United States to work with a famous coach in preparation for the next Olympics. The family stopped to see me in New York on their way to the training program because she had "minor knee pain." When I took the history, Tania's knee pain had begun over a year previously. At first it occurred only when she worked out, but with time it had become more persistent. Her family was very proud. "She works out six days a week, many hours each day despite the pain." Unfortunately, careful evaluation revealed that Tania had permanently damaged the bone in her leg (proximal tibia). Her dedication in continuing to practice despite the pain did not lead to the Olympics; it led to surgery and the end of her career. Had Tania stopped and been properly evaluated sooner, the diagnosis of benign hypermobile joint syndrome could have been made, the permanent injury could have been prevented, and her athletic career might have been saved.

Many of the children with enthesitis-associated arthritis have been misdiagnosed as having chronic sports injuries by physicians who are unfamiliar with childhood arthritis (see Chapter 9). It is often easy to make the correct diagnosis if the physician takes a complete history and examines the entire child. However, if you go to a physician complaining about your left ankle and the physician never examines the rest of your body, there is little likelihood he or she will recognize that you have problems in other joints as well. I often see children with arthritis in multiple joints who came to me complaining only about their knees or ankles. Not they, their families, nor their physicians had recognized that they were suffering from arthritis and not multiple independent injuries. With proper treatment we can often make many problems go away and allow the resumption of full activity.

SPECIFIC INJURIES

The emphasis in this book is on children with chronic or recurring problems. The proper evaluation and differential diagnosis of these conditions are discussed in the following sections. This book does not deal with specific fractures or acute injuries. However, it is important to realize that some problems that seem to begin as acute injuries are in fact chronic conditions. A child with Lyme disease may first be noticed to have a swollen knee when he or she complains of pain after a soccer game. Everyone's initial thought is that it must have been twisted. It is important that medical as well as orthopedic conditions be considered when, after an "injury," a child's pain is not resolving as expected.

Stress fractures

Stress fractures are one of the most common chronic injuries associated with sports activities in children and adolescents. They occur because of overuse and abuse of the bones. Typically, these fractures are caused by repeated impact. Stress fractures of the metatarsals (bones of the foot) are a common injury in runners, tennis players, and other athletes. However, stress fractures may occur in many different locations. Most often they occur in the legs, but tennis players and baseball players may experience stress fractures in the arms and shoulders as well. Most often stress fractures occur early in the athletic season because the child tries to do too much too soon. But older children who are participating in team sports may overuse their bones with continued efforts and develop more severe stress fractures later in the season.

Stress fractures usually first become evident when a child reports pain in a specific location following activity. If ignored, the pain will gradually become more severe and begin to occur earlier in the course of activity. Children with severe stress fractures of the metatarsals may have pain with walking. Because the pain of a stress fracture is right at the location of the fracture, it is often easy to diagnose on physical examination. However, other conditions can also cause the gradual onset of worsening bone pain at a specific site and proper radiographic evaluation (X rays) is important. Most stress fractures occur in the shaft of the bone and not near the ends. But in growing children there can be stress fractures at the growth plate. These can be diagnosed by characteristic changes on the X rays. Immediately after the injury, the X rays may be negative, but in any child with chronic pain the X rays should indicate the diagnosis. MRI studies are more sensitive and will help to exclude other possible causes of pain. Although much less common than stress fractures, both infections of the bone and bone tumors may begin with similar symptoms. Some children with arthritis are also initially misdiagnosed as having stress fractures that "did not show up on the X ray." If the child has complained of pain for more than two weeks and the X ray does not show a fracture, it is very unlikely that there is one.

Children with stress fractures who are diagnosed quickly often will recover with ten to fourteen days of rest. However, it is recommended that children not begin to resume activities until they have had no symptoms for three weeks or more. Full activity should be avoided for several months. Continued participation despite pain may result in permanent disability. In more severe cases, casting is necessary. If rest and casting do not provide relief, surgery may be required. Any child with a presumed stress fracture who does not begin to recover as expected should undergo a thorough evaluation to exclude other causes of bone pain.

Tendonitis and sprains

Tendonitis is inflammation of the tendon usually occurring at its point of attachment to the bone. Sprains are partial tears of ligaments. A tendon attaches a muscle to a bone. A ligament attaches two bones to each other and holds them in proper alignment. Tendonitis is usually the result of recurrent pulling on the bone when there is overuse of the muscles or an imbalance between the strength of the muscles and the bones. Bones and the attachments of tendons to bones strengthen only slowly with growth and activity. Muscles are able to strengthen much faster. As a result, children who begin vigorous activity at an early age strengthen their muscles and are able to put excessive force on the bones and tendons before the bones and tendons are able to adapt. This results in inflammation at the site where the bone and tendon join (see Fig. 11). This should be treated with rest and, if necessary, nonsteroidal anti-inflammatory drugs (NSAIDs). Continued activity may result in damage to the tendon or bone.

Most commonly, tendonitis occurs in the shoulders and elbows of children who are participating in throwing sports (e.g., baseball, basketball,

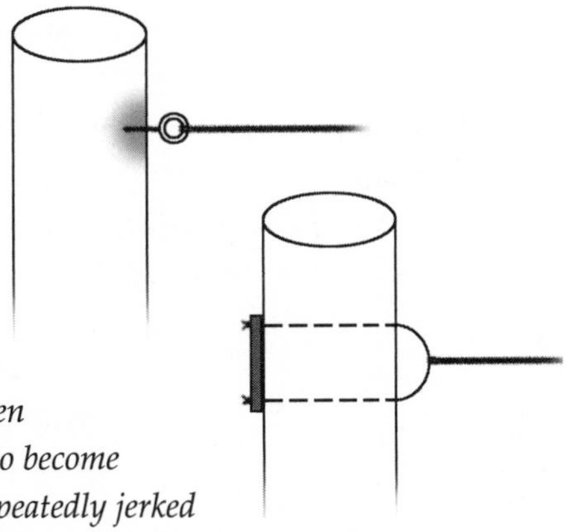

FIG 11. *On a working farm or ranch you will never find a rope attached to a post by a single screw. Because the rope is often yanked on, it has to be carefully secured. Most often there is a U-shaped attachment through the post with solid supports on the other side. A rope attached to a fence post by a simple eyelet screw will rapidly be pulled out. As children are growing, it takes time for the tendons to become firmly anchored to the bones. If they are repeatedly jerked with physical activity such as jumping or kicking a ball, the insertion becomes irritated and may never develop normally.*

football) or around the ankles of children who are participating in activities that involve a lot of running. Tendonitis around the knee is relatively rare, with the exception of Osgood-Schlatter disease (see Chapter 3). In this condition, there is inflammation of the insertion of the patellar tendon (which transmits all of the force from the muscles in the thigh to forward motion of the lower leg) where it attaches to the lower leg (anterior tibial tubercle). In children who are beginning to develop rapidly in the ten- to fifteen-year-old age group, the muscles often strengthen more rapidly than the bones. Lots of running and kicking exercise leads to inflammation at the tendon insertion. As a result, the anterior tibial tubercle (bump just below the knee) becomes swollen and tender. The key to resolving this situation is to enforce relative rest so the inflamed tendon and bone can heal and the relative strength of the bone can catch up with the muscles.

Since tendonitis is most often associated with overuse, its occurrence should be regarded as a warning to decrease the intensity of training until the child's body is able to mature further. In older children who are skeletally mature, it is a clear indication of overuse. Although the inflammation can be reduced by local injections of corticosteroids, this does not correct the fundamental problem. Reduction of the activity causing the inflammation is the wiser approach.

Children with enthesitis-associated arthritis (spondyloarthropathy; see Chapter 9) have excessive tendonitis as part of their disease. Any child with multiple episodes of tendonitis or tendonitis in multiple joints should be carefully evaluated to exclude these conditions.

BACK PAIN

Back pain is not a common complaint in childhood. Children with back pain should be carefully evaluated, and chronic back pain should never be dismissed as growing pains (see Chapter 3). The most common cause of chronic back pain related to sports in adolescents is **spondylolysis**. This is a stress fracture of the pars interarticularis (see Fig. 12). It is often the result of excessive stress on the low back with dancing, running, weight lifting, or other activities. Female participants in gymnastics are prone to this injury. As with stress fractures in other locations, the complaint of pain is usually exacerbated by activity and relieved by rest. X rays may reveal the fracture, but in some cases an MRI or bone scan may be required. Children with this type of pain should be carefully questioned about pain in other joints or stiffness when they arise in the morning. Children with involvement of other joints or morning stiffness may have arthritis.

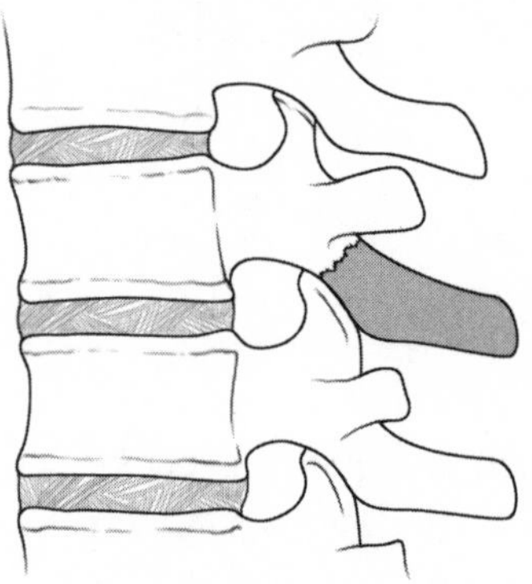

FIG 12. *Stress fracture of the pars interarticularis (darkened segment) causing back pain.*

Other causes of back pain that may become evident in association with physical activity are **disc herniation** or **spondylolisthesis.** Significant disc herniation is readily apparent on proper physical examination. Any child with pain when the straight leg is raised while the child is lying flat on his or her back requires a prompt medical evaluation (see Fig. 13).

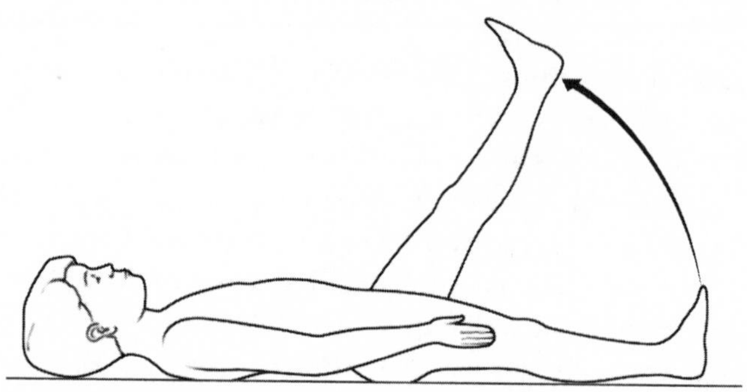

FIG 13. *Any child with pain when the straight leg is raised while lying flat on his or her back requires prompt medical evaluation.*

Spondylolisthesis is a progression of a spondylolysis to the point where the vertebral body slides forward. This causes chronic back pain and is readily evident on X rays of the spine. Many other chronic back conditions are not the result of sports injuries but may become more obvious when they limit a child's ability to participate in sports. These conditions are discussed in the general section on back pain in Chapter 3.

ELBOW PAIN

Chronic elbow pain often results from overuse. Younger children are very vulnerable to damage to the ligaments and growth plate of the elbow. Excessive pitching or throwing exercises and climbing on overhead bars (such as monkey bars) are common causes of elbow pain in children. All parents should be aware that their desire to see their child excel in sports today must be balanced against the risk of injury that will make him or her unable to perform in the future. Even if a child is well within the recommended level of activity for his or her age (e.g., 200 pitches per week for Little League), pain is an indication of ongoing injury. The child should be allowed to stop and rest the joint. If the pain recurs after a period of rest, full medical evaluation should be obtained. Other causes of elbow pain are discussed in Chapter 3.

Osteochondritis dissicans is the development of a dense area of damaged bone along the edge of the joint line. This may be the result of direct trauma or overuse. It is a common injury in children who have continued throwing activities despite pain. It may respond to extended rest and immobilization of the limb, but in some cases the fragment of damaged bone will fall into the joint. If this happens, the elbow may lock and surgery may be required to remove the fragment.

SHOULDER PAIN

Overuse is again the most common cause of pain in the shoulders. The shoulder is a relatively unstable joint that has a large range of motion. This is because there is relatively little bony reinforcement. The lack of bony reinforcement puts significant additional stress on the muscles and tendons of the shoulder. **Little Leaguer's shoulder** is the result of repeated stress to the growing bone of the arm (humerus). Chronic pain and weakness in the shoulder are accompanied by widening of the growth plate on X rays. Rest, enforced by immobilization in a sling or cast in more severe cases, will usually result in full recovery.

Rotator cuff inflammation and **impingement syndromes** often result from excessive stress to the shoulder. Acute tears are typically sudden in onset and easily recognized. Chronic inflammation may come on more slowly. Over time these children experience increasing pain with activity, especially with overhead throwing or swimming activities. The overuse syndromes are best treated with rest and modification of activity. Some children require NSAIDs. Every child with chronic pain of this type should be carefully evaluated for symptoms in other joints. Children with spondyloarthropathies may first come to medical attention because of chronic shoulder pain. Only when specifically questioned will they admit to pain in other joints. Even then, they often attempt to "explain away" these pains.

WRIST AND HAND PAIN

Wrist and finger injuries are common in sports activities. Fractures are usually immediately apparent. However, fractures of the scaphoid bone may not be immediately recognized because this bone is deep in the middle of the wrist. These fractures usually occur after a fall on the outstretched hand. Following the fall there is continued pain in the wrist, but no pain at the ends of the long bones in the forearm (radius and ulna). If there is a fracture of the scaphoid, pressure at the bottom of the extended thumb (see Fig. 10, p. 55) produces a dramatic increase in pain.

Another fracture that may not be immediately recognized is the **boxer's fracture**, which occurs at the first knuckle of the little finger (end of the fifth metacarpal). This fracture frequently occurs when the adolescent strikes something hard, often a wall or a locker. There is marked pain over the base of the finger. This fracture should be identified and properly treated, as failure to correct the injury may result in significant deformity.

Swollen and "jammed" fingers should be regarded with suspicion. A diffusely swollen finger is often thought to be due to an injury in basketball or other sports. However, these are a common finding in children with psoriatic arthritis and other spondyloarthropathies. A swollen finger that is not improving within ten to fourteen days should be thoroughly evaluated from both medical and orthopedic viewpoints.

HIP PAIN

Acute fractures and dislocations of the hip are immediately evident. The hip and pelvis are also the location of numerous avulsion fractures, in which a tendon pulls off its attachment to the bone. These injuries are usually associated with the sensation of a snap or pop and immediate pain. X rays typically confirm the diagnosis. Stress fractures in the femur or pelvis may come on more slowly. The athlete complains of progressively increasing groin pain with activities. Although stress fractures in the femur are not always evident on X rays, most often they are obvious on bone scan. MRIs may also be helpful to confirm the diagnosis.

Stress fractures of the pelvis are typically an injury of adolescent runners. This is an uncommon injury that is indicated by steadily increasing pain in the lower groin with activity. The pain usually becomes apparent with activity and is relieved by rest. As with stress fractures elsewhere, they may be diagnosed by bone scan before they become evident by X ray. The treatment is rest.

There are a number of chronic conditions in the hip that may initially become evident during physical activity. These are described in detail in the section in Chapter 3 on hip pain. Hip pain is a common complaint of children with spondyloarthropathies. Any child with chronic or recurrent hip pain that does not resolve with a period of reduced activity should be carefully evaluated. Continued activity in a child complaining of hip pain may result in permanent disability.

KNEE PAIN

The most common cause of knee pain in athletic children is **Osgood-Schlatter disease**, discussed at the beginning of this chapter and in the section in Chapter 3 on general knee pain. **Sinding-Larsen-Johansson disease** is similar in its cause to Osgood-Schlatter disease. This condition is common in the early teenage years as well as among teenagers who are doing a lot of jumping in sports such as basketball and volleyball. Jumping increases stress on the knee with sudden pulling on the tendon that attaches to the bottom of the kneecap (patella). As a result, these children complain of knee pain whenever they jump. On examination, they have pain when the bottom of the kneecap is pressed (see Fig. 14). This condition should be treated by resting the knee and avoiding

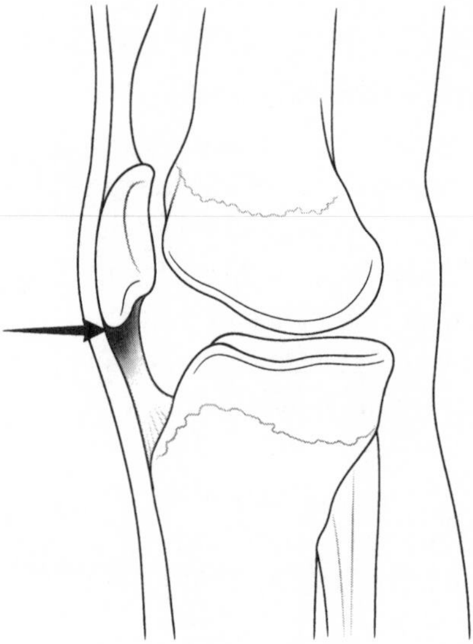

FIG 14. *Irritation where the tendon attaches to the bottom of the knee cap (patella) causes pain with jumping, which can be reproduced by pressing on the bottom of the patella in teenagers with Sinding-Larsen-Johansson disease.*

jumping activities. It is caused by the relative imbalance between the strength of the muscles and the strength of the bone. **Jumper's knee** is a more severe injury occurring in older children. The mechanism of the injury is the same. Excessive jumping repeatedly jerks the tendon where it joins to the bottom of the kneecap. In jumper's knee there is a deep tear of the tendon itself that may ultimately require surgery to relieve the pain.

Knee pain with sports may also be the result of **osteochondritis dissicans**. Just as in the elbow, osteochondritis dissicans in the knee is the development of a dense area of damaged bone along the edge of the joint line. This may be the result of direct trauma or overuse. It is a common injury in children who have continued running and jumping activities despite pain. It may respond to extended immobilization, but in some cases the fragment of damaged bone will fall into the joint. If this happens, the knee may lock and surgery may be required to remove the fragment.

Another common condition is **chondromalacia patella** or **patellofemoral dysfunction**. Knee pain with activities that is much worse when going downhill or downstairs is a very common problem. Despite the large number of children and young adults who suffer from this condition, it is poorly understood. You will hear many explanations in the doctor's office about "fragmentation of the underside of the kneecap" or "poor tracking of the patellar mechanism because of imbalance of the muscles." In truth, no one has been able to demonstrate convincingly the cause of this condition. I have been told of one athletic physician who was so frustrated that he actually consented to surgical removal of the kneecaps, only to have the pain continue.

Careful and complete medical and orthopedic evaluations are the most important aspects of treatment for these conditions. Many children incorrectly labeled with chondromalacia patella or patellofemoral dysfunction have easily treated problems that are discovered only when a proper evaluation is done. Although there are many proposed treatments for patellofemoral dysfunction, only two are generally agreed upon. The first is to avoid the activities that aggravate the condition. The second is a program of straight-leg raising exercises, which increase the strength of the muscles around the knee without bending it. Many patients find that several weeks of properly done straight-leg raising exercises are followed by the ability to resume normal activities without pain.

The iliotibial band is a band of tissue that runs along the outside (lateral) edge of the leg and anchors to the knee. If the band becomes tight, it will produce pain along the outside edge of the knee and in the outer aspect of the thigh. Although they most commonly occur in joggers, iliotibial bands may occur in children who are active in sports. Typical findings are chronic pain along the thigh and the outer edge of the knee. The pain comes on with running, but only after an extended period. It is often aggravated by climbing stairs, in contrast to chondromalacia patella, which is made worse by going downstairs. A program of proper stretching and leg-strengthening exercises is often sufficient to correct this problem.

Plicae are folds of synovial tissue that may be seen in the knee on MRI. They are a normal finding and not usually a cause of pain. If a child has vague unexplained knee pains and a plica is noted on MRI, orthopedists may suggest arthroscopic surgery. However, there is a good chance that the plica is not the cause of the pain. Proper treatment of children with plicae centers on excluding other causes of the pain. Once that has been done, most children are advised to avoid the activities causing pain. If the pain persists despite these measures or the activity cannot be reasonably avoided, the family may wish to consider surgery. Since early arthritis is accompanied by thickening of the synovium, it is not rare for a child with arthritis to be misdiagnosed as having plicae.

The menisci are button-shaped cartilage shock absorbers found on top of the tibia that absorb the downward pressure from the femur during activities. Meniscal tears are typically acute injuries when the foot is fixed in position and the leg twists excessively, compressing the meniscus. Meniscal injuries during sports activity often are associated with damage to the cruciate ligaments and dramatic pain and swelling. These injuries are promptly brought to medical attention and diagnosed. Chronic knee pain due to meniscal injury usually is the result of a fall or twisted knee that initially responded to rest. These are less severe injuries that may not have come to immediate medical attention. Children with these injuries often report a grinding sensation or a sudden catching feeling deep in the knee. (This is not the same as the grinding or catching under the kneecap that is felt in patellofemoral syndromes.) If the cruciate ligaments have been injured, there will also be instability of the knee. Instability of the knee often results in complaints of the knee suddenly giving out or locking. These symptoms always necessitate a thorough orthopedic evaluation and may require an MRI to properly evaluate the internal structure of the knee.

True meniscal tears and cruciate ligament tears often require surgical intervention. Partial tears may be treated conservatively or operatively, depending on their severity. When MRI testing first became routinely available, some children were found to have irregularities in the meniscus that did not extend to the surface. The explanation for these MRI findings remains controversial, but most authorities agree that surgery is not indicated.

LOWER LEG PAIN

There are relatively few conditions that cause pain in the bone itself. The two primary bones in the lower leg are the tibia (shinbone), which provides the bulk of the support, and the fibula (a small thin bone running alongside the tibia). Overuse may result in stress fractures in either of these bones. These stress fractures result in chronic pain that recurs whenever the child attempts to resume active physical activity. Infections and tumors can also occur in these bones. Since these conditions most often are easily detected by X rays, routine X rays should be obtained whenever a child has persistent complaints.

Shin splints are a common complaint of children who are doing a lot of running. They typically occur in children who are trying to do too much too fast. Often the problem disappears with additional conditioning. Children with continuing pain in the shin area (tibia) should be evaluated with X rays to be sure there is not a more serious problem (stress fractures, infections, etc.). Arch supports and orthotics may be helpful in chronic cases.

Chronic compartment syndrome may be a cause of pain in the calf that recurs whenever the child is very active in sports. These children often feel well but complain of pain in the calf region after playing on the field for a significant period. The pain disappears with rest but recurs with activity. Often these children complain of tenderness when the calf is squeezed. Typically, the problem is one-sided and occurs in the dominant leg (i.e., the right if the child is right-handed). If the problem does not resolve with a period of rest, surgery may be required. The pain results from enlargement of the muscles with exercise to the point that they are constricted by the surrounding tissues.

Blount's disease is a condition in which the growth plate of the tibia becomes damaged along its inner aspect. This damage results in unbalanced growth. The outside edge grows more than the inside edge, resulting in a curvature at the knee ("bow legs," or genu varum). This condition seems to occur more often in children who are heavy and may be related to the stress this places on the growing bone. The diagnosis can usually be made on a routine X ray. Surgery may be necessary to correct the condition. (See the section on knee pain in Chapter 3.)

ANKLE PAIN

The ankle is particularly vulnerable in growing children. Missteps and falls that place excessive force on the ankle joint are common injuries. Most ankle sprains are easily recognized and treated. More severe injuries should be evaluated by a physician to determine whether X rays are necessary to exclude the possibility of a fracture. This is especially true if there is evidence of bruising. Chronic or recurrent ankle injuries require careful medical evaluation. Some of these are due to partial tears of the ligaments that support the ankle. Others may be due to damage to the growth plates of the bones.

A child with recurrent ankle pain without obvious injury should be investigated fully. Some children with recurrent ankle sprains in fact have inflamed tendons from arthritis. Children with enthesitis-associated arthritis may have marked tendon swelling and tenderness, especially around the ankle. On careful examination, many of these children have tendon inflammation (enthesitis) around multiple joints that has been overlooked. With appropriate diagnosis and treatment, they are often able to resume full activity.

FOOT PAIN

There are many bones and joints in the foot. All are subjected to substantial stress with normal walking and running that is greatly increased by competitive athletic activities. Because the foot is heavily reinforced mechanically and typically protected by shoes, acute injuries are relatively uncommon. When they do occur, they usually are the result of obvious direct trauma (i.e., someone stepped on the foot or something fell on it). Chronic foot pain may result from a variety of conditions.

The most common serious cause of chronic foot pain in athletes is a **stress fracture of the metatarsals**. These are overuse injuries found in many different sports, ranging from football and soccer to dance and gymnastics. These cause severe local pain, often over the lateral aspect of the foot. They are typically treated with casting and rest. Although the initial X ray may not show the fracture, follow-up X rays should demonstrate healing bone to confirm the diagnosis.

Mild **mechanical foot pain** with activities is quite common. Many children are found to have flat feet, and their pain is attributed to this finding. However, "flexible" flat feet are a common normal variation and not thought to be a cause of significant foot pain. Some children obtain relief from the use of pads and other shoe inserts. A physician should evaluate all children with chronic foot pain. Although relatively uncommon, there are more serious causes of flat feet that do require surgical correction. (See Chapter 3.)

Tarsal coalition is a condition in which there is fusion of two of the tarsal bones. This condition may cause frequent foot pain, ankle sprains, and other foot discomfort. Although the condition has its onset early in life, many children become symptomatic only in the teenage years. This is also a time when children may become symptomatic with enthesitis-associated arthritis (see Chapter 9 for a full discussion). Children with chronic foot or ankle pains should be carefully evaluated for this condition. Tarsal coalition should be easily recognized on CT scan.

Heel pain is another symptom that can have multiple causes. *Children with enthesitis-associated arthritis often have heel pain that has been unsuccessfully treated as a sports injury.* A proper history and careful physical examination of the entire child are the keys to making the proper diagnosis. Many children with heel pain are given the diagnosis of **Sever's disease**. Sever's disease may be clinically diagnosed in children with pain at the sides of the heel but not at the base of the heel. X-ray diagnosis of Sever's disease on the basis of darkening of the growth plate at the back of the foot (calcaneal apophysis) is unreliable. Many children without heel pain have identical findings. (See Chapter 3.)

Part II

THE RHEUMATIC DISEASES AND RELATED CONDITIONS

6

Why Do Children Get Rheumatic Disease?

One of the questions parents ask me as they come to grips with their child's diagnosis of rheumatic disease is: "Why did this happen?" Medical research has made great strides over the past fifty years, but we still can't really answer this question. It is frustrating to think that all of that time and effort has not given us the answers. The following paragraphs detail some of my own thoughts. Some of it is proven. Some of it is conjecture.

Most of the rheumatic diseases clearly occur with increased frequency in relatives of people with the diseases, not so much that a mother needs to be concerned that her child will have the disease, but enough that investigators have to notice. Fill a football stadium with 100,000 random children, and the rheumatic diseases are rare. Fill that same football stadium with 100,000 children who have relatives with rheumatic disease, and children with rheumatic disease would be ten or twenty times as common. *So there must be a genetic contribution.*

Since it is not good for your health to have rheumatic disease, *why don't genes that contribute to them go away over time*? Imagine, if you will, a bank of ten switches that regulate the power to your town. Each switch provides 10 percent of maximum power. If all the switches are turned off, nothing works. One switch on helps, but two or three switches turned on are better. Everything works very well if five or six switches are turned on. However, maximum power is too much and things will start to overheat or short out if seven switches are turned on, especially if there is a thunderstorm. Eight switches on causes many more problems if it is too hot or too cold or there are storms. Things always go wrong if nine or ten switches are on. Now imagine if the number of switches that are turned on for any given town is controlled by rolling dice. Most towns will do fine. Some towns will have problems only in special situations, such as thunderstorms. However, a few towns will have trouble all the time. But since each switch is independently controlled and you need to have some turned on or there is no power, everyone has to take the chance that too many switches might be turned on.

Now think about the same story and imagine that instead of power switches we are discussing genes that regulate the ability to fight infection. You are born with them either on or off. If you are born with none turned on, you are very likely to get an infection and die. Too many turned on and you get a rheumatic disease if the wrong things happen. Most people end up in the middle and do fine. You can't get rid of the switches because you never know which ones will be turned on in any given child at birth.

How does the body's ability to fight infection relate to autoimmune disease? Rheumatic diseases appear to be the result of the immune system causing damage to normal tissues as if there was an infection. Does this mean the immune system is too strong or too weak? Imagine that your work requires you to go into a bar in a tough part of town. You were selected for this job because you are big and strong. If someone starts a fight, you will win, but if the person who attacks you is also big, there may be damage to the bar and some of the innocent patrons might be injured. That wasn't because you wanted to hurt them. The damage to the other patron is "bystander damage"—an inadvertent side effect of what you had to do to protect yourself. So a strong immune system can cause unintended damage.

If someone is weak and he has to go into a tough bar, he is in big trouble. Either he will be quickly done away with or he will carry a shotgun for backup. If someone picks on him and he starts firing the shotgun, lots of people will get hurt and lots of furniture will be damaged. Again, a lot of bystander damage. People with weak immune systems who survive do so because the immune system "overreacts" to any threat.

There is scientific evidence that this crude bar story is actually a good framework for understanding how autoimmune diseases come about. From the immune system's point of view, there are all sorts of bad guys out there. We need a strong immune system, but not too strong. That's why the drugs we use for serious cases of rheumatic disease are immunosuppressive drugs. Survival depends on maintaining the delicate balance between overreacting to an infectious agent and not reacting adequately to protect yourself from the infection.

7

Juvenile Arthritis

Juvenile Rheumatoid Arthritis (JRA), Juvenile Chronic Arthritis (JCA), Juvenile Idiopathic Arthritis (JIA)

THINGS YOU NEED TO KNOW

Two important points always must be remembered whenever considering the diagnosis of juvenile arthritis. *First, fever and rash should not be present except in children with systemic onset arthritis.* If a child with arthritis has fever or a rash, an extensive effort must be made to exclude infectious causes. Fever and rash may be present in Lyme disease, reactive arthritis, and a variety of other diseases that are not juvenile arthritis.

Second, it is important to differentiate between arthritis with painful swollen joints and bone pain. Children are sometimes thought to have arthritis because they hurt all over. As a general observation, *children with arthritis do not cry in pain when you are not touching them* or not touching an inflamed joint. This level of distress usually indicates a fracture, an infection, or a malignancy (leukemia, lymphoma, neuroblastoma, among others).

NOMENCLATURE

Names may not seem very important, and indeed in many ways they are not. It does not matter what you call a disease. It's still the same disease. You really don't care what I call your child's illness, as long as I "fix it." However, having the correct name for a disease is very important when you are trying to learn more about it or when two doctors are trying to discuss the care and treatment of a child (see the case history below). While most of the orthopedic conditions are well defined and only occasionally have more than one name for the same condition, the nomenclature of the rheumatic diseases of childhood is less clear.

According to the criteria of the American College of Rheumatology, juvenile rheumatoid arthritis (JRA) is the proper diagnosis for any child with the onset of arthritis before sixteen years of age if the arthritis lasts at least six weeks in more than one joint or three months in a single joint, without other explanation. *Thus, every child with chronic arthritis has JRA. However, it is very clear that not every child with arthritis has the same condition.* Imagine if you went to a rheumatologist specializing in adults and told him that every adult with arthritis lasting at least six weeks in more than one joint or more than three months in a single joint had rheumatoid arthritis. The adult rheumatologist would tell you that you were poorly informed. There are more than fifty causes of chronic arthritis in adults, only one of which is rheumatoid arthritis. Nothing magic happens at age seventeen. There are probably just as many different causes of arthritis in childhood. However, we haven't worked out the details because everyone is used to lumping all children with arthritis together as having JRA. This has resulted in a lot of confusion and misinformation.

Children with JRA are traditionally divided into three major groups: **pauciarticular onset** (less than five joints involved during the first six months), **polyarticular onset** (five or more joints involved during the first six months), and **systemic onset** (daily spiking fevers and rash; the number of joints does not matter). *This system of nomenclature is unsatisfactory because a little girl with a swollen knee and inflamed eyes does not have the same disease as a teenage boy with a swollen knee and ankle pain.* It is important to recognize that they do not have the same disease because they have a *different prognosis* (probable outcome in the future), *different responses to medication* (the best medicine for the little girl is unlikely to be the best medicine for the boy, and vice versa), and *most likely a different cause.* Yet both fit the official criteria for pauciarticular JRA. This is very troublesome when doctors study whether or not a medicine is effective. It may work for the little girl but not the teenage boy. If both are grouped together in a study as cases of pauciarticular JRA, the study may conclude that a drug does not work because it did not make enough people better. However, if the study had been done only with little girls, the doctors might have found the drug worked very well.

I would like to describe a common fruit. It begins green, and while some remain so, many varieties turn red or yellow in color as they ripen. It has a prominent stem, is somewhat juicy, and has an obvious core with seeds that people normally discard. Some eat this fruit with the skin on, while others prefer to peel and section it before eating. This sounds like a clear description of an apple, and we are all familiar with apples. However, this would also describe a pear. To those of us who are familiar with these fruits, the distinction is obvious when we have one in our hand. However, for someone unfamiliar with these fruits, this description could easily lead to misidentification of a pear as an apple, or vice versa. Imagine attempting to follow an apple pie recipe using pears or a constantly varying mixture of apples and pears. Not only would you never get the expected results, but if you had a constantly varying mixture you would never get the same results twice. Now imagine the confusion that happens when doctors think all children with arthritis have the same disease and should be treated the same way.

CLASSIFICATION

Arthritis is defined as pain, swelling, or limitation of motion in a joint. The official definition of JRA is any arthritis starting before sixteen years of age that persists as above without other explanation. (The persistence is important because many viral and bacterial illnesses can cause arthritis that lasts only a few weeks; see section on reactive arthritis below). The arthritis may not necessarily have been noticed by a doctor for the six weeks or three months prior; there simply has to be convincing evidence that it has been present for at least that long.

Most children with arthritis do not have a disease that is in any way related to the rheumatoid arthritis seen in adults. To reflect this difference, it has been proposed that the terms juvenile chronic arthritis (JCA) or juvenile idiopathic arthritis (JIA) replace JRA. However, children suffer from many different forms of arthritis with many different causes and courses. *It must be clearly recognized that these names refer not to a single disease but to a variety of diseases that share arthritis as a prominent symptom.* To minimize confusion, I use the following nomenclature in this text. **Juvenile arthritis (JA)** will refer to "idiopathic" inflammation of the joints in a child. (*Idiopathic* simply means unexplained, as opposed to inflammation caused by an infection or other obvious cause.) I use this term as JRA was originally used, that is, to refer to *all* children with unexplained arthritis beginning before the age of sixteen, with the requirement that the arthritis is present for an extended period, as described above. *JA does not refer to a single disease with a single cause. JA is not a disease at all; it is a group of signs* *and symptoms with many different causes and outcomes.* Thus, to say that a child has juvenile arthritis is no more meaningful than to say a child has a broken bone. Much depends on which bone and how badly it is broken. In JA, much depends on the type of JA and how severe it is.

In our efforts to distinguish the different types of JA, a number of subgroups have been proposed. None of these is truly definitive and there may well be several distinct diseases within each of the subgroups. I indicate the generally accepted subgroups in each section, but I also make distinctions based on my personal experience. Three important points must be remembered. First, unless we attempt to identify and investigate subgroups, we will never advance our current knowledge. In the end, some of the subgroups may need to be divided further, while others may be incorporated into the larger group. Second, if we insist on lumping groups together until someone has proven they are different, we risk attempting to make apple pie with varying combinations of apples and pears, and wondering why our results are inconsistent. Virtually every published article on the treatment of JRA suffers from this fault. Third, while it may be possible to memorize the entire American Kennel Club classification of breeds of dogs, there will still be dogs that are mixed breeds and do not fit any classification. We are dealing with biologic phenomena occurring in nature, not a predetermined system. *Diseases do not read or write textbooks and are not bound by what is written in them.*

PAUCIARTICULAR ONSET JUVENILE ARTHRITIS

The first key distinction made by physicians evaluating children with arthritis is between children with arthritis in a few joints (pauci- or oligoarticular onset JA) and children with arthritis in many joints (polyarticular onset JA). As originally defined, this categorization refers to the number of joints involved during the first six months of illness. Thus, a child who originally has only one joint involved but develops arthritis in four more joints during the next three months has polyarticular onset disease. But a child who originally has only one joint involved and slowly develops more joint involvement, but not until eight months later, still has pauciarticular onset disease.

The distinction between pauciarticular onset and polyarticular onset JA is made only on the basis of the number of joints involved six months after onset. This is both confusing and of limited utility. After all, who knows exactly when the arthritis started and can accurately date the six months? However, the classification persists because it is generally useful. The flaws are easily dealt with by recognizing that *children with involvement of the small joints of the hands and feet, with or without involvement of the large joints, have a different prognosis (and probably different disease) than children with only large joint involvement*. Since there are not that many large joints (JA tends to spare the hips at the beginning), children with only large joint involvement typically have pauciarticular onset JA. In contrast, involvement of the fingers or toes rapidly becomes polyarticular. *Further, even if children have only one finger involved (two or three joints), they have an entirely different prognosis (and different disease) from children with two or three large joints involved.* Understanding this flaw in the nomenclature makes it clear why a child who had pauciarticular onset JA may have disease that does not behave like the textbook or pamphlet said it would. The proper classification should be onset with only large joints versus onset with small joints involved, with or without large joints.

Pauciarticular onset arthritis may take a variety of different forms. This is most often a disease of young girls and some boys that starts between one and seven years of age. (Older children with disease only in large joints often have a spondyloarthropathy. This is a completely different group of diseases with different outcomes and different best therapies. Thus, they are discussed separately in Chapter 9. Children with involvement of fingers or toes [*dactylitis*] also must be considered separately, even if there are fewer than five joints involved during the first six months of disease.)

In the most typical cases of pauciarticular disease, there is a single swollen knee. Frequently, there is no history of pain and the parents have been unaware of the problem until a friend or relative pointed out the swollen joint. When asked, the parents cannot tell you when the problem began. There may be awareness that the child walks funny when he or she first gets up, but because he or she walks normally after a little while, the parents often think he or she "just sleeps on it funny." Some physicians have referred to this as "painless JRA" because the child does not complain. However, if you squeeze the joint or attempt to range it fully, it is painful. The child is not complaining because the child does not recognize that this is not the way it is supposed to be.

Children with the acute onset of a painful swollen knee should not be considered as having pauciarticular JA. Among the conditions that may cause the acute onset of a painful swollen knee are infections (including Lyme disease), reactive arthritis, foreign body synovitis, and injuries. On rare occasions a child with a chronic swollen knee (i.e., pauciarticular arthritis) that has gone unnoticed will be brought to the doctor complaining of acute pain in conjunction with an infection. The chronically swollen knee was noticed only with the increased problems brought on by the infection. This can be recognized by careful history and physical examination. Frequently, bony overgrowth is present. This is a clear indication that the disease has been going on for a prolonged period, since bony overgrowth takes months to develop.

Children who begin with pain in the hip also should not be considered as having pauciarticular JA. Although polyarticular arthritis and systemic onset arthritis may ultimately involve the hip, it is never the first joint involved and the hip is never involved in pauciarticular arthritis. I have seen cases of toxic synovitis, Lyme disease, osteoid osteoma, occult fractures, and tumors misdiagnosed as juvenile arthritis starting in the hip. Spondyloarthropathies may start in the hip, but these are most often in children over the age of ten years. Any young child with hip pain must be thoroughly investigated and an explanation other than pauciarticular onset arthritis should be found. *(There are exceptions to every "rule," but never accept the idea that you are the exception without very careful evaluation.)*

Laboratory findings in children with pauciarticular onset disease are usually entirely normal. They should have a normal complete blood count (CBC), normal metabolic panel, and normal sedimentation rate. Rheumatoid factor (RF) should be negative, but antinuclear antibody (ANA) may be present (see Chapter 24 for a full discussion of these tests). Mild abnormalities of the CBC and erythrocyte sedimentation rate (ESR) are common. But children with significant laboratory abnormalities during the first six months of treatment should be regarded with suspicion.

During the first six months of disease, children with "true" pauciarticular disease should not have a hemoglobin level below 11 gm/dl without explanation or a sedimentation rate greater than 40 mm/hr. Those who do are more likely to have further arthritis in the future. Other findings that increase the risk of continuing or recurrent arthritis are immunoglobulin A (IgA) deficiency or presence of the genetic marker HLA B27. A family history of psoriasis or inflammatory bowel disease also increases the risk of further arthritis. It is most likely that these children do not have the same disease as the "true" pauciarticular onset children. The prognosis for children with well-defined pauciarticular onset disease is good. This is the form of JA responsible for the myth that "most children grow out of it." Children who do not do well with pauciarticular onset disease are usually recognized by the exclusions I indicated above.

Complications

There are two well-known complications of typical pauciarticular onset disease that must be watched for. These are limb length discrepancy (one leg grows longer than the other) and eye inflammation. Limb length discrepancy in children with pauciarticular arthritis is most often seen if the inflammation is in one knee and is not brought under control quickly. The inflamed knee develops increased blood flow as a result of mediators produced by the inflamed synovium. This increased blood flow brings more nutrients to the bones around the knee and they will grow more rapidly, causing the leg to be longer on that side. (This is just as if you were growing carrots and gave one row of carrots more water and fertilizer.) Thus, the arthritic leg will actually grow longer. This is not always easy to see, but it is easy to detect by properly measuring the leg. This is best accomplished by doing a special radiograph called a **scanogram**. This is simply an X ray in which a ruler that can be seen on the X ray is included so the bones can be directly measured.

Just by watching a child walk, one may not be aware of a difference in leg length. This is because children with arthritis in the knee often develop a flexion contracture that makes the leg appear shorter. A flexion contracture of the knee is a shortening of the tendons around the knee that prevents the knee from moving into a fully straight position. The flexion contracture comes from holding an inflamed knee in a bent position. Children do this because bending the knee decreases the pressure in the inflamed joint and it hurts less. Unfortunately, at the same time, the pain is causing the muscles around the knee to spasm (they are trying to protect the joint). As a result of prolonged muscle spasm, the tendons around the knee become tight. Unless the child is receiving anti-inflammatory medications and doing physical therapy to prevent the problem, it becomes impossible to completely straighten out the leg (this is the definition of a contracture).

As the inflammation improves with treatment, the physician and therapists may become concerned that the flexion contracture is not resolving as expected. However, if a child has developed a leg length discrepancy, the child will need to continue to hold the longer leg bent in order to keep both legs functionally the same length when walking. This can be corrected by putting a lift in the shoe on the normal (but shorter) side. Many parents don't like to put a lift in their children's shoes. However, failure to properly correct the situation makes it difficult to correct the flexion contracture and may lead to hip damage in later life. Occasionally, children

Testing for a knee flexion contracture

If you as a parent are concerned that your child may have a knee flexion contracture, you can easily evaluate this by having your child sit on the floor. A normal child can put his or her knee flat on the floor so that you cannot even slip a piece of paper underneath it. If you can see a space under the knee or slip your fingers under it, there is a flexion contracture (see Fig. 15).

with involvement of the elbow may develop a discrepancy in the length of the arms or a flexion contracture at the elbow. In these children it is noticed when they cannot fully extend the elbow.

When evaluating a child with pauciarticular onset disease for joint swelling or a limb length discrepancy, you may be fooled by the fact that in addition to the leg growing longer, the knee (distal femur and proximal tibia) will also grow larger in diameter. When the arthritic leg is compared with the normal side, muscle atrophy will make the situation look even worse. Just as children with arthritis develop flexion contractures if they do not get physical therapy, they also develop muscle atrophy. Although the muscles initially spasm to protect the joint, over time the child is not using the leg that hurts and the muscles atrophy (grow smaller). Any child with muscle atrophy or flexion contractures will benefit from physical therapy.

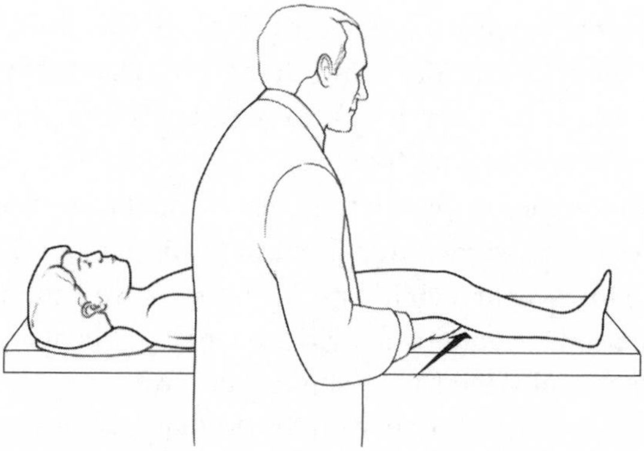

FIG 15. *You should **not** be able to slip your hand under the child's leg when he or she is lying flat on the bed.*

When both muscle atrophy and bony overgrowth are present, the knee appears even larger than it actually is. You need to examine the knee carefully to differentiate between bony overgrowth and continued swelling. Bony overgrowth makes the knee look bigger, but excessive joint fluid is not present. This does not require a change in medication. If the knee is swollen because of extra joint fluid, then it does need to be treated. Sometimes a knee with bony overgrowth becomes inflamed and there is extra joint fluid, as well. The key to preventing muscle atrophy, limb length discrepancies, and flexion contractures is to bring the inflammation under control quickly. Once these problems have developed, the child should be given extensive physical therapy to correct the weakness and contracture as quickly as possible. Leg length discrepancy may not persist if the inflammation is brought under rapid control. If the leg length discrepancy does persist, it should be corrected as the child nears adult height (see below).

Eye involvement is the other significant complication of pauciarticular JA. Although the explanation has never been determined, the presence of a positive ANA is strongly correlated with the risk of eye disease (see Chapter 8). *Children with pauciarticular onset disease who are ANA-positive are much more likely to have eye disease than those who are ANA-negative.* The eye disease takes the form of inflammatory cells in the anterior chamber of the eye. This may be referred to as uveitis or iridocyclitis. The inflammation can lead to damage to the iris with scarring and irregularity of the pupil. These scars are called *synechiae* (see Fig. 16). *Because the eye disease is usually painless and may go unnoticed for a long period, it is recommended that an ophthalmologist screen such children every three months.* ANA-negative children should be screened every six months. Although the risk of eye involvement is lower in ANA-negative children and in children with polyarticular onset disease, it may still occur. For more information, see Chapter 8.

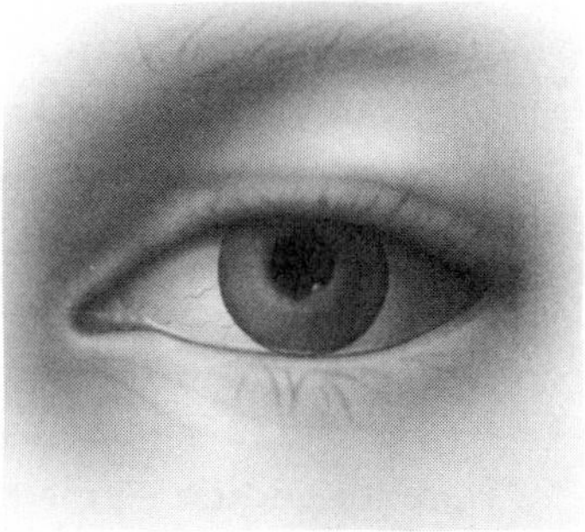

FIG 16. *Synechia in the eye of a child with uveitis.*

On occasion I see children who were diagnosed with pauciarticular onset disease many years before who now have stiff necks. It is well recognized that children with polyarticular onset disease may develop cervical fusion over time that causes a stiff neck. Often there is no real complaint from the child, and the finding is noted only on X rays. Usually at the time I see these children, it is because they have developed more arthritis. It is unclear whether cervical fusion is a complication of "true" pauciarticular onset arthritis or whether these are children who should have been characterized as polyarticular initially.

Medical treatment

Treatment for pauciarticular onset arthritis usually consists of nonsteroidal anti-inflammatory drugs (NSAIDs). These drugs are discussed in detail in Chapter 22. Since this is primarily a disease of young children, medications that are available in liquid form are preferred. Ibuprofen and naproxen preparations are widely available in liquid form. Indomethacin is also available in liquid form but has a greater frequency of side effects and should be reserved for difficult cases. Rofecoxib is a selective COX 2 inhibitor (see Chapter 22) that is also available in liquid form. Nabumetone comes only in pill form but dissolves easily in warm water and can be drunk by children who do not know how to swallow pills.

I often use diclofenac for children with pauciarticular onset disease that does not respond adequately to the readily available liquid medications. Although it is not stocked in liquid form, a compounding pharmacist can easily provide liquid diclofenac. This will cost extra, but a compounding pharmacist will also prepare the medication in your choice of flavors. Not having to struggle with a child to get him or her to take medication is a major benefit. Naproxen, nabumetone, and diclofenac also have the advantage of being given less frequently than ibuprofen.

For children who meet my definition of pauciarticular arthritis, it is rare for additional medications to be necessary. Corticosteroids (prednisone), methotrexate, cyclosporine, and other immunosuppressive drugs should not be needed (remember, there are exceptions to virtually every rule, but they are rare). Occasionally, there are children who have persistent swelling of one or two joints despite an adequate trial of NSAIDs. This is the point at which it is reasonable to consider intra-articular (directly into the joint) injection of corticosteroids.

Intra-articular corticosteroids rarely have side effects and often provide rapid and dramatic relief (see Chapter 22). Unfortunately, it is impossible to predict who will respond and for how long. However, the majority of children get a good response for months, if not longer. Some physicians will inject multiple inflamed joints in an effort to avoid increasing the medications. I will consider injecting two joints, but if more than two joints are persistently inflamed, I prefer to alter the medication rather than subject the child to multiple injections.

If only one joint is to be injected, the majority of children can be easily talked through the procedure without requiring anesthesia and without undue distress. If multiple joints are to be injected, anesthesia may be necessary. Most pediatric rheumatologists believe that appropriate use of intra-articular corticosteroids will decrease the frequency of leg length discrepancy by bringing resistant inflammation under control more rapidly. Intra-articular corticosteroids in conjunction with **night splints** or **serial casting** (see the Glossary) and physical therapy often make it easier to correct flexion contractures. Physical therapy is a valuable adjunct for children with arthritis. In children with pauciarticular onset disease, physical therapy can help to rebuild lost strength and to correct or to prevent flexion contractures. In many cases, children with flexion contractures will benefit from night-resting splints or serial casting without intra-articular injections.

Surgery

Surgical therapy for "true" pauciarticular onset arthritis is rarely necessary. Surgical therapy may be required to correct leg length discrepancy. Fortunately, this is a minor procedure. Most small children who develop leg length discrepancies as a result of pauciarticular onset arthritis will self-correct with growth and remodeling over time. However, the arthritis must be under good control for this to happen.

In children who reach the age of ten with a significant persisting leg length discrepancy, an orthopedic appointment should be scheduled. With the special X rays called scanograms and an X ray called a "wrist for bone age," the orthopedist can predict the amount of future bone growth using standard tables. In general, they will not intervene unless they expect a leg length difference of greater than one inch. If it is likely that there will be a significant difference, the orthopedist will monitor the child to determine how long it will take the short leg to catch up to the long one. The child is then taken to the operating room and under anesthesia a small incision is made and a staple placed in the growth plate (distal epiphysis) of the leg that is too long. This signals the bone to stop growing. Now the bone that is too long has stopped, and the one that is too short keeps growing. If the child follows the predictions in the table, there will be no or only a slight difference in the length of the legs once full size is attained.

There are two other situations in which surgery is considered for children with pauciarticular onset arthritis. If a very severe flexion contracture has developed and it cannot be corrected with physical therapy and intra-articular corticosteroids, the orthopedist may consider doing tendon releases. This is virtually never necessary for children who have received appropriate care early in the course of their disease, but nonetheless may be needed. In addition, there are exceptional cases of children with chronic active synovitis unresponsive to multiple medications or intra-articular corticosteroids. These children probably do not have "true" pauciarticular onset arthritis. It may be necessary for the surgeon to explore the joint to determine what is going on, to remove some of the excess tissue (this is called doing a synovectomy), and to obtain appropriate tissue for examination by the pathologist (a biopsy) to exclude other diseases such as plant thorn synovitis (see Chapter 3).

Prognosis

The prognosis for the typical child with "true" pauciarticular arthritis is very good. Most children respond as expected to therapy and are well within a few months. My normal standard is to treat a child until there has been no evidence of active disease for six months. This often means nine months to a year of treatment. At that point, I will discontinue the NSAIDs and watch carefully. Most of the children (about 80%) will remain well without medication. In a few children, the disease will flare up shortly after stopping medication, and a few more children will develop new episodes of arthritis over the next few years. The explanation for this is unclear.

When pauciarticular onset arthritis flares up in a child, he or she should be carefully reinvestigated to exclude other problems. Children with a well-documented history of JA may nonetheless develop Lyme disease, bone infections, or other problems that at first look like a recurrence of the JA. If other problems have been excluded, but the child does not respond quickly to reintroducing NSAIDs, they probably did not have "true" pauciarticular onset arthritis. This is true even though they fulfilled all of the initial criteria. Children who do not fulfill my definition of "true" pauciarticular arthritis are less likely to recover completely in six months and much more likely to flare when the medication is discontinued (see the next section).

There is no reason to expect that children with "true" pauciarticular onset disease will not be able to carry out fully functional lives in every way. There is nothing about pauciarticular onset disease that should limit their ability to play sports, have families, or participate in all other normal activities. The prognosis for children with significant eye disease will depend on their ultimate visual status. This is best discussed with the treating ophthalmologist (see Chapter 8). It should be noted that it is rare for children with pauciarticular arthritis to develop new eye disease after ten years of age.

Children who do not have "true" pauciarticular arthritis may ultimately be recognized as having several different diseases. As previously indicated, any child with a hemoglobin level below 11.0 gm/dl, an ESR greater than 40 mm/hr, IgA deficiency, HLA B27, a family history of psoriasis, or a family history of inflammatory bowel disease should not be considered as having pauciarticular arthritis. Many will develop arthritis in additional joints before six months and fulfill criteria for polyarticular onset disease. However, the parents may have been given false expectations at the beginning. It is common for me to see children for a second opinion because the parents were told that the child had pauciarticular onset disease and would grow out of it. A few months later the disease is spreading and their physician is recommending aggressive therapy. The family looks at the possible side effects and says, "Why should we take these risks if our child is going to grow out of this?" If the physician had recognized that the child was at increased risk, this situation could have been avoided.

Not all children who fulfill the criteria for increased risk do poorly. Many children who fulfill these criteria do just as well as the children with "true" pauciarticular onset disease. However, the percentage of children who have continuing problems is higher. If the parents and physicians are aware of the increased risk, they will not be lulled by false expectations. They will know to monitor the child more carefully and recognize that for these children it is appropriate to intervene more aggressively to prevent additional damage. They should be treated like children with polyarticular onset disease (see next section).

POLYARTICULAR ONSET JUVENILE ARTHRITIS

Polyarticular onset disease is defined as arthritis involving more than four joints during the first six months of disease, without other explanation. In my opinion, any involvement of small joints indicates polyarticular type disease even if initially there are fewer than five joints involved.

Polyarticular onset disease may occur in any age group but is found more often in girls than in boys. This is a very heterogeneous group of diseases. There are two major peaks in the age at onset of disease; young children with the onset of disease between eighteen months and eight years of age and teenagers with the onset of disease after eleven years of age. Some children start with only one or two arthritic joints, with the arthritis slowly spreading to other joints, while other children rapidly develop arthritis of multiple joints.

Most pediatric rheumatologists make distinctions based on the presence or absence of rheumatoid factor (it is normally absent). These children may also be subcategorized according to whether the disease is symmetric (both elbows or both knees, etc.) or asymmetric (only one elbow or one knee, but there still must be more than four joints involved, according to the official nomenclature). Children with tendon insertion inflammation (enthesitis), a family history of psoriasis, a family history of inflammatory bowel disease, or the presence of HLA B27 are included in this group by some physicians but are excluded by others. I exclude children with these findings because I believe most of them have spondyloarthropathies that behave differently (see Chapter 9). Even when all the children with these findings are excluded, the remaining children are a diverse group and most likely have several different diseases.

Laboratory findings in children with polyarticular onset arthritis are highly variable. Some have entirely normal laboratory tests, while others have elevated ESR and low hemoglobin. A small percentage of children with polyarticular onset are rheumatoid factor (RF)-positive and should be considered as having an early onset of adult-type rheumatoid arthritis. However, RF may be found in a number of other conditions (see Chapter 24) and should not be relied on to establish this diagnosis. *A positive test for rheumatoid factor (RF) in a child less than ten years of age is far more likely a false positive result or an indication of another illness than a sign of early-onset RF-positive polyarticular arthritis.* The test for ANA may also be positive in children with polyarticular onset disease. Although their risk of eye disease is lower than that of ANA-positive children with pauciarticular onset disease, ANA-positive children with polyarticular disease also have an increased risk of uveitis and should be sent to the ophthalmologist for screening examinations every three months.

Several diseases need to be distinguished from polyarticular onset arthritis. Children with rheumatic diseases such as systemic lupus erythematosus, dermatomyositis, polyarteritis nodosa, sarcoidosis, and mixed connective tissue disease often have polyarticular arthritis in addition to their other symptoms. There are a variety of less frequent diseases that also may begin with polyarticular arthritis. These diseases should be excluded by appropriate history, physical, and laboratory evaluation.

The disease most often confused with polyarticular onset JA is **reactive arthritis** (also called **infection-associated arthritis**). Reactive arthritis often begins with the rapid onset of disease involving the large and small joints (see Chapter 9). The key to suspecting this diagnosis is a history of an infection usually ten to fourteen days before the onset of arthritis. Children who rapidly develop polyarthritis should be evaluated carefully for evidence of either a recent infection or an infection that is still present and may need to be treated. Parvovirus B19 infection and Lyme disease are just two examples of many infections that cause an acute reactive arthritis with an elevated sedimentation rate and an ill-appearing child. Often reactive arthritis can be differentiated by the history or the laboratory findings. This is important because reactive arthritis typically resolves over a period of a few weeks to several months. In some cases it appears that an infection that is known to cause reactive arthritis initiates chronic polyarticular arthritis in a susceptible individual (this arthritis is discussed in detail in Chapter 9).

Children with early onset of polyarticular disease often seem to improve, then worsen repeatedly over a period of years. As a result of repeated episodes, they progressively develop more joint involvement and are a difficult group to bring under continued control. It is usually possible to bring their arthritis under reasonable control with medications, but it is unlikely that their arthritis will ever be completely gone, never to return.

Children with early onset of polyarticular onset disease who have continuing smoldering disease activity should be treated relatively aggressively. Often the parents and children become tired of all the medicines and doctor appointments. However, the outcome is generally much better for children who are consistently treated than for those who just take the pills when they are uncomfortable (see Chapter 26). Children with the later onset of polyarticular disease are highly varied in their outcomes. Some seem to have arthritis that resolves without explanation, while others with no apparent risk factors progressively develop more severe joint involvement.

Complications

The complications of polyarticular onset arthritis are primarily those of the arthritis itself. Pain, swelling, and limitation of motion may result in weakness, bone loss (osteoporosis), and difficulty in activities of daily living. This type of arthritis may spread to involve the hip in some children, and hip replacement surgery is sometimes necessary to maintain function (see section on surgery below). Involvement of the wrists and fingers may also limit function. Cervical spine fusion and foot deformities are additional complications that are seen in some children with chronic active disease.

The key to minimizing complications in children with polyarticular disease is early and aggressive medical intervention. Once it is recognized that a child has progressive polyarticular disease, every effort must be made to suppress the inflammation. While any parent reading this list of possible complications might become depressed, it is important to recognize that the vast majority of children who receive proper treatment do very well. If families follow my advice, I can keep 90 percent of the children at least 90 percent of where they want to be, 90 percent of the time. With the newer biologic agents, the statistics are even better.

> An excellent example is a young woman who came to me seven or eight years ago with polyarticular onset disease and an elevated sedimentation rate. Over the years she has had persistent arthritis in her wrists and knees despite multiple medications. However, she played in her high school orchestra, participated actively in student government, and graduated high school to attend a prestigious Ivy League college. She has now graduated college and gone on to graduate school. She has every potential to lead a full and happy life and be a beautiful wife and mother in the future. I can tell she still has arthritis and so can she. She takes a lot of medications, but no one passing her on the street or sitting next to her in class would ever notice until they had known her for a long time.

Medical treatment

Medical therapy for severe arthritis has progressed dramatically in the last twenty years. The potential side effects and appropriate monitoring for each of the medications are discussed in detail in Chapter 24. A few children with mild polyarticular onset arthritis will respond well to NSAIDs. Most need the more effective NSAIDs (diclofenac is often my first choice), but some find nabumetone, naproxen, or ibuprofen adequate. For children with more severe disease, sulfasalazine is often an effective second-line agent. If further medication is necessary, the standard answer is to proceed to methotrexate. However some families and physicians prefer to use the biologics early in the disease course. The majority of children do well on these medications, but they may be difficult to withdraw.

Doxycycline and hydroxychloroquine are useful adjunctive agents. Neither drug is striking if given alone, but in study after study patients given either drug in addition to their standard regimen do better than patients who are not given the extra drug. Note that doxycycline's use is limited by the associated upset stomachs and photosensitivity in some patients. In addition, *doxycycline should not be given to children under ten years of age* because it will permanently stain their teeth (see Chapter 24).

For children who do not do well enough on methotrexate even after the addition of doxycycline or hydroxychloroquine, there are a variety of alternatives. Etanercept has been the most dramatically effective, providing rapid and near complete relief for many children. Infliximab has been very beneficial for others. Adalimumab is a newer biologic agent that also is very effective. I have had good results with leflunomide in some older children, but the experience in younger children is limited. Additional agents continue to be developed and investigated. For some drugs such as kinaret, the appropriate usage remains to be determined. When these drugs fail, it becomes a matter of careful testing to determine what will help. Cyclosporine is effective for some children, and azathioprine for others. A few centers still use intravenous immunoglobulin G (IVIgG), but it has few lasting effects and most have discontinued its use for polyarticular onset arthritis.

> *I am often confronted by parents who are concerned that their children are on too much medicine.* "Why can't we just wait and see what happens?" they ask. If the disease is mild and the child appears to be doing well, this is a perfectly sensible question. However, the reason for being a specialist in a field of medicine is to gain greater experience in that area and then bring that experience to bear on the problem. As a practicing pediatric rheumatologist, I pay a lot of attention to my sense of whether or not things are going right. If they are not, I will strongly encourage families to move forward before the damage is obvious. Imagine if you are having a party and a guest reports they smell smoke. No one will be too concerned if no one else smells smoke, but you'd better investigate, just in case. However, at the first indication that there really is smoke you want to quickly call the fire department. Imagine explaining to the firemen that you did not call sooner because you did not want to upset everyone or disrupt your party. They will then explain to you that they can put out fires,

but once the fire has gotten out of control they cannot repair what has already been damaged. Anti-inflammatory drugs work the same way. They can suppress inflammation to prevent joint damage, but they cannot repair joint damage once it has occurred. Don't let your child accumulate a lot of permanent damage before deciding to accept more aggressive therapy. The whole point of aggressive therapy is to prevent the damage.

Prednisone or corticosteroids must be regarded with caution in polyarticular onset arthritis. Steroid-containing drugs will make a child feel better rapidly, but if they are used for a prolonged period, they are frequently associated with major side effects. For children with polyarticular onset arthritis, corticosteroids should be viewed like a fire extinguisher next to the stove. They may be very useful if things suddenly flare out of control, but they certainly are not intended for repeated or continuing use. That doesn't mean we never use them—only that we try to minimize their use.

In earlier times corticosteroids were the only treatment available for children with severe disease. When significant doses of corticosteroids were used extensively to control arthritis, the result was a large collection of short, obese children with artificial hips (steroids interfere with growth, cause obesity, and predispose patients to avascular necrosis of bone, which may necessitate hip replacement surgery). It is important to remember that prednisone is useful for emergencies, but it is not a good long-term answer. I reserve steroid-containing drugs primarily for children who cannot get out of bed to go to school in the morning. I will nearly always begin a second-line agent shortly after I begin the corticosteroids with the intent that the second-line agent will aid me in stopping the steroids as quickly as possible. With the ready availability of the newer biologic agents that block tumor necrosis factor alpha (TNF-α) activity, the use of steroids is rarely necessary.

I occasionally see children with arthritis who are taking "pain killers." Excessive use of codeine and its derivatives or similar drugs is often associated with abnormal behavior and in some cases can lead to addiction. Some physicians feel that judicious use is warranted. Unfortunately, everyone's definition of judicious is different. I was trained never to use them. My attitude is that I should fix the problem, not simply mask the pain. The correct answer is a matter of opinion. For most children with arthritis, acetaminophen is an appropriate and adequate addition to help control pain. I have not written a prescription for a codeine derivative in over ten years. However, I do have a few patients who require tramadol or propoxyphene on occasion.

Surgery

Surgical therapy for children with polyarticular onset arthritis is primarily limited to joint replacement surgery. Children with severe involvement of the shoulder may benefit from replacement of the head of the shoulder (glenoid). This is the one joint replacement surgery in the upper extremity that is useful. Upper extremity joint replacement below the shoulder is generally unsatisfactory. However, children with fused elbows may benefit from elbow replacement surgery to restore some movement. If a child loses significant range of motion in both elbows, it becomes very difficult to carry out daily activities, such as eating and dressing.

Children with severe involvement of the wrist or fingers may benefit from fusion of particularly troublesome joints. Replacement of finger joints is not generally helpful. When there is significant subluxation (downward slipping) of the wrist, surgery to fuse the wrist in a functional position is often helpful. In addition, it is sometimes necessary to remove the tip of the bone at the end of the forearm (distal ulna) if it is causing damage to the tendons that extend the fingers, as the tendons pass over the bone.

Joint replacement surgery for the lower extremity is much more effective. If a child is losing the ability to walk because of hip pain, it is important to replace the hip. Twenty-five years ago a child with severe hip pain was given a wheelchair, and most are still in them. Now we replace the hip joint, and arthritic children in wheelchairs are no longer frequent in major treatment centers. *The time to replace the hip joint is as soon as it is preventing the child from walking outside the house.* Many parents are worried and want to wait. This does not make sense. As soon as the child is limiting the amount of walking around he or she is doing, strength and range of motion are being lost. This makes recovery after surgery much more difficult and complete functional recovery much less likely. I have many children who have had total hip or total knee replacements (usually because of damage done before they came under my care). They could walk right by you in the hall and you would never notice (see Chapter 25).

Physical and occupational therapy

Physical and occupational therapy play an important role in children with polyarticular onset disease. Exercises and stretching play an important role in maintaining strength, endurance, and range of motion for children. Parents often complain that their children do all sorts of physical and occupational (not to mention medical) therapy and never seem to get better. It is important to realize that children with arthritis who are left untreated steadily get worse. Sometimes in the face of very active disease, successful therapy is slowing down the problem until new medications take effect or the disease itself slows down. These children are much better off because of their therapy, even though they may have gotten worse while being treated.

Splinting is an important part of physical and occupational therapy. Children with pain often hold their joints in the position of maximum comfort. This is not the position of maximum function. Over time the tendons contract and the child progressively loses range of motion and function. Knee flexion contractures can be sharply reduced or prevented by the appropriate use of night-resting splints. These are splints that are strapped around the leg at night. Often these are fabricated from casting material as if the child had broken the leg. The cast is allowed to dry, then cut off and used as a splint at night. Children do not like them because they cannot walk with the splint on and it is uncomfortable to sleep with your leg held straight all night. Nonetheless properly used they are an important part of your child's therapy. Imagine what the doctor will say when he measures that a flexion contracture has gotten worse, if you tell him you didn't use the splints because the child did not like them.

Splints are also important to prevent flexion contractures at the wrist. Children often resent these because a properly made wrist splint interferes with hand function. However, they prevent further wrist subluxation and substantially improve the long-term outcome. Parents are often concerned because the children complain about wearing the splints. In addition, the children's wrists or knees are often stiffer in the morning after they take the splints off. However, these are minor inconveniences that are more than offset by the prevention of subluxation. The problem is that as parents, you will not see the problem that was prevented unless you take the splints off and allow it to happen. Parents who use the splints properly will hear only the complaints and wonder why they are putting the splints on. A year later, however, their children will function better than the children of parents who listened to their children's complaints and took the splints off. Who was truly more concerned about their child's welfare?

Prognosis

The long-term prognosis for children with polyarticular onset disease is highly variable. The list of possible complications is quite long and disturbing. The key to remember is that most of the long-term complications can be prevented or corrected with proper therapy. As with many other conditions in childhood, the majority of children and families who keep their appointments and comply with medications and recommendations to change medications will do well. It is the children whose families miss appointments for months at a time and often refuse advice for more aggressive therapy who frequently do poorly.

SYSTEMIC ONSET JUVENILE ARTHRITIS

Things you should know

- The fever must fall back to normal at least once each day. If it does not, the diagnosis is probably wrong.
- The rash should have the characteristic salmon pink appearance. The rash is never ecchymotic or purpuric (it doesn't look like bruises).
- ANA and eye disease are both rare in systemic onset juvenile arthritis.
- Rheumatoid factor should not be present.

Systemic onset juvenile arthritis refers to the onset of arthritis with fever and a characteristic rash. Systemic onset juvenile arthritis has no relationship to adult-onset rheumatoid arthritis and most likely no relationship to the other forms of juvenile arthritis, either. It is best considered an entirely separate disease.

Although all of the children with systemic onset arthritis share key characteristics, the outcome of systemic onset disease is so varied that it is difficult to believe it is in fact a single disease. There are several key points when making the diagnosis of systemic onset arthritis. First, the fever must fall back to normal at least once each day. Second, the rash should have the characteristic salmon pink appearance. The rash is never ecchymotic or purpuric (it doesn't look like bruises). It is occasionally itchy (pruritic). Occasionally, there are children with the onset of fever and rash before the arthritis becomes evident. These children should always be followed carefully for the possibility of another diagnosis, especially an infection.

Pauciarticular onset arthritis and polyarticular arthritis affect more frequently girls than boys. In systemic onset arthritis, the sex ratio is equal. In pauciarticular and polyarticular onset disease, ANA is commonly present and eye disease is frequent. ANA and eye disease are both rare in systemic onset juvenile arthritis. Rheumatoid factor should not be present in children with systemic onset arthritis. If RF is found in a child being investigated for systemic onset disease, it is more likely that the cause of the symptoms is an infection.

The typical presentation of systemic onset arthritis in a child is one who has recurring fevers and a rising ESR, WBC count, and platelet count, but falling hemoglobin. Often the child looks extremely ill. Most often the child is thought to have an infection, and the possibility of systemic onset arthritis is considered only when there has been no response to antibiotics. Many diseases can look like this.

The first real indication that the diagnosis is systemic onset arthritis may be the appearance of the characteristic rash. Children with recurrent fevers that fall back to normal should be examined carefully. If the rash is not obvious, parents and physicians should look for it under the arms (in the axillae) and around the belt line. The rash is often visible only when the child is hot. If the child is left with his shirt off, the rash may disappear before you can show it to someone else. It is often possible to make the rash more evident with a warm bath. Textbooks describe the Koebner phenomenon, in which a line made by pressure on the skin will spread beyond the initial area that was touched (after you scratch the skin, the area you touched turns red, but then red spots appear around the area that you touched). In clinical practice, this test is rarely positive or useful. *Arthritis may be present even at the earliest stages of the disease. Often it is present but has been overlooked.* But sometimes it is absent until later in the course of the disease.

A key finding in establishing the diagnosis of systemic onset arthritis is the child's dramatic improvement during the period when the fever is gone each day. Often I will be called in the afternoon to see a child who looks very ill and might have systemic onset arthritis. The child has been in another hospital and was not getting better. After transfer to my hospital, pediatric rheumatology has been called as part of the evaluation. Typically, after evaluating the child carefully for other explanations, we discuss the possibility of systemic onset arthritis and wait for new test results. While everyone is waiting for the new results, it is common for the physicians on the ward to change to new antibiotics.

The next morning, the ward physicians are happy to announce that the fever is gone, the child looks much better, and by changing the antibiotics they are curing the infection; pediatric rheumatology isn't needed. In the late afternoon I get a phone call saying, "Please come back right away." The fever has returned and the child looks awful again. This is typical for systemic onset arthritis. *Children with reactive arthritis, infections, or leukemia may be misdiagnosed as having systemic onset disease. However, these diseases rarely have periods without fever, during which the child looks nearly normal.*

In children with reactive arthritis, the fever usually does not return to normal at least once every day. Infections also tend not to have normal temperatures during the course of every day. Children with infections may have a rash, but it is not the classic salmon pink rash of systemic onset disease. Children with leukemia also may appear very ill and in pain, with elevated sedimentation rates suggesting the possibility of systemic onset JA.

Children with diseases other than systemic onset JA can often be differentiated by their laboratory findings, in addition to their failure to look better at any point during the day . Systemic onset arthritis is characteristically associated with a significant elevation of the platelet count. Reactive arthritis, leukemia, and infections are more likely diagnoses in children with decreased platelet counts. If a child is thought to have severe systemic onset arthritis, a low or even low-normal platelet count should be considered suspicious.

Until the diagnosis of systemic onset arthritis is clear, it is far better to continue to look for infections and treat with antibiotics if necessary. It is also far better to have done a bone marrow aspiration to exclude the possibility of leukemia than to delay that diagnosis, thinking the child has systemic onset arthritis. Children sent to me for possible systemic onset arthritis have had cancers, infections, polyarteritis nodosa, Kawasaki's disease, and many other illnesses.

In addition to the high white blood cell (WBC) count, high platelet count, high ESR, and low hemoglobin, laboratory evaluation of the child with systemic onset arthritis may show mild elevation of the liver enzymes (AST/ALT; see Chapter 24). Significant elevation of these tests in a child with systemic onset arthritis is a cause for concern. It may signal the beginning of a severe complication called macrophage activation syndrome (MAS; see below).

Complications

The complications of systemic onset arthritis may take many forms. In addition to the problems of fever, rash, and arthritis, virtually every child will have a small **pericardial effusion** on an echocardiogram. These are often insignificant, but if they become large they may cause difficulty. An enlarged liver or spleen (hepatomegaly or splenomegaly) may be found. **Proteinuria** is a major cause for concern, as there is a strong association between systemic onset arthritis and **amyloidosis**, but this has become rare.

There are reports describing systemic onset arthritis with damage to the heart or heart valves, lung involvement including pleural effusions, central nervous system problems such as seizures, and a number of vasculitic complications. Whether these are true complications of systemic onset arthritis is uncertain, because many times what is reported as an "atypical complication" of systemic onset arthritis is really a typical complication of systemic vasculitis with arthritis or another disease in a child mistakenly thought to have systemic onset arthritis. Children with systemic onset arthritis must have a fever that falls back to normal every day and must have the characteristic rash. Many other illnesses can cause fever, high ESR, and rash, leading to a mistaken diagnosis. It is important to remember that even information published in medical journals and textbooks may be incorrect.

Macrophage activation syndrome (MAS) is the most worrisome acute complication of systemic onset arthritis. If a child with typical systemic onset arthritis seems to be responding to therapy but the ESR, platelet count, and WBC count begin to fall rapidly while the liver enzymes are increasing, this should spark great concern. When seeing the ESR come down and the WBC count and platelet count decreasing, many physicians assume that the patient is getting better. The physician may suspect the elevated liver enzymes are an indication of mild liver irritation caused by the medicine. However, this may instead be the beginning of MAS. This is especially true if the child appears ill.

Most often the onset of MAS occurs early in the course of systemic onset arthritis. However, it may occur later. The typical presentation is in a child with systemic onset arthritis who rapidly appears ill with fever, abnormal liver enzymes, and liver enlargement. MAS frequently occurs shortly after a change in medication or in conjunction with a viral illness. However, the cause is not always evident. In the early stages of MAS, the fibrin degradation products (FDP) or fibrin split products (FSP) test may become abnormal and the prothrombin time (PT) may be prolonged (see Chapter 24 for an extended discussion). This will not be the case if the child's systemic onset arthritis is improving.

A definite diagnosis of MAS is made by demonstrating the presence of macrophages that are destroying erythrocytes in the bone marrow (the macrophages are eating red blood cells and their precursors). This requires a bone marrow aspiration. However, it is rarely necessary to perform this test as the clinical picture is quite striking. This can be a severe and life-threatening problem because of the clotting abnormalities and liver damage that occur. It is treated with high doses of intravenous corticosteroids and fresh frozen plasma. Some children with MAS have improved with cyclosporine therapy. MAS has been reported infrequently in children with other types of arthritis. New research suggests there may be predisposing genetic factors. Under the right circumstances, MAS may occur in any child with the genetic predisposition, even if he or she doesn't have systemic onset arthritis.

Severe arthritis and the complications of chronic corticosteroid therapy are the major long-term problems for children with systemic onset arthritis. While some children have little or no residual arthritis, as noted above, those who progress to chronic destructive disease may have severe damage to both large and small joints. Hips and knees are frequently affected and may require replacement. The cervical spine is another frequently affected area, and fusion of the vertebrae in the neck may occur. In some children the wrists are also significantly involved.

As is true for children with polyarthritis, the physician's first goal must be to prevent joint destruction. When this cannot be accomplished, total joint replacement and reconstructive surgery for systemic onset arthritis is similar to reconstructive surgery for children with polyarticular onset arthritis (see Chapter 25). Many children with systemic onset arthritis receive corticosteroids to control the fever and rash. As a result, osteoporosis is a common complication and avascular necrosis of the hips may also occur (see the Glossary). This can be corrected by total hip replacement.

Short stature is another common complication of prolonged use of corticosteroids. This cannot be corrected by surgery and may lead to a lifetime of social difficulty. However, short stature has been reported in children with severe systemic onset disease who never received corticosteroids.

Medical treatment

The medications used in the treatment of systemic onset arthritis are essentially the same as those used to treat polyarticular onset disease. However, there are a number of key differences. It is important to remember that virtually all of the medicines used to treat JA may irritate the liver. In children with systemic onset arthritis, the disease itself often causes irritation of the liver as well. But it is difficult to avoid these medications, as corticosteroids are the only readily available alternative. As a result, children with systemic onset arthritis must be monitored carefully for signs of liver irritation, especially after any change in medication (see Chapter 22 for recommendations regarding monitoring).

Indomethacin is uniquely effective in treating the fever of systemic onset arthritis and may be effective when other NSAIDs have not been helpful. However, indomethacin is associated with irritation of the stomach, the kidneys, and the liver more often than the other NSAIDs. It also may cause headaches and depression. In small children, indomethacin is associated with an increased incidence of inexplicable temper tantrums. Experienced physicians frequently use indomethacin in children with severe systemic onset juvenile arthritis when none of the other NSAIDs has been adequate. If a child is very ill, it may be necessary to use corticosteroids to provide immediate relief, but they are not desirable long-term treatment.

For children who fail to respond adequately to NSAIDs, methotrexate is the traditional next choice. Children with continuing active disease, despite methotrexate, are problematic. A few children with severe systemic onset arthritis can be controlled only with long-term use of corticosteroids, but every alternative should be considered. None of the remaining medications is consistently effective, but there are several, and it is rare for a child not to respond to any of them. Cyclosporine, etanercept, and infliximab have all been used with success in some children. Adalimumab may also be beneficial for these children. There are early reports that a biologic agent which blocks IL-6 is useful, but this agent is not yet available for routine use.

I have cared for children who failed to improve with every medication I tried until I added cyclosporine. The fever and rash subsided and the child was "perfect" in ten days. However, the next child who seemed identical did not respond to cyclosporine at all. Leflunomide, azathioprine, mycophenolate mofetil, and cyclophosphamide have all been used with limited success. All have significant potential risks (see Chapter 22). Thalidomide has been beneficial for the rare children with systemic onset arthritis for whom all other medications have failed.

As with medical treatment for all forms of arthritis, the key to care of the child with systemic onset arthritis is to eliminate the symptoms and relieve the inflammation associated with the disease with the least possible toxicity. Many parents are disturbed by the possible side effects of immunosuppressive medications recommended for the treatment of systemic onset arthritis. The key is to remember that significant side effects of the medications are rare. In contrast, everybody gets side effects from corticosteroids. Children who are short, obese, and have suffered fractures and joint replacements secondary to steroid-induced osteoporosis often become very discouraged (see Chapter 26).

Bone marrow transplantation and other new "cures"

Bone marrow transplantation and other dramatic therapies have been proposed for children with the most severe disease. When parents hear that children with severe disease have been "cured" by these treatments, they get very excited. There are a number of interesting experimental therapies for children who have failed to respond to all alternatives.

We can eliminate systemic onset arthritis if we eliminate the immune system. However, the immune system is how we fight infection. Elimination of the immune system for even a short period (as is done in bone marrow transplantation) carries a high risk. Nearly one-fifth of the children who underwent bone marrow transplantation for systemic onset arthritis died. It is true that some of the others remain well without taking medication, but others have relapsed. This is not a miracle cure. It is an experimental procedure that should be reserved for the very worst cases. That doesn't mean bone marrow transplantation is wrong. One of my most severe systemic onset arthritis patients underwent bone marrow transplantation at my suggestion.

Good results have been reported for small numbers of patients with a variety of very potent medications. Again, unless you are one of the very worst cases, you do not want to take the risk until these new medications have been proven safe and effective. We will have better therapy for children with arthritis in the future. Some of the new treatments you hear about will turn out to be major advances. But some will be failures, and the children will not benefit. Until we know more about new therapies, they should be reserved for only the most severe cases, and these children should be receiving their care at the most advanced centers.

Physical therapy and surgical treatment

Physical and occupational therapy are very important in maintaining strength and range of motion for children with systemic onset arthritis, just as they are in each of the other subtypes of JA. Without proper therapy, these children may develop widespread weakness, muscle atrophy, and flexion contractures.

Surgery has little direct role in the treatment of children with systemic onset arthritis. But once the systemic manifestations have come under control, these children may be left with significant polyarthritis. Reconstructive surgery as discussed for children with polyarticular onset arthritis is appropriate for children with systemic onset arthritis. Because many of these children have required extended periods of therapy with corticosteroids, they often have avascular necrosis of bone and require joint replacement surgery (see Chapter 25).

Prognosis

The normal course of systemic onset arthritis is highly varied. Some children make a complete recovery in a short period of time and never have further problems. Other children have chronic debilitating disease that leaves them with permanent limitations. There are three key groups of children with systemic onset arthritis, but not all children fit one of these descriptions. The first group consists of children who have an acute onset of fever, rash, and arthritis that responds quickly to treatment with NSAIDs. Because these children have a fever that falls back to normal every day and the characteristic rash, they are classified as systemic onset arthritis. However, in many cases the duration of disease is less than three months. Some have argued that these are unusual viral infections mimicking systemic onset arthritis. An outbreak of what was initially thought to be an epidemic of systemic onset arthritis in a boarding school was found to be due to parvovirus infection when it was carefully investigated. All of these children recovered. Perhaps all of the children who rapidly recover never really had systemic onset arthritis. We don't know.

The second group of systemic onset arthritis patients consists primarily of teenage boys. Although their disease may be significant initially, they most often come under control with NSAIDs. A few require the addition of a second-line agent, but their primary problems are fever and rash with relatively little arthritis. Many of these teenagers find that they do well except for the recurrence of rash whenever they are very hot in physical education class or other activities. Some have mild persisting arthritis or limitation in their wrists, but they do not have major arthritic problems.

The third group is a much more problematic group of children who begin with systemic onset disease early in life. Many of these children come under control with multiple medications, but some require continuing treatment for years. Most of these children are brought under good control long before there is significant damage to the bones and joints, but a few suffer from chronic destructive arthritis. Others are ultimately limited by the side effects of the chronic corticosteroid therapy used to control their fever and arthritis. The key to an improved prognosis for this group is early recognition and aggressive intervention while avoiding chronic high-dose corticosteroid therapy whenever possible.

The long-term prognosis for most children with systemic onset disease is very good. The systemic symptoms usually disappear over a period of time, and the remaining problems are those of polyarthritis. Only a small percentage of children develop prolonged unresponsive arthritis or life-threatening complications of the disease itself. With the advent of newer therapies and increasing recognition of the importance of intervening early to minimize use of corticosteroids, the long-term complications of corticosteroid usage are becoming less frequent. Most children with systemic onset arthritis will be able to go on and live full and productive lives. To get the best possible outcome, the small group of children with severe resistant disease should be shifted to the care of very experienced specialists as soon as they are recognized.

STATE-OF-THE-ART CARE FOR CHILDREN WITH JUVENILE ARTHRITIS

State-of-the-art care for children with pauciarticular onset, polyarticular onset, and systemic onset juvenile arthritis requires that physicians and families make sure that the inflammation is promptly brought under control and not allowed to cause continuing joint damage. In the past physicians believed that children who had evidence of "low-grade" active disease but were "doing okay" should not be treated aggressively. We now know this is wrong. Smoldering disease means continuing bone and joint damage and a continuing risk of further disease flares.

Children whose disease comes under good control within six months of starting therapy will generally do well. Children with any type of juvenile arthritis whose disease is not under good control within six months of starting *appropriate* therapy are at increased risk of a poor outcome. While this may seem obvious, it is a very reliable guideline. Appropriate therapy means the right NSAID in the right dosage. It also means monitoring carefully and changing the NSAID if it does not appear to be having the desired effect.

Because there are studies that indicate that NSAIDs may not reach their full effectiveness until they have been taken consistently for three months, some physicians will not consider changing therapy until three months after the first dose. Indeed, some physicians will prescribe an NSAID and then not see the child for several months. We must not allow growing children to have continuing joint damage for any longer than is absolutely necessary. *If a child is not beginning to improve within three or four weeks of starting an NSAID, another should be tried.*

Any child who is not clearly improving after six months of disease may need to be on a second-line agent. However, before I regard a child as needing a second-line agent, I want to have tried two or three first-line agents (see Chapter 22). Different children have different responses to these medications. This means I want to see the child at least monthly at the beginning, and more frequently if he or she is not making good progress. You do not want to change NSAIDs at every visit to the doctor. If the child is clearly improving, you want to stick with the medication. But if the child has obviously stopped improving or is getting worse, appropriate changes should be made. The best possible care requires careful monitoring by both the parents and physician so any problems are promptly dealt with and appropriate adjustments are made as needed.

In addition to routine checkups, every child should be carefully reevaluated six months after starting therapy. Is the disease under good control? Are the remaining problems simply weakness, contractures, or bony overgrowth? These require physical therapy and time, not more medicine. However, if there is evidence of active disease with an elevated sedimentation rate, unexplained anemia, morning stiffness, joint swelling, or pain, more aggressive therapy with a second-line agent should be considered. For children with pauciarticular onset arthritis, this might be the time to consider an intra-articular corticosteroid injection.

For children with continuing active polyarticular or systemic onset JA six months after diagnosis, a second-line agent should be added, if one has not been added already. Sometimes I'll wait a little longer if the child still seems to be almost completely better. These are not absolute rules—there are not any. But if the fire is not clearly out, there is ongoing bone and joint damage. This should not be tolerated for an extended period. You cannot rely on X rays to detect joint damage early in the disease in childhood. The earliest damage is to the rapidly growing cartilage, which does not show up on X rays. These changes may not show up as bone damage visible on X rays until years later.

The second-line agents most commonly used for resistant JA are methotrexate, sulfasalazine, and etanercept. Adalimumab is a newer drug that may play an important role. More experience is necessary to define when it is best used. Cyclosporine, leflunomide, infliximab, and azathioprine are less commonly used. Oral corticosteroids should be avoided except for children who are having serious problems and cannot function without them. With appropriate use of second-line agents, the need for corticosteroids is becoming rare. All of these medications are discussed in detail in Chapter 22, on medications. Few children fail to respond adequately to some combination of these agents. Those who do should be under the care of experienced pediatric rheumatologists in major centers, where they have access to ongoing investigation of the newest therapies.

MEDICATIONS NO LONGER ROUTINELY USED FOR JUVENILE ARTHRITIS

The medications used in the treatment of children with arthritis have changed dramatically in the last thirty years. There are three medications that were commonly used in the past that are no longer routinely used by pediatric rheumatologists in the United States. When I began my career, aspirin and "gold shots" were the mainstays of therapy. In the intervening years, other medications have replaced them. Aspirin remains a useful medication for children with arthritis. It is very inexpensive. However, it needs to be given three or four times a day and has a very high frequency of side effects. Aspirin remains a mainstay of therapy only when the expense of other medications is a major barrier to care (mostly in Third World countries).

Gold shots are injections of gold-containing compounds given initially once each week. They are extremely effective for some children but are given much less often now (see Chapter 22). Many other medicines are as effective as gold shots and available in more convenient form. The exception is the small group of children with RF-positive polyarticular onset arthritis. Gold shots still seem to be very effective for this group.

D-penicillamine is another medicine that is now rarely used. Although this medication was beneficial for some children, it has been replaced by other medications that have a lower incidence of side effects.

8

Uveitis

Eye Complications of Juvenile Arthritis and Related Conditions

Virginia was a nine-year-old girl who had pauciarticular onset JA. Her arthritis began when she was two years old but came under good control with medication. She had a flare-up of arthritis in her knee at six that was easily controlled. Because she was antinuclear antibody (ANA)-positive, her family had her eyes checked every three months, as recommended. There were never problems with her eyes. Shortly after her eighth birthday, her parents separated and Virginia moved out of state with her mother. Her father brought her in for a routine check of her arthritis when she returned to visit him two years later. Virginia said she was doing fine and had had no problems with her arthritis. However, when I went to examine her I could not see into her right eye. It was quickly apparent she could not see out of the eye. When asked, she admitted she had slowly noted decreasing vision with the right eye, but she had not said anything because she did not want to upset her mother. Her mother had had too many other things on her mind after the divorce and had not arranged for a new ophthalmologist to monitor Virginia. By the time I discovered the problem, the vision in the right eye could not be saved.

It is important that the parents of children with JA and related conditions understand that the eyes may be involved even when there is no evidence of active joint disease. Ocular complications may take several forms. Children with pauciarticular onset, polyarticular onset, and psoriatic JA are all at risk of developing chronic anterior uveitis (silent painless eye inflammation). In this condition, inflammatory cells accumulate in the eye and the resultant irritation may cause damage to the iris (the colored part of the eye that forms the pupil), the lens, and other structures (see Fig. 16

above). The most worrisome aspect of this inflammation is that it does not produce pain. As a result of its gradual, painless progression the inflammation may produce serious eye damage without being detected.

The key to preventing serious eye damage in children with JA is careful screening for the presence of inflammatory cells by an ophthalmologist (a medical eye doctor). This is done with a special instrument called a slit lamp, which is not regularly available in the office of physicians who do not specialize in eye disease. The specialized examination done by the ophthalmologist is called a slit lamp exam. A trained ophthalmologist can detect the earliest signs of inflammation in the eye and begin treatment.

Since we cannot rely on children to tell us when there is inflammation, pediatric rheumatologists insist on routine screening as described in the box. An additional quick and easy test recommended by some ophthalmologists is for parents to shine a flashlight in the child's eyes at bedtime one night each week. If you shine a light in a normal child's eye, you will see the pupil (black center) shrink dramatically. It should shrink in a perfect circle. If one eye does not shrink or the circle is irregular, this might be evidence of eye involvement. Whatever the cause, any child whose eyes do not shrink equally when you shine a light in them should be evaluated by an ophthalmologist. This test may detect the onset of inflammation in the eye occurring between screening tests, but it is not a substitute for the screening tests.

Frequency of routine screening ophthalmologic examinations for children with JA

Pauciarticular onset JA, ANA-positive
- Screening every three to four months until eleven years of age, then every six months

Pauciarticular onset JA, ANA-negative
- Screening every six months

Polyarticular onset JA, ANA-positive
- Screening every three to four months until eleven years of age, then every six months

Polyarticular onset JA, ANA-negative
- Screening every six months

Systemic onset JA
- Screening yearly (eye involvement is rare but not unheard of)

Physicians do not understand why some children get eye disease and others do not. There are certain genetic factors that seem to increase the risk. However, many children with these factors do not get eye disease, and some children without these factors do get eye disease. Attempts to understand why having ANA increases the risk have failed.

If you look carefully at the joint of a child with arthritis, the inflammation is centered in the synovium. This is the lining tissue the normal function of which is to keep the joint clean of debris. Examination of the eyes of children with uveitis has shown that the inflammation is centered in the ciliary body. This is a tissue in the eye that serves to keep the fluid in the eye clean of debris. Since the two tissues serve a similar function, it is easy to understand how the same disease process might involve both. But if it were that simple, we would expect all children with arthritis to develop eye involvement. In fact, less than half ever have any evidence of eye inflammation.

If uveitis is present, it should be treated aggressively. The normal first-line therapy is steroid eye drops. Often a short course of this treatment is enough to bring the disease under control. Unfortunately, steroid eye drops will damage the eye if used for an extended period. The prolonged use of steroid eye drops is associated with an increased risk of both cataracts and glaucoma. Because of these complications, if it appears that a short course of treatment with steroid eye drops is inadequate, many ophthalmologists will recommend switching children with severe eye disease to immunosuppressive medications taken by mouth. Often methotrexate is the first medication used after corticosteroids have proven inadequate. Adalimumab and infleximab are also used.

Many children with JA are found to have mild uveitis, but treated aggressively they do very well. However, if the uveitis is very severe, very resistant to therapy, or not found until very late, there is a risk of permanent blindness. Uveitis may occur in only one eye or in both eyes and may occur at a time where there is no evidence of active arthritis. This is why routine monitoring is so important. Routine monitoring will find eye disease that you do not suspect is present, and it is hoped that it will allow the doctors to begin therapy before too much damage accumulates. *Do not put off your child's eye doctor appointments because you have not noticed any problem.*

Eye involvement may also occur in children with spondyloarthropathies. However, these children usually get acute and painful eye disease (see Chapter 9). Because it is painful, it is usually rapidly detected.

Frequent monitoring of children older than ten years of age with spondyloarthropathies who do not have symptoms in their eyes is not required. In contrast, young children with psoriasis-associated arthritis are at high risk of inflammatory eye disease and must be monitored just as if they had typical JA.

Eye disease may also complicate the other forms of rheumatic disease in childhood, including sarcoidosis, systemic lupus erythematosus, and Sjogren's syndrome. Children with each of these conditions should have their eyes checked by an ophthalmologist at least every six months. In some cases, they will have symptoms of their eye disease; in other cases the eye disease may occur without the parents or child being aware of it. This is why routine checkups by the ophthalmologist are so important.

Some children develop uveitis without evidence of a rheumatic disease. Since this eye disease looks the same as the eye disease in children with JA, it is treated the same way. However, the first step in evaluating a child who is found to have uveitis is a careful evaluation to make sure he or she does not have a rheumatic disease. Sometimes I find children who cannot bend one knee all the way or who have one leg longer than the other. Although there are other possible explanations, these findings suggest the child may have had arthritis at one point that was "never noticed." Physicians evaluating children with eye disease must also remember that there are a variety of diseases unrelated to rheumatology that must also be considered in caring for these children.

9

Spondyloarthropathies

Enthesitis-associated Arthritis

Fifteen-year-old Samantha initially began to complain of hip pain after a skiing accident. When repeated evaluations of her injury were negative, she was told the hip was "bruised." Although she improved with physical therapy, the family became concerned when she awoke a few months later with pain in the opposite hip. A family friend assured them these were all the symptoms of Lyme disease. However, visits to several doctors confirmed that all of her tests for Lyme disease were negative. Samantha began experiencing intermittent pain in both hips and occasional knee pain. When she went for long car rides, she could barely get out of the car. When she did, she walked like "a little old lady" for ten to fifteen minutes until she loosened up. She was diagnosed with fibromyalgia by an adult rheumatologist. On physical examination, she was tender in several fingers. She nearly jumped off the table when I tapped on her sacroiliac joints. She had pain in the tendons around her knees and in her ankles.

Spondyloarthropathy does not describe a specific disease. Instead, it describes a pattern of arthritis that may occur in adults or children with a variety of underlying conditions. Conditions that are associated with this pattern of arthritis in childhood include enthesitis-associated arthritis, ankylosing spondylitis, juvenile ankylosing spondylitis, SEA syndrome, reactive arthritis, infection-associated arthritis, Reiter's syndrome, psoriatic arthritis, arthritis associated with gastrointestinal diseases (including inflammatory bowel disease [IBD] and celiac disease), and a variety of miscellaneous conditions (e.g., recurrent "toxic synovitis" hypogammaglobulinemia-associated problems or immunoglobulin A [IgA] deficiency).

Spondyloarthropathy merely means "arthritis involving the back." Adult rheumatologists first used the term "spondyloarthropathy" when they began to recognize different forms of arthritis in adults. In adults, rheumatoid arthritis rarely involves the back, while spondyloarthropathies often involve the back and sacroiliac joints.

Children with spondyloarthropathies confuse some physicians and parents because often damage to the back and sacroiliac joints does not become obvious on X rays until the children reach adulthood. For many years, children with spondyloarthropathies were included in JRA. The current official term for this group is enthesitis-associated arthritis. (Although enthesitis-associated arthritis is a subtype of JA or JIA in the newest nomenclature, it is important to recognize that this is a very different disease from typical JRA. Remember, JA and JIA are being used as umbrella terms encompassing a large number of different conditions.) In contrast to typical JRA, the spondyloarthropathies have a different pattern of joint involvement, a different prognosis, a different best medication, and a different cause. Nonetheless, until recently, these children were commonly included in reports discussing JRA. This has caused a lot of confusion.

The first widely recognized group of children with spondyloarthropathies were teenage boys with swollen knees and low back pain. They stood out because under the old nomenclature they were classified as pauciarticular onset arthritis. However, typical pauciarticular onset arthritis occurs in young girls. Teenage boys with spondyloarthropathies differ in many ways. Unlike the young girls, who usually get better, the boys often have persistent chronic arthritis. The boys are rarely antinuclear antibody (ANA)-positive, and if they get eye disease, it is acute and painful, not the silent eye disease seen in younger children. In addition, their disease may start in the hip and is often associated with back pain.

When rheumatologists began to look more carefully at this group of teenage boys they discovered that they often had inflammation in the tendons around the joint (enthesitis) as well as in the joint. Recognition that these boys, were different was hastened by the discovery of HLA B27. This is a genetic marker that is found in about half of this group (discussed later in this chapter) but only infrequently in young girls with arthritis. Once this group was recognized, pediatric rheumatologists realized that spondyloarthropathies are common in childhood.

Spondyloarthropathies do occur in girls, but rarely in severe form. They typically begin in the early teenage years and are often mistaken for recurrent athletic injuries. Many of the children who come to me have been treated extensively for repeated ankle or knee sprains with exercise, casting, and in some cases even surgery. Other children with spondyloarthropathies who have a lot of tendon pain but no swollen joints or abnormal laboratory tests have come to me after having been labeled "complainers." Unlike typical pauciarticular arthritis, in which it is uncommon for there to be another affected family member, other family members of children with spondyloarthropathies are frequently found to be symptomatic. *However, the affected relatives often do not know they have this problem.* They have had chronic back or knee problems since they were teenagers that they attribute to many different causes.

The key findings in children with spondyloarthropathies often relate to tendon inflammation rather than arthritis. Enthesitis often causes pain around the wrists, knees, ankles, or heels. Frequently, physicians are confused because the child is complaining of a lot of pain, but nothing is broken and the joint is not swollen. Careful palpation around the joint will often reveal the painful tendonitis. Sometimes the tendons are very swollen and easily noticed on examination. In other cases the tendonitis is obvious only when the child complains of pain when the tendons are compressed.

Periarticular pain (pain around the joint), is the hallmark of spondyloarthropathies. The key to recognizing that the child is not suffering from recurrent athletic injuries lies in careful examination that often reveals multiple tender joints are present. Discovering that there are similarly affected family members when taking the family history also may speed recognition of a spondyloarthropathy.

If they are questioned carefully, most of these children have pain and inflammation in at least two locations. It is common for them to have low back pain or stiffness. Surprisingly, asking about this often produces resistance. "Why are you asking about my back? It's my knee that hurts!" Or, "Of course my back is stiff for ten to fifteen minutes every morning. Isn't everyone's?" Another common finding is pain at the Achilles tendon insertion on the back of the heel or at the insertion of the plantar fascia on the bottom of the foot (see Fig. 17). This can be detected by percussion or deep palpation at either point.

Dactylitis (sausage digit) may be the first manifestation of a spondyloarthropathy in both young children and teenagers. Instead of the joints, the entire finger or toe appears swollen, like a sausage. This is because of swelling around the inflamed tendons as well as the joint. At first, the

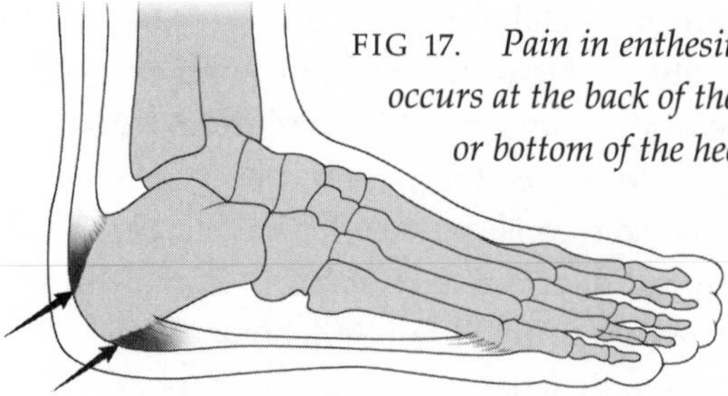

FIG 17. *Pain in enthesitis-associated arthritis commonly occurs at the back of the heel (Achilles tendon insertion) or bottom of the heel (plantar fascia insertion).*

child is complaining of only a single finger or toe and is initially thought to have injured it. However, on careful examination, periarticular involvement is often evident in multiple joints. Often there is unrecognized inflammation in toes on the same side as the finger (or in fingers on the same side as the toe that was noticed) that can be found by careful examination. It is also common to find unsuspected wrist involvement on the affected side. These children do very well when properly treated for their arthritis, but I have seen a number who have undergone unnecessary surgery for suspected tumors or torn tendons, among other things. These children may be ANA-positive and may have unsuspected uveitis. It is important that they be properly screened for eye disease.

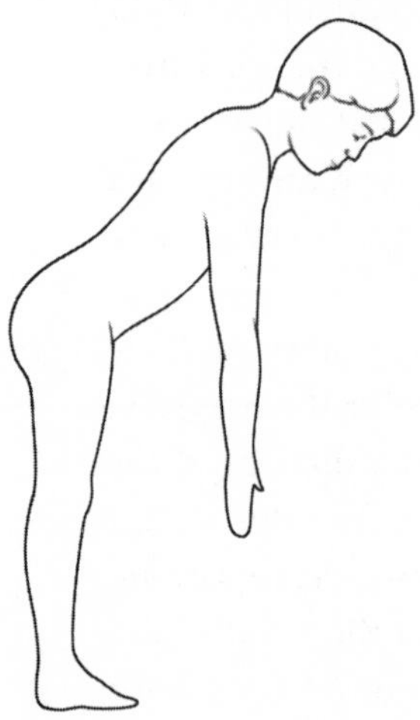

FIG 18. *Flattening of the back with limited anterior forward flexion in a child with enthesitis-associated arthritis.*

In teenagers, limited anterior forward flexion is an additional finding that assists in making this diagnosis. Typically, these children are unable to touch their toes (see Fig. 18). Frequently, the parents and physical education instructors have noted that they are not flexible. Sacroiliac joint tenderness is another common finding. Laboratory findings may not be helpful. Although severe cases may have an elevated sedimentation rate, all tests are often normal in children with mild spondyloarthropathies. HLA B27 is present in about one-half. Rheumatoid factor (RF) should never be present. ANA is present in some (see Chapter 24).

Once a child is diagnosed with a spondyloarthropathy, it is important to recognize that this pattern of joint involvement may be associated with ankylosing spondylitis, reactive arthritis, Reiter's syndrome, psoriatic arthritis, infection-associated arthritis (including Lyme disease), and the arthritis associated with gastrointestinal diseases (including IBD and celiac disease). Many children have a nonspecific spondyloarthropathy, meaning there is no associated condition. However, the associated condition may not become evident until years after the arthritis begins.

Parents of children with spondyloarthropathies should not be excessively concerned that their children are going to have other problems; most do not. But if new problems occur, everyone should be aware of the conditions associated with spondyloarthropathies so that the child can be evaluated appropriately. This is particularly true of children who develop recurrent abdominal pain that might be IBD. While most children with IBD develop arthritis after their bowel disease is recognized, this is not always the case. The associated findings and long-term prognosis for each of these conditions are different, so each is discussed separately below.

FORMS OF SPONDYLOARTHROPATHIES

Nonspecific spondyloarthropathy, enthesitis-associated arthritis, SEA syndrome, ankylosing spondylitis, and juvenile ankylosing spondylitis are discussed together because it is rarely possible to separate them reliably in childhood. Most children have a nonspecific spondyloarthropathy. SEA syndrome (seronegative enthesitis-arthritis syndrome) and enthesitis-associated arthritis are just different names for the same condition. About half of the children with spondyloarthropathies are HLA B27-positive, as noted above. Often the HLA B27-positive boys are labeled as having juvenile ankylosing spondylitis. However, many and most likely most of these children will *not* go on to have ankylosing spondylitis and should *not* be labeled juvenile ankylosing spondylitis. This is discussed in detail in the section on prognosis below.

Nonspecific spondyloarthropathies are very common. These children have the typical findings of a spondyloarthropathy without a recognized associated condition. The majority of these children who have enthesitis but little if any joint swelling rarely experience significant problems. Their primary complications are related to the arthritis. But the discomfort and stiffness associated with the enthesitis may result in poor sleep patterns and fatigue. It is not uncommon for these children to be mislabeled as having fibromyalgia. For children with abnormal laboratory findings or persistent pain and joint swelling, long-term joint damage is a significant concern. Most often the damage can be minimized by appropriate medical treatment, including second-line drugs.

Complications

Complications that do not involve the joints (extra-articular complications) are most common in children who have the associated conditions that are discussed below. However, a few specific complications are well recognized to occur in children with nonspecific spondyloarthropathies. **Acute anterior uveitis** is the most common complication. This is painful eye disease involving the front of the eye. Often the eye appears very red and the vision may be affected. This is very different from the silent eye disease of children with pauciarticular onset arthritis. Although it may be mistaken for "pinkeye" (conjunctivitis), it will not respond to antibiotic drops and requires care by an ophthalmologist. Acute anterior uveitis may occur in both HLA B27-positive and B27-negative individuals.

Cardiac involvement in adults with spondyloarthropathies is well recognized. Fortunately, it occurs in only a small number of children. The most common form of cardiac involvement is inflammation of the root of the aorta (the vessel carrying blood out of the heart), which is called **aortitis**. This inflammation can result in damage to the heart valves and a condition called **aortic insufficiency**. Children with aortic insufficiency complain of loss of energy and increasing shortness of breath with activity. The condition is easily detected by echocardiography, which is a painless and simple test where sound waves are bounced off the heart to monitor the motion of the heart valves and muscle. Less frequent complications include involvement of the lungs or kidneys. These cardiac complications have been described in teenagers but are very rare. Most often these complications occur in adults with definite ankylosing spondylitis.

Medical treatment

Treatment for children with spondyloarthropathies must be appropriate to their level of discomfort and their risk of developing severe disease. Girls who are at low risk of significant long-term complications rarely require second-line agents (with the exception of sulfasalazine) unless they have obvious swollen joints or an elevated erythrocyte sedimentation rate (ESR). Within the nonsteroidal anti-inflammatory drugs (NSAIDs), it is important to remember that diclofenac, nabumetone, piroxicam, tolmetin, oxazepram, and indomethacin are generally more effective for enthesitis than ibuprofen or naproxen. (Sulfasalazine is often remarkably effective for children with spondyloarthropathies, but it contains sulfur and is associated with an increased frequency of allergic reactions.) The majority of children can be treated successfully with these

NSAIDs. For children with more severe disease, methotrexate, etanercept, adalimumab, infliximab, cyclosporine, azathioprine, and leflunomide all have been used with varying success (see Chapter 22).

Physical therapy

Physical therapy is important in caring for children who do not fully respond to NSAIDs. The major concern is their progressive loss of flexibility over time. This loss of flexibility can be slowed if not completely prevented by a program of anti-inflammatory medications, exercises, and strengthening with attention to good posture (see Fig. 19). Local inflammatory changes in the wrist may be helped by the use of wrist splints to protect against subluxation and to reduce discomfort. For children with plantar fascia insertion pain or heel spurs, the use of gel-filled heel cups placed inside the shoe may provide substantial relief.

Surgery is rarely necessary for children with spondyloarthropathy. In the small subgroup of children with severe disease, it may become necessary to replace a damaged hip. Occasionally, children develop severe wrist arthritis and may require surgical fusion. Chronic active arthritis may require a synovectomy. With proper physical therapy, it is uncommon for children to need tendon releases.

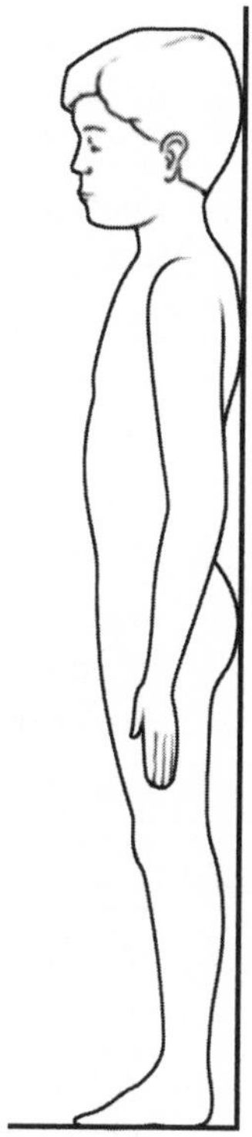

FIG 19. *Children should practice standing with their heels, butt, shoulders, and head flat against the wall.*

Long-term prognosis

The majority of children with spondyloarthropathies do well. When considering prognosis, it is important to consider boys separately from girls, the HLA B27-positive children separately from those who are HLA B27-negative, and those with an elevated sedimentation rate separately from the others. Girls who are HLA B27-negative with a normal sedimentation rate do well in the long run but may have recurrent complaints. Many require NSAIDs on a consistent basis, especially in the wintertime, but it is rare for this illness to have a major negative impact on their lives. Most of these children have recurrent enthesitis, but swollen joints are rare. HLA B27-positive girls with a normal sedimentation rate tend to have a higher frequency of complaints and more frequently recurring disease but again have a good long-term prognosis.

Girls who have an elevated sedimentation rate or recurrent joint swelling are more worrisome. Some of these girls have significant arthritis that will require continuing care and may necessitate the use of second-line drugs. Nonetheless, I expect these girls to grow up to have solid jobs and families of their own. The prognosis is a little more guarded for the girls who have elevated sedimentation rates and swollen joints and are HLA B27-positive. This group is more likely to require second-line agents and to have persisting problems into adulthood. However, with proper care they should still have a very acceptable outcome and enjoy a full life.

Most HLA B27-negative boys with a nonspecific spondyloarthropathy also do well. However, their complaints tend to be more frequent and more severe than the complaints of HLA B27-negative girls. They also tend to have more persistent problems with heel pain and back pain. This group may require chronic medication. They generally function well as adults but are typically excluded from the armed forces and emergency services.

Boys with an elevated sedimentation rate and swollen joints are at greater risk of an unsatisfactory outcome. They may have more difficulty over the long term and often require second-line agents. Although their outcome is usually quite acceptable, there are HLA B27-negative boys with chronic and persistent arthritis lasting into adulthood. Nonetheless, most have jobs and families and are not limited by their arthritis, with the exception of athletic activities and occupational limitations as above.

There are two distinct groups of HLA B27-positive boys. Some have normal sedimentation rates, no swollen joints, and only mild complaints. It appears that they have only minimal genetic predisposition toward arthritis (see Chapter 24). Like the others in this group, these children do well. Boys who are HLA B27-positive and have swollen joints with an elevated ESR are at greater risk. Some will go on to develop definite ankylosing spondylitis or another associated condition (see the next section).

JUVENILE ANKYLOSING SPONDYLITIS AND ANKYLOSING SPONDYLITIS

In the 1970s the genetic marker HLA B27 was a new discovery. Since virtually all adult men with ankylosing spondylitis (AS) were HLA B27-positive, there was great concern that all of the HLA B27-positive boys who came to the attention of rheumatologists would ultimately develop ankylosing spondylitis. However, since most individuals with AS do not fulfill criteria for the diagnosis until after they reach thirty years of age, you need at least fifteen years of follow up to know which teenage boys ultimately develop AS. Keeping track of teenagers is very difficult. Further, the ones who have trouble are more likely to keep in touch with their doctors than the ones who do not.

No one is sure how great the future risk of developing AS is for HLA B27-positive teenage boys with mild or moderate complaints. Diagnosing all HLA B27-positive boys with a spondyloarthropathy as having juvenile ankylosing spondylitis (JAS) is predicting the future without the benefit of a crystal ball. Not only does it cause undue worry for many parents, but it also makes life and health insurance difficult to obtain. Although some will develop AS, labeling all of these children with JAS is unnecessary.

I recommend that the term "juvenile ankylosing spondylitis" be avoided. Certainly, an HLA B27-positive boy who has swollen joints and an elevated sedimentation rate is at risk of progressing to definite AS and should be treated aggressively, but there is no accurate information about how likely he is to develop definite AS. To be diagnosed with definite AS, a child must fulfill a set of criteria that were developed for adults. The specific degree of radiographic evidence of sacroiliitis required by these criteria is rarely present in childhood. Careful studies of adults who were ultimately diagnosed with AS have determined that they often did not fulfill the required radiographic criteria until they reached their thirties. That does not mean that these men did not have arthritic complaints earlier in life. However, they were not diagnosed with definite AS because many individuals with arthritic complaints do not develop full-blown disease. The same is true of children.

Occasionally, I see HLA B27-positive teenage boys who have obvious sacroiliac joint involvement on their X rays and can be labeled definitively as having AS. However, this is uncommon. Parents of a child who is HLA B27-positive must remember that the child inherited the gene from them. If you did not develop AS, why should you assume your child will? Further, even if you have AS, we know the penetrance of the disease is highly variable. That means it is not a sure thing that your child will develop the disease. These children should all be under the care of an experienced rheumatologist who appropriately treats whatever problems develop. This will assure them the best possible outcome, whatever the ultimate diagnosis. Prematurely labeling the child with a diagnosis of juvenile ankylosing spondylitis does not benefit anyone.

REACTIVE ARTHRITIS: INFECTION-ASSOCIATED ARTHRITIS AND REITER'S SYNDROME

Bruce was a sixteen-year-old passenger on a large cruise ship. Due to circumstances beyond control, one of the dishes served on the ship was contaminated by a bacterium that causes gastroenteritis (vomiting or diarrhea). Some 500 passengers who ate the contaminated food became ill. Most passengers recovered completely within a few days. But 10 percent of the passengers who became ill developed aches and pains in their joints one to two weeks after being sick. Only five of the ill passengers developed persistent arthritis that required treatment. Bruce was one of them. Fortunately, he recovered over a six-month period. However, two other passengers never fully recovered from their arthritis. Although only forty of the passengers who became ill were HLA B27-positive, four of the five passengers who required treatment for their arthritis were HLA B27-positive. (HLA B27 is indicative of a genetic predisposition to arthritis.)

Reactive or infection-associated arthritis and Reiter's syndrome are important special cases of spondyloarthropathy. Affected children are often very ill, with fever, rash, and widespread arthritis. Sometimes the arthritis is in only one large joint, but at other times it may be widespread in large and small joints. It was originally termed **"reactive arthritis"** because the arthritis frequently begins shortly after a significant viral or bacterial infection. The name was changed to infection-associated arthritis to remind physicians that in some cases the infection is still present and may require treatment.

The most common infectious agents that cause these forms of arthritis are bacteria—shigella, salmonella, neisseria, and chlamydia—and viruses, especially parvovirus B19. The arthritis associated with Lyme disease is also a form of infection-associated arthritis. Mild and brief arthritis following a variety of infections is very common. Once the episode has passed, most children recover completely. A typical episode of infection-associated arthritis resolves in three to six weeks. However, some children develop arthritis that lasts for a longer period, as exemplified by the case history above. Occasionally, children have lingering disease that may persist for many months. If the arthritis persists for a year or more, then it is considered arthritis that was initiated by an infection, but it is no longer considered reactive or infection-associated arthritis.

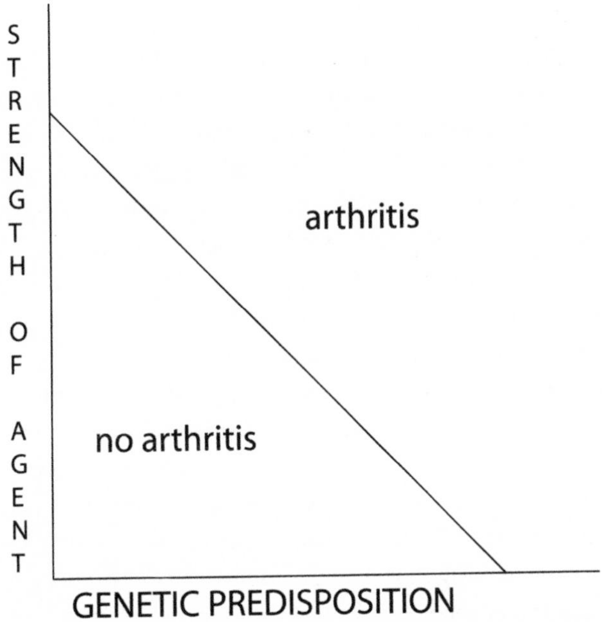

FIG 20. *A child with very little genetic predisposition but affected by a strong environmental agent is much less likely to ever have arthritis again than a child who has a strong genetic predisposition. That person may develop arthritis following infection with any number of weaker agents.*

Although many children with infection-associated arthritis look very ill at the beginning, the majority of children recover completely. Some are initially misdiagnosed as having systemic onset arthritis, but the fever pattern and rash of reactive arthritis and systemic onset arthritis are different. Recurrences of reactive arthritis are rare (if the underlying infection has resolved), but there are children with a substantial genetic predisposition to arthritis that develop repeated episodes of arthritis following exposure to different infectious agents. HLA B27 is just one example of genetic predisposition. There are many people with a genetic predisposition to arthritis who are not HLA B27-positive (see Fig. 20).

Complications

Since, by definition, infection-associated arthritis resolves within a year of onset, long-term complications are infrequent. There may be complications related to the initial infection, but most children recover fully and do well.

Reiter's syndrome

Reiter's syndrome is a special case of reactive arthritis. It is distinguished from other cases of reactive arthritis by the occurrence of arthritis, urethritis, and conjunctivitis. (Urethritis is irritation of the urinary tract and is typically evident because of pain or white blood cells in the urine.) Children with Reiter's syndrome sometimes have rashes particularly on their hands and feet. They may also have severe, painful, acute anterior uveitis. When evaluating a child for the diagnosis of Reiter's syndrome, it is important to remember that the arthritis, urethritis, and conjunctivitis do not have to all be present on the same day. They may occur one after the other without ever overlapping in time. Incomplete Reiter's syndrome is just another term for reactive arthritis. Although Reiter's syndrome with all of the findings is common in adults, it is rare in childhood.

Treatment. The most important step in the treatment for children with infection-associated arthritis including Lyme disease and Reiter's syndrome involves making sure the infection is properly treated. Once it is clear that the infection associated with the arthritis is no longer active, these children should be treated just like other children with spondyloarthropathies. Most respond well to easily tolerated NSAIDs, but some may require indomethacin during the early phase of their arthritis. In most cases, the arthritis resolves completely over a period of a few months. Second-line agents are rarely required, but some children benefit from the addition of sulfasalazine. Although intra-articular injection of corticosteroids may be useful if a single joint remains troublesome after the infection has been fully treated, oral corticosteroids are rarely necessary.

Physical therapy and surgery. Physical therapy to maintain strength and range of motion is often necessary during the acute phase of the disease. Surgery should not be necessary for a child with infection-associated arthritis unless it is necessary for treatment of the infection.

Prognosis. Once the infection is properly treated and has resolved, the long-term prognosis for children with infection-associated arthritis is very good. Occasionally, children have recurrent episodes of arthritis with subsequent infections. Rarely children may have an episode of infection-associated arthritis, recover, and then develop persistent spondyloarthropathy years later.

PSORIATIC ARTHRITIS

> Susan is a delightful girl who initially was seen by her pediatrician at the age of two for a stubbed toe that just did not get better. There was no obvious explanation for the diffusely swollen toe, and it finally went back to normal over a four-month period. Susan then did well until she was six years of age. At that time she had a swollen knee and was noted to be ANA-positive. She was diagnosed with pauciarticular JA. Her sedimentation rate was elevated to fifty but returned to normal after several months of treatment. Her knee slowly improved, and by age eight she was off all medications. She became my patient at age twelve when she presented with pain and swelling in both knees and the right wrist. Over the ensuing years she has had continuing polyarthritis controlled by sulfasalazine, methotrexate, and etanercept. Despite aggressive treatment, she has lost some range of motion in her wrists. Nonetheless, she is currently a successful college graduate in her mid-twenties, working for a prestigious firm on Wall Street. Only a careful physician would recognize that she continues to have limitations due to her arthritis. However, she remains on multiple medications.

Psoriatic arthritis is another spondyloarthropathy that requires special attention. Pediatric rheumatologists continue to debate exactly who belongs in this group, since one does not have to have psoriasis to have psoriatic arthritis and one might have another form of arthritis and coincidentally have psoriasis (see below). The situation is further complicated by recognition of two distinct subsets. One group is made up of young children, mostly girls, who are often ANA-positive and may have pauciarticular onset. However, these are often the children who have the elevated sedimentation rates or low hemoglobin values. Many of these children start with a swollen finger or toe (dactylitis). The confusion about this group results from a lack of long-term follow up for many children. This is a disease that evolves over a period of years, just as Susan's did. *Most of the children in this group do not have psoriasis.* So, why is it called psoriatic arthritis? I often think it would be easier to simply call this Joe's disease. However, if you follow children who have this type of arthritis for a long period, ultimately (it may be ten or fifteen years later) many of them will develop psoriasis.

There are varied criteria for the diagnosis of psoriatic arthritis. They require that the child have arthritis plus dactylitis or changes in the fingernails of a type often seen in children with psoriasis (onycholysis), as well as a close relative with psoriasis. Some physicians argue over how close the relative must be and how sure you are that the relative has psoriasis. These arguments fail to recognize that this arthritis has a characteristic appearance and behavior.

If a child presents with dactylitis or obvious swollen tendons, it is most likely psoriatic arthritis. It does not really matter whether there is a relative with psoriasis or whether the child ultimately develops psoriasis. What matters is that the physician recognizes that children with this pattern of arthritis require more aggressive treatment. The same is true for little girls with only a single swollen joint, if they have an elevated sedimentation rate or low hemoglobin, as noted in the discussion of pauciarticular JA.

The young children with this form of arthritis need to be treated more aggressively than children with typical pauciarticular arthritis. Most often they are girls, but there are some boys in this group. Except for the laboratory criteria discussed above, they may look just like other children with pauciarticular onset arthritis. However, they are often more difficult to bring under control with NSAIDs, and their disease recurs much more frequently. Interestingly, they are often ANA-positive and as much at risk of eye disease as the true pauciarticular onset children. Some will have a family history of psoriasis and others will have a swollen tender finger or toe that might not have been noticed. In some cases, the swollen toe may have been noticed several months before the knee became swollen and then cleared up.

Despite the fact that only a few joints are affected at the beginning, over time these children often develop polyarticular disease. A typical child might have had a swollen toe that rapidly improved at eighteen months of age, then a swollen knee at thirty-six months of age that improved over six months, then swollen wrists at six years of age that are still causing trouble at age twelve. The key to obtaining a good outcome for these children is aggressive therapy to bring their disease under control, followed by prolonged suppressive therapy with a medication such as sulfasalazine. I have cared for children who had no evidence of arthritis while being maintained on sulfasalazine for several years, only to flare within a few months when the sulfasalazine was discontinued.

The second group of children with psoriatic arthritis is made up of children who often first see a rheumatologist when they are between twelve and sixteen years of age. Again, girls are more common than boys in this group. Often they give no history of earlier problems. Their problems may begin with a swollen finger or toe and they are invariably thought to have suffered recurrent athletic injuries. Some present with a swollen wrist without evidence of any other joint involvement. They often have an elevated sedimentation rate and about half have a family history of psoriasis. Sometimes the arthritis is difficult to control. In other children it seems to come under control easily, but it keeps coming back. It is unlikely that this form of arthritis is ever truly gone in the sense that you can be sure it will not come back again. A significant number of these children develop widespread arthritis over time. However, most respond well to aggressive therapy. As with all forms of arthritis in childhood, early intervention is essential to prevent the accumulation of significant long-term joint damage. Since it frequently recurs, continued follow up even when the child seems well is also important. I frequently have parents return after having skipped appointments for a year or two because the child recently had begun to complain of pain. On careful examination, there are often long-term changes that take months to appear. If the family had kept the scheduled follow-up appointments when the child was not complaining, the problem could have been detected sooner and much of the damage prevented.

Because of its destructive potential, it is important that this form of arthritis be recognized promptly. This is the most likely diagnosis for any child presenting with dactylitis or predominant upper extremity involvement (i.e., elbows, wrists, and shoulders). Although the neck is rarely the first joint involved, it frequently becomes involved over time. Involvement of the jaw is also more frequent in these children than in children with other forms of spondyloarthropathy.

Complications

The primary complications of psoriatic arthritis are related to recurrent arthritis. Some children develop significant joint damage over the course of their disease. Serious eye involvement can occur in young children, and children with ANA-positive psoriatic arthritis must be monitored just as carefully as children with ANA-positive pauciarticular onset JA. Fortunately, eye involvement is less common in teenagers but still possible. Persistent wrist and finger involvement is often prominent. In some children this seems to be the only evidence of disease. However, children may begin with only wrist involvement but years later develop problems in other joints. Elbow, neck, and jaw involvement is more common in children with this form of arthritis and must be looked for. However, hips, knees, ankles, and toes may also be involved. Because the arthritis can become widespread, it is important to do everything possible to bring it under control quickly and, if possible, to prevent it from returning.

Medical treatment

Initial treatment for this group is the same as the treatment for other children with spondyloarthropathies. Again, it is important to remember that diclofenac, nabumetone, piroxicam, tolmetin, oxazepram, and indomethacin are generally more effective for enthesitis than ibuprofen or naproxen. I am much quicker to use sulfasalazine for children in this group. It is often remarkably effective. Children may promptly improve on sulfasalazine who did not improve with any of the other NSAIDs. I have cared for a number of children who did very well for several years on sulfasalazine, but then had recurrent disease within a few months of stopping the drug. As a result, in the absence of side effects, I continue sulfasalazine as long as possible. As with all medications, children on long-term therapy with sulfasalazine require routine monitoring of their laboratory tests (see Chapter 22). Most often problems with sulfasalazine occur at the beginning of treatment.

While the majority of children are treated successfully with NSAIDs and possibly sulfasalazine, some children have arthritis that is more difficult to control. In different children I have had excellent success with methotrexate, etanercept, adalimumab, infliximab, cyclosporine, azathioprine, or leflunomide. None of these medications works for every child, but it is rare for a child to fail to respond to any of them. Thalidomide has been effective in children who have failed all other therapies, but it must be used only by physicians with extensive experience with this medication (see Chapter 22 for more details). Except for occasional intra-articular injections, corticosteroids are rarely necessary and should be avoided if at all possible.

Physical therapy

Physical therapy plays an important role in maintaining strength and range of motion for these children. Since this form of arthritis has a propensity to involve the wrists and fingers, occupational therapy is often an important part of their care as well.

Surgery

Surgery is rarely necessary for children with psoriatic arthritis. For children with severe disease it may be necessary to replace a damaged hip.

Occasionally, children develop severe, painful wrist arthritis that may require surgical fusion. With proper physical therapy it is uncommon for children to need tendon releases or any other surgical procedures.

Prognosis

The long-term prognosis for children with psoriatic arthritis is more guarded than for children with a nonspecific spondyloarthropathy or typical pauciarticular onset JA. Young children who have only dactylitis that resolves quickly may nonetheless years later develop arthritis in other joints. With aggressive therapy and careful monitoring, most of the children with psoriatic arthritis will have a very acceptable, if not perfect, outcome. Over a period of years some children with this arthritis develop progressive changes in their fingers and wrists despite aggressive therapy.

Children with psoriatic arthritis and significantly elevated sedimentation rates should be treated aggressively even if it appears that there is involvement of only a single joint. It is common to see a teenager who initially complained of only a single swollen finger or tender wrist with an elevated sedimentation rate ultimately developing widespread polyarthritis. This group of children frequently requires NSAIDs, sulfasalazine, methotrexate, etanercept, or adalimumab. Leflunomide may also be useful. With aggressive therapy, the majority of these children are able to function normally as adults.

ARTHRITIS ASSOCIATED WITH BOWEL DISEASE

Ulcerative colitis and **regional enteritis** are collectively referred to as **inflammatory bowel disease** (IBD). It is well known that some children with these diseases have arthritis. This arthritis typically takes the form of a spondyloarthropathy. It is also well recognized that the arthritis may become evident before the IBD. The complete explanation for this association is unclear. Careful studies have demonstrated that many individuals with spondyloarthropathy have an unusual appearance to their gastrointestinal mucosa (lining). Exactly how this relates to developing arthritis is uncertain. Children with IBD are often on strong immunosuppressive medications for the IBD. They also may be receiving corticosteroids. In most cases the therapy for their IBD is sufficient to control their arthritis. However, occasionally, children require NSAIDs in addition to the therapy for their IBD. Infliximab and adalimumab are beneficial for children who don't respond to NSAIDs.

In evaluating a child with a spondyloarthropathy who has gastrointestinal complaints, testing for the antibody pANCA may speed recognition of the child with IBD. Two skin findings, erythema nodosum (large, tender, painful, red or purplish bumps over the shins) and pyoderma gangrenosum (large areas of skin breakdown with weeping sores), in a child with a spondyloarthropathy should spark careful consideration for possible IBD. Many of the children with arthritis and IBD are HLA B27-positive. Children with IBD who are HLA B27-positive are more likely to have significant and persistent arthritis than those who are HLA B27-negative.

Complications

The long-term complications of children with IBD are primarily related to their gastrointestinal disease and its treatment and are not discussed here. Complications of the arthritis of IBD are similar to those of children with spondyloarthropathy. With the exception of hip and sacroiliac joint involvement the arthritis rarely is of long-term significance.

Physical therapy

Physical and occupational therapy for these children is the same as for other children with other spondyloarthropathies.

In addition to IBD, children who have abdominal pain, rash, and arthritis might have **reactive arthritis, Henoch Schoenlein purpura, Kawasaki disease, polyarteritis nodosa, dermatomyositis, systemic lupus erythematosus, or other vasculitic diseases,** as well as many other conditions (see the appropriate chapters). Most often the correct diagnosis is evident, but I have seen children with IBD initially misdiagnosed with these illnesses, and vice versa.

One special situation that deserves attention is the child with a complaint of severe abdominal pain, fever, arthritis, and limp. If a child has been ill with severe abdominal pain and developed a limp on the right side, the physicians should remember to consider the possibility of undiagnosed **appendicitis**. Most children with appendicitis develop fever and severe abdominal pain and are promptly diagnosed. However, over the years I have seen several children referred for evaluation with a limp. On careful examination these children had right lower abdominal pain on deep palpation.

The limp and the findings "in the right hip" were the result of abdominal pain because there was an abscess around a ruptured appendix that was not diagnosed at the time it occurred. This situation can often be suspected from a careful history and physical examination. It can be confirmed by a CAT scan of the abdomen or perhaps abdominal ultrasound.

Celiac disease (gluten-sensitive enteropathy) is another gastrointestinal disease associated with arthritic complaints that typically takes the form of a spondyloarthropathy. Celiac disease most often begins with poor growth during the first years of life. However, celiac disease is being increasingly recognized in teenagers with nonspecific joint complaints or spondyloarthropathies and chronic upset stomachs. When questioned, many of these children complain of disliking pasta, pizza, and other high-gluten foods. A definite diagnosis of celiac disease requires the characteristic findings on small intestinal biopsy, but the diagnosis is strongly suggested by the presence of anti-endomyseal antibodies (IgA anti-tissue transglutaminase) in the blood. Treatment for celiac disease is a gluten-free diet. With this the arthritic complaints will normally subside. Untreated celiac disease is associated with a number of autoimmune conditions, including thyroiditis, and may be associated with a positive ANA.

Nonspecific arthritic complaints may also be seen in children who have recovered from a severe insult to the gastrointestinal tract. The most common examples are children who suffered **necrotizing enterocolitis** during the neonatal period. "Bypass arthropathy," in which individuals with surgically induced short-bowel syndromes developed arthritis, was well recognized when this surgery was briefly popular for the treatment of morbid obesity. Because of the very high rate of complications associated with this procedure, it is now done only rarely.

Since there are a variety of conditions that affect the gastrointestinal tract and cause arthritis, it is natural to wonder how the two problems are associated. There are no studies that answer this question to everyone's satisfaction. It appears that a damaged or "different" intestinal tract will allow elements from the diet to get into the bloodstream. In some people (perhaps because of genetic predisposition), these elements may reach the joints and initiate arthritis. If the damage to the intestinal tract can be corrected, the arthritis may go away. This association has led to the hope that dietary changes may relieve the arthritis. This is true for children with celiac disease who improve if they avoid foods containing gluten. However, it does not appear to be true for other conditions (see Chapter 23).

MISCELLANEOUS CONDITIONS RELATED TO SPONDYLOARTHROPATHIES

Hypogammaglobulinemia-associated problems

IgA deficiency. IgA deficiency is a low level of immunoglobulin A (see Chapter 24 for a full discussion of immunoglobulins). Children with IgA deficiency develop rheumatic diseases much more frequently than the normal population. While this often takes the form of a spondyloarthropathy, studies have shown an increased frequency of children with IgA deficiency in virtually every rheumatic disease. There are two important problems to be aware of regarding a child who is recognized to have IgA deficiency. The first is to recognize that this is a permanent condition that makes recurrent arthritis more likely, even in a child who otherwise appears to have pauciarticular onset disease.

The second problem is that individuals who are IgA-deficient are vulnerable to "transfusion reactions." These are not due to incompatibility with the transfused red blood cells, but are the result of a reaction to the IgA in the serum transfused with the red blood cells. Routine laboratory cross-typing will not detect this. Parents of children who are IgA-deficient should be sure that they inform any treating physician of this condition. A clue to the presence of IgA deficiency is a strong history of recurrent ear infections or similar problems. However, many children who have had lots of ear infections do not have any identified abnormality.

Common variable hypogammaglobulinemia. This is a condition in which children with immature immune systems do not have fully normal levels of immunoglobulin. As the immune system matures, the problem frequently corrects itself. Children in the three- to seven-year-old age group who limp whenever they have a viral infection often have low immunoglobulin levels. This group is not well described in the literature. On evaluation they often have a very mild degree of periarticular pain and no other obvious findings. The complaints typically disappear in a day or a few days, when the infection has resolved. However, the limp or other joint pains may recur with subsequent infections. I have seen a number of children with six, seven, or even eight such episodes.

Routine laboratory evaluation of these children is usually completely normal. When serum immunoglobulin levels are measured, the children have values that would clearly be abnormal for an adult but are considered at the low end of normal for their age. I have cared for several dozen of these children over the past twenty years. As their immune system matures, the immunoglobulin levels rise and the problem ceases. No detailed reports of the long-term outcome for these children are available. None that I have cared for has developed significant rheumatic disease. Since these children are at the low end of normal for their age, they are not officially immunodeficient. Many have been misdiagnosed as having JRA.

Children with definite common variable hypogammaglobulinemia and IgG subclass deficiencies may also have an increased incidence of arthritis. These are children with low immunoglobulin levels of varying specific types. The arthritis these children get also generally follows the pattern of a spondyloarthropathy. Many investigators feel that this situation is similar to the situation for children with abnormal gastrointestinal tracts. In children with mild immune deficiencies, proteins or other molecules that are normally kept out of the body by the immune system are able to get in and cause mild arthritis. In most children these episodes are short-lived and without serious complications, but there are exceptions. In addition, it is important to recognize that the defect in their immune systems leaves them vulnerable to bone or joint infections that require treatment with antibiotics.

Children with more severe forms of immunodeficiency are occasionally found to have arthritis. For these children, the immune deficiency and the resulting infections are usually a more significant problem than the arthritis. However, these children may benefit from treatment with NSAIDs. Often the underlying immunodeficiency is treated with intravenous immunoglobulin (IVIgG), and this leads to resolution of the arthritis as well.

"Recurrent" toxic synovitis

Toxic synovitis is a transient inflammation of the hip that most often occurs in young children (see Chapter 3). I occasionally see children diagnosed with "recurrent" toxic synovitis. These children should be regarded with suspicion. Some have Legg-Calve-Perthes disease that has not been recognized. In other children, recurrent episodes of synovitis in the hip may be the first manifestation of what ultimately becomes an obvious spondyloarthropathy. Toxic synovitis should never be diagnosed in a child over nine years of age. Isolated synovitis of the hip in children over the age of nine is usually the initial manifestation of a spondyloarthropathy. However, other causes of hip inflammation must be excluded.

Post-streptococcal reactive arthritis and rheumatic fever

Post-streptococcal reactive arthritis is another form of infection-associated arthritis. It differs in that we know this form of infection-associated arthritis is initiated by a group A streptococcal infection. Post-streptococcal reactive arthritis behaves just like the other forms of infection-associated arthritis. Sometimes the arthritis is in a single large joint such as the hip, and at other times it can affect multiple joints.

There is a lot of confusion regarding the relationship of post-streptococcal reactive arthritis to acute rheumatic fever. Since acute rheumatic fever is associated with possible damage to the heart and requires penicillin prophylaxis, this is an area of great concern. **Acute rheumatic fever** is defined according to the Jones criteria (see box). Children who develop a nonmigratory (not moving from joint to joint) arthritis after a streptococcal infection do not fulfill these criteria. As a result, many physicians do not treat these children with penicillin prophylaxis. However, some of these children have gone on to develop heart damage of rheumatic fever following a later streptococcal infection.

Medical therapy. Since no large-scale studies have been carried out to determine how much risk there is for children with post-streptococcal

Jones criteria for the diagnosis of acute rheumatic fever

Major criteria

- Carditis (inflammation of the heart valves or muscle)
- Migratory polyarthritis (swollen and tender joints with involvement shifting from one joint to another)
- Sydenham's chorea (a type of uncontrollable movements)
- Subcutaneous nodules (bumps under the skin)
- Erythema marginatum (a red rash with dramatic red outlines)

Minor criteria

- Raised CRP, ESR, or leukocytes (laboratory results)
- Arthralgia (joint pain without swelling or limitation)
- Fever

The diagnosis of acute rheumatic fever requires two major criteria, or one major and two minor criteria, and evidence of a recent streptococcal infection.

reactive arthritis who do not fulfill Jones criteria, there is no definite right answer regarding penicillin prophylaxis for these children. In families where there is a history of acute rheumatic fever or in children where the arthritis associated with the streptococcal infection was severe, *I prefer to treat with penicillin prophylaxis to prevent recurrences and reduce the risk of future rheumatic fever-related heart damage.* Some physicians insist this should not be done unless the child fulfills Jones criteria. I would point out two facts to these physicians. First, Jones criteria are guidelines, not laws—they were drawn up by a committee. Second, if you talk to physicians who were practicing medicine when rheumatic fever was common, many of them freely acknowledge treating many children who did not definitely fulfill the Jones criteria. *Our concern should be for preventing children from developing heart disease, not slavishly applying written guidelines.* However, this must be balanced against the risks of penicillin allergy and the appearance of bacteria that are resistant to penicillin.

The arthritis in children with post-streptococcal reactive arthritis is treated with NSAIDs, just like other forms of spondyloarthropathy. Although aspirin was the old therapy for acute rheumatic fever, the other NSAIDs are safer, more convenient, and equally effective.

Prognosis. The prognosis for children with post-streptococcal reactive arthritis and children with acute rheumatic fever is primarily related to heart involvement. By definition, children with post-streptococcal reactive arthritis do not have heart involvement. If they have heart involvement, they fulfill criteria for rheumatic fever. (Our concern is that they will develop heart involvement with a future streptococcal infection.) For children with acute rheumatic fever, severe inflammation of the heart can lead to permanent heart damage or even death. However, the arthritis is short-lived and rarely of long-term significance. Any child with heart damage secondary to acute rheumatic fever should be under the care of a cardiologist.

10

Lyme Disease

Frankie was a delightful twelve-year-old who loved to play sports. Halfway through football season, he began to complain of knee pains. When his symptoms didn't improve, he was taken to his pediatrician. At first the pediatrician thought Frankie simply "twisted it." When Frankie was unable to continue football because the knee was swollen and painful, he was referred to an orthopedist. Three months later Frankie continued to have pain in the knee that prevented him from playing sports. With activity the knee often became swollen but would improve over a week to ten days. He was sent to me to treat his "JRA." The father was sure he had been tested for Lyme disease, but careful review of the records revealed that the test had never been done. The orthopedist was sure the pediatrician had checked, and the pediatrician was sure the orthopedist had. When I did the Lyme test, it was strongly positive and Frankie improved dramatically when we treated him with antibiotics.

Samuel was a five-year-old from an area where Lyme disease was quite common. Although he had played happily outdoors all summer, he seemed to be dragging in the fall. When he began to complain of pain, his mother took him to the pediatrician. The blood tests were negative for Lyme, but the erythrocyte sedimentation rate (ESR) was moderately elevated. Since Lyme was common in the area where Sam lived, the pediatrician simply treated him for Lyme despite the negative test. When Sam didn't get better with the oral antibiotics, he got intravenous antibiotics for two more months. He still didn't seem better. Finally, Sam was sent to me for treatment of his difficult Lyme disease. X rays revealed that Sam had a large tumor in his pelvis, necessitating surgery, radiation, and extensive chemotherapy. Sam was left with permanent bone damage after the surgery. He never had Lyme. Had the tumor been found sooner, he might have done better.

Lyme disease is a chronic infection by *Borrelia burgdorferi*. This is a spirochetal organism that is carried by mammals such as deer and deer mice and spread by very small deer ticks (*Ixodes scapularis*). The ticks bite an infected animal and pick up the spirochete with their blood meal. They then transfer the spirochete to people or animals they feed on, infecting them with Lyme disease.

Lyme disease in humans is often only an acute flu-like illness. However, some adults and children develop rash and arthritis. The key to understanding Lyme arthritis in children is to recognize that it is in many ways a typical infection-associated arthritis. The major difference is that Lyme disease follows a much more protracted course. Typical infection-associated arthritis develops within a few weeks of the original illness. The fever and rash (erythema chronicum migrans, or ECM) of Lyme disease also occur early. However, the arthritis of Lyme disease usually does not appear until two to four or more months after the initial infection.

Ticks found in the spring and early summer are young ticks (nymphs) that are not as likely to carry Lyme disease. But as they feed repeatedly on different animals, the likelihood of their being infected dramatically increases. Many of the children I see in my office seem to have become infected during late August or early September. They develop arthritis in November, December, or January, when parents and physicians are not thinking about Lyme disease. Children who present with arthritis in the early summer often have been infected the previous fall. (It is rarely possible to prove exactly when a child was infected. The Western blot test detects a specific number of bands, which gradually increases over time as the infected individual mounts an immune response to the spirochete. A child diagnosed with Lyme disease in the early summer who has more than ten positive bands on the Western blot was most likely infected the previous year.)

Some parents know their children are at risk because they live in areas where deer are common. Other families have visited such areas but never found a tick on their child. It is important to realize that the deer tick that carries Lyme disease is extremely small. It is no larger than the head of a typical pin. Ticks are often recognized only after the area around where they have bitten becomes red and irritated, or when a parent notices a "moving freckle." While it is a disadvantage that these ticks are so small, parents who find a larger dog tick on their child (about the size of lentil) can be confident that these ticks do not carry Lyme disease. Even parents who live in areas where Lyme disease is common are often surprised to learn that arthritis that appeared in January is the result of a tick bite the previous summer.

In children the flu-like symptoms of early Lyme disease are often dismissed as a virus. The child may develop the characteristic rash of ECM a few weeks after the original illness. This is most often a series of large circles the size of a quarter or even much bigger. The outer edge of the circle is red and inflamed looking, while the center of the circle is usually pale. Anyone with the characteristic appearing rash should be tested and treated for Lyme disease. (There are other illnesses that may produce a rash with central clearing. If the Lyme test is negative, make sure other possible explanations are carefully considered.) Children do not usually have arthritis when the rash first appears. However, the rash can recur later in the illness at a time when the child does have arthritis. This rash does not come and go rapidly like the rash associated with systemic onset arthritis. In addition, in children with Lyme disease the individual lesions are typically far fewer, but much larger.

A number of nonspecific symptoms, such as headaches, are often seen at the beginning of Lyme disease. Their significance is uncertain. It is clear that Lyme disease does involve the nervous system in some children, although most children with headaches do not have central nervous system Lyme disease. Bell's palsy, one symptom of Lyme disease, is an irritation of the facial nerve, which is responsible for moving the side of the face. If this nerve is not functioning properly, the child cannot open the mouth to smile or close the eye tightly on the involved side. While there are many possible causes of Bell's palsy, it is well recognized that Lyme is a common cause in Lyme-endemic areas.

Lyme arthritis usually begins dramatically. It can affect any large or small joint and often suddenly affects many joints. Children with Lyme disease are often in significant pain. This is very different from typical childhood arthritis, which comes on gradually. Although ECM is a typical manifestation of early Lyme disease, it is rarely present when the arthritis develops.

Since the arthritic symptoms develop months after the initial tick bite, children with Lyme disease are easily diagnosed only if the physicians remember to check a Lyme titer. Some children with Lyme disease present with only a single swollen joint. These children differ from children with typical JA in that the arthritis often comes on rapidly. In addition, like other forms of infection-associated arthritis, Lyme arthritis can begin in the hip. (However, I have never seen dactylitis due to Lyme disease.)

Children with Lyme disease who have gone untreated for a long period of time may have recurrent episodes of joint swelling. This most often takes the form of recurrent knee swelling, which may have been dismissed as an athletic injury or sprain. It is important that any child with swollen joints who lives in or has visited an area where Lyme disease occurs be appropriately tested. This is particularly important for children who may be known to have JA. I have had several children under my care for JA who unexpectedly developed a dramatic worsening of their symptoms. When tested, they had become Lyme-positive even though when I initially began treating them several years previously, they had been Lyme-negative. This is not JA due to Lyme disease. This is a child with JA who, because they lived in an endemic area, also developed Lyme disease. Most children who develop Lyme disease are detected because of the new onset of symptoms. Because the children I follow have chronic arthritis, I systematically check Lyme titers in the fall each year.

DIFFERENTIAL DIAGNOSIS

Lyme disease is a typical infection-associated or reactive arthritis. As a result, it may be confused with any other infection-associated arthritis. The key differences in children with arthritis due to Lyme disease are the absence of a recent infection (most children develop infection-associated arthritis two to three weeks following a recognized illness) and the presence of a positive Lyme titer. In any child being evaluated for Lyme arthritis, it is important to consider the other causes of infection-associated arthritis, including streptococcal and other bacterial infections and parvovirus and other viral infections.

Systemic lupus erythematosus and other forms of collagen vascular disease may also begin with the rapid onset of arthritis involving the large and small joints. The key to distinguishing these diseases is their different clinical appearance and use of appropriate laboratory testing. I have seen many children with these illnesses misdiagnosed as "seronegative" Lyme disease. In areas where there is a high frequency of exposure to Lyme disease, the situation may be complicated by a positive Lyme test in a child who is suffering from another illness. All children with positive Lyme tests should be treated for Lyme disease, but if there is not a quick and dramatic response, physicians should be sure to investigate carefully for other possible causes of the child's symptoms.

There is much debate about the occurrence of Lyme disease in children who do not have positive titers (see Chapter 24). Most of this debate stems from the period when Lyme testing was not well standardized. At present, it is extremely unlikely that a child with a negative Lyme titer has the disease. While it is always possible for the laboratory to make a mistake in reporting a result, this can be easily resolved in a suspicious situation by simply repeating the test, perhaps using a different laboratory. I have seen many children treated extensively for "Lyme test negative" Lyme disease. More unfortunate than the fact that they were treated with unnecessary antibiotics is that they were not properly treated for what was really wrong with them. In the case of children with bone or joint pains due to infections, JA, or cancer, this can have tragic consequences.

LABORATORY FINDINGS

Children with Lyme disease almost invariably have a positive Lyme titer and a positive Western blot (see Chapter 24 for a discussion of these two tests). In addition, they have elevated ESRs and white blood cell counts. While these findings are commonly present in children with polyarticular onset arthritis, they are infrequent in children with pauciarticular onset disease. Some children with Lyme disease have positive tests for antinuclear antibody (ANA). They should not have rheumatoid factor (RF), antibodies to double-stranded DNA (dsDNA), or complement abnormalities.

Some physicians and laboratories have developed specialized tests for the detection of Lyme disease. If these tests had stood up to careful evaluation, we would all be using them. However, strategies such as giving a child antibiotics and then collecting the urine to look for evidence of spirochete antigens are unlikely to detect subtle Lyme disease that did not show up in regular testing. It is important to understand that all humans have normal spirochetes in their mouths. That is why the Western blot test was developed. Screening tests for spirochete antigens do not distinguish between the response to the spirochetes that are normally present in the body and the Lyme spirochete. Only the Western blot does this.

COMPLICATIONS

Fortunately, serious complications of Lyme disease are rare. The vast majority of children with Lyme disease–related arthritis recover promptly (within a few weeks) and completely with treatment (see next section).

In children with Lyme who have large numbers of bands on their Western blot (e.g., nine or more), it is likely the infection has been present for a prolonged period. Some of these children will have continuing arthritis after the first thirty days of antibiotics. It is important to recognize that like other causes of infection-associated arthritis, Lyme tends to provoke arthritis in those who have an underlying "arthritic predisposition." If the arthritis persists after appropriate treatment for Lyme disease, the emphasis must be on treatment of the arthritis, not continued antibiotics. As is typical of infection-associated arthritis, the majority of these children are well within a year of diagnosis. Any child with arthritis persisting after a year must be treated with the assumption that Lyme provoked an underlying arthritic disease that must be treated. There is no evidence that further antibiotics are beneficial.

The Bell's palsy and other neurologic symptoms of Lyme disease typically respond well to antibiotics. There are some who argue that Lyme has many chronic symptoms in childhood, including attention deficit disorder and other unexplained conditions. It is important to recognize that Lyme disease is common. Therefore it will be found in a significant number of children with a wide variety of coincidental problems that are unrelated to Lyme disease. The issue seems clear-cut, if the child's problems resolve with treatment of the Lyme disease. However, if the problems are not related to Lyme, months or even years of antibiotics are unlikely to provide real relief. While every child with positive testing for Lyme disease deserves appropriate treatment, it should not be allowed to deflect attention from other potential causes of the child's complaints.

Another possible complication of Lyme disease is the **Jarisch-Herxheimer reaction**. This was initially described in the treatment of syphilis (another spirochete infection) when penicillin first became available. When the first dose of penicillin was given to a patient who was heavily infected, a very large number of spirochetes would die and release their contents into the blood. This would produce an acute toxic reaction with fever, rash, and severe malaise. Although it could occur in someone with a large number of Lyme spirochetes as well, I have never seen this reaction in a child under my care.

MEDICAL TREATMENT

Optimal treatment for Lyme disease is dependent on the age of the child, the manifestations of the disease, and whether the child has any allergies to drugs. Young children are typically treated with amoxicillin, while children over the age of ten are typically treated with doxycycline. Doxycycline is not used in younger children because it will become incorporated in the enamel of developing teeth and may cause a permanent grayish stain. Some physicians feel it is acceptable to use doxycycline in children as young as eight years of age, if the adult teeth appear to be fully formed in the gums. In children who are allergic to these drugs, consideration may be given to cephalosporins or erythromycin derivatives. This should be discussed carefully with your physician because these drugs differ in how well they reach the central nervous system. Ceftriaxone is a potent cephalosporin that may be given as intramuscular injections.

The duration of therapy for Lyme disease also depends on the manifestations of disease. The majority of the medical community is in agreement with the recommendations shown in the box.

One of the least settled questions in the treatment of Lyme disease is the response to children found with an embedded deer tick. The correct answer is to obtain a Lyme titer. It will not reflect infection from the tick just found, but may indicate that there is a preexisting infection that requires treatment. If this titer is negative, it needs to be repeated in six weeks to determine whether it has turned positive. If it has, the child should be treated appropriately.

Some physicians recommend an alternative approach. If a child is found with an embedded tick, a Lyme titer is performed, but two weeks of oral antibiotic therapy are begun immediately. If the titer is negative, treatment is stopped at two weeks. If the titer is positive, then treatment is continued for an additional week. It has been shown that this may prevent Lyme infections and is more cost-effective than repeated testing. One new study suggests one day of treatment may work as well as two weeks. However, if a child lives in an area where Lyme is common, how often are we going to treat him or her? There is no answer to this question that everyone agrees with.

How do I know if my child gets infected again? This is another of the questions for which there is no satisfactory answer. In most infections, the assumption is that either the bacteria can be cultured if it is present or, in the case of viruses, a single infection provides immunity that prevents further infection. In the case of Lyme disease, it is virtually impossible to culture the spirochete from tissues to prove an infection is present. At the same time, it appears that a single Lyme infection does not provide

Duration of antibiotic therapy for the manifestations of Lyme disease

- Children with positive testing for Lyme disease in the absence of arthritis or neurologic symptoms should be treated with *twenty-one days* of an appropriate antibiotic. The vast majority will respond well to oral antibiotics.
- If a child has arthritis, *thirty days* of antibiotic therapy are recommended. Again, this may be done orally. However, therapy is often begun intravenously for a possible bacterial infection of the joint and switched to oral only after bacterial infection has been excluded. This judgment will depend on the clinical situation and how strongly the physicians suspect that a bacterial infection might be present. The children should also be treated with NSAIDs for as long as the arthritis continues. This will control the inflammatory response in the joint, minimizing the damage from inflammatory enzymes and providing significant pain relief.
- Children with *neurologic manifestations* of Lyme disease also require *thirty days* of antibiotic therapy. However, in this situation many physicians prefer to begin with intravenous therapy, since this provides better assurance of a high level of drug reaching the central nervous system. The majority of children who do not have a long-standing infection (as evidenced by the number of bands on the Western blot) respond completely within thirty days. Further treatment of children with neurologic manifestations that have not completely resolved after thirty days of intravenous therapy will depend on the nature of the manifestations and the degree of improvement that has occurred.
- Children who have arthritis that has not fully resolved with thirty days of oral therapy represent a challenge. Since this is infection-associated arthritis, it is well recognized that the arthritis may persist long after the infection is gone, and thus further antibiotics may not be necessary. For children who have only a moderate number of bands on the Western blot, I recommend a month of continued nonsteroidal anti-inflammatory drug (NSAID) therapy. Almost all are well at the end of an additional month.
- Children with a large number of bands on the Western blot may be difficult to bring under complete control. Most often these are children who have had arthritic symptoms for months before being recognized as having Lyme disease and did not receive appropriate treatment. Since the arthritis frequently lingers in this group, I recommend an additional thirty days of intravenous therapy so that both the parents and I can be assured that the Lyme has been adequately treated. Some of these children will continue to have active arthritis after the additional thirty days of antibiotics are completed. I do not treat these children with further antibiotics. Over time they will respond to NSAIDs.

lifelong protection. The Lyme vaccine was recently withdrawn from the market because it had side effects and did not guarantee protection from future infection.

In my patients, I periodically monitor the Lyme titer and Western blot. During the first few months after diagnosis and treatment, both the Lyme titer and the number of Western blot positive bands may increase. This represents "immunologic recruitment" (the immune response is gathering strength over time), not continued infection. After six or more months, the Lyme titer should begin to decrease. The number of positive bands on the Western blot may not. If a child develops signs of possible repeat infection a year or more after initial treatment, I will compare the results with those found six months after the initial treatment (to account for the immunologic recruitment). If the response is stronger, I will retreat with oral antibiotics. There is no proof and there are no controlled studies to guide us. Each physician must recommend what he or she thinks makes the most sense in this situation.

There are some physicians who firmly believe that Lyme is a more chronic infection and may require years of therapy. There is no convincing evidence that they are correct, and prolonged antibiotic therapy has been associated with serious side effects. Many children come to me after long periods of antibiotic therapy without sustained improvement. Often it is because Lyme disease is not the cause of their complaints. Once a proper diagnosis is made and they are begun on appropriate therapy they often promptly improve. I have seen children who came to me after many months of antibiotics for "Lyme disease" who turned out to have tumors, infections, and arthritis.

11

Systemic Lupus Erythematosus

Margaret was fourteen years old when I met her. She did well in junior high school but seemed lazy over the summer before starting high school. When high school began she did not seem to be making new friends and complained of being tired. School was hard. Her family just assumed she needed to get used to high school. As the semester progressed she seemed to be spending more time in her room. Her parents got phone calls that she was not performing well in school and her grades were poor. She was losing weight, irritable, and disinterested. By December there were questions about drug use, difficulty adjusting to the new school, and so on.

In January the school requested a psychiatric evaluation. The psychiatrist asked for a pediatric evaluation. Fortunately, the pediatrician ran a full set of blood tests and found that she was anemic, with an elevated sedimentation rate and a positive test for antinuclear antibody (ANA). She was referred to my office. When I walked into the room and shook her hand, she cried because her hands hurt when I squeezed. She had not realized that she had arthritis. She had no rash but had confirmatory findings of SLE on her blood and urine tests. As I write this, I saw Margaret yesterday. It's eight years later and she is finishing college and doing very well. She wants to teach English.

WHAT IS SYSTEMIC LUPUS ERYTHEMATOSUS?

In textbooks, SLE is defined as a complex autoimmune disease with protean manifestations. That does not translate into plain English very well. Typically, SLE is a disease that affects teenage girls and young adult women. Less frequently, SLE occurs in both older and younger individuals and in boys. SLE often begins with fevers, rash, joint pains, and fatigue. Although these symptoms are worrisome, it is the ability of SLE to affect many different internal organs that makes this a serious illness. Serious involvement of the lungs, brain, or kidneys in cases of SLE can lead to permanent disability or even death. It is important that children who have SLE be promptly recognized so that they can be treated and internal organ damage prevented whenever possible. Some children are discovered to have evidence of internal organ damage without ever complaining of obvious symptoms.

The key to understanding SLE is to recognize that the disease begins with a breakdown in regulation of the immune system. In a normal immune response, the immune system identifies "an invader" and mounts a response against it. To protect itself, the body uses every possible type of immunity (e.g., antibodies, complement, and cell-mediated immunity). Once the invader has been controlled, the system turns off and everything goes back to normal. In children with SLE, the immune system is constantly responding to "an invader." No one has found an indication of what the invader is. Because decades of research have failed to find an invader (despite many false leads in the past), we now believe that in SLE the regulatory system breaks down and the body is unable to turn off the immune response after the initial attack (by any one of many different invaders) is over.

Because in children and adults with SLE the body fails to turn the immune response off, SLE patients get fevers, ache all over, and often have a rash. When one gets these symptoms as part of a normal infection, the infecting virus or bacteria does not directly cause the problems. The fever and aches and pains are the result of the body's immune response that is trying to fight the infection. Just as different infections can damage different parts of the body, in children with SLE, the uncontrolled immune response can produce all sorts of different damage. There can be problems anywhere: in the brain, heart, lungs, muscles, kidneys, skin, joints, liver, or intestine.

Whenever the areas damaged by SLE are examined, doctors find the type of damage they would expect if there had been a serious infection. Antibodies are present, complement is present, inflammatory cells are present, and the local tissue has been damaged by the inflammation. All these findings are signs that the body has been trying to fight an infection. We are beginning to understand more about why the immune system fails to turn off in children with SLE, but we do not understand why certain children develop one set of problems and other children develop completely different problems. In animal models, genetics seem to be an important factor that determines which problems develop.

DIAGNOSIS: WHEN TO SUSPECT SLE

SLE most often affects girls in the teenage years, but it may affect boys and girls at any age. *Although the typical butterfly rash on the face is considered a characteristic feature of the disease, it is found in only one-third of children when they first come to the doctor's office.* Since many doctors do not think of SLE unless they see the butterfly rash, many children have symptoms of SLE for months before the proper diagnosis is made. *The key to a prompt diagnosis of SLE is for primary-care physicians to consider this diagnosis whenever they are evaluating children who appear chronically ill or have unexplained damage in organs that are frequently affected by SLE (e.g., the kidneys).*

Many physicians are confused by the American College of Rheumatology criteria for a definite diagnosis of SLE (see box on next page). They often assume that these criteria are the most common symptoms of SLE. This is completely incorrect. The criteria were written to help distinguish SLE from other diseases. They are intended to make sure everyone included in a study of patients with SLE really has SLE, not to aid in making the diagnosis. The most common symptom of SLE is fever. The second most common symptom is a chronic complaint of not feeling well (malaise). The third common symptom is arthritis of the small joints of the hands and feet that is often described as "hurting all over."

Prompt diagnosis of children with SLE requires parents and physicians to consider SLE whenever a child is not doing well. For very young children who are "failing to thrive" there is a standard evaluation to look for problems such as cystic fibrosis and hypothyroidism. Physicians also need a standard work-up for older children who are failing to thrive (see Chapter 4). Although SLE is only one of many possible causes, it is important to include ANA testing in this evaluation. Many diseases may be associated with a positive ANA test in children and teenagers (see Chapter 24 on diagnostic testing). However, SLE should be carefully excluded when evaluating any child with a positive test. A negative test for ANA makes SLE very unlikely.

American College of Rheumatology criteria for a diagnosis of *definite* SLE

1. Malar rash: a red rash over the cheeks (often crossing over the nose)
2. Discoid rash: a scaly red rash (uncommon in children)
3. Photosensitivity: easy sun burning and sensitivity to light
4. Mucosal ulcers: sores in the mouth or nose
5. Serositis: inflammation of the lining of the chest or abdomen producing pain
6. Arthritis: pain swelling or limitation of motion of a joint
7. Renal involvement: abnormalities on the urine tests or blood tests (see this chapter)
8. Neurologic involvement: problems with seizures or difficulty thinking normally
9. Hematologic involvement: abnormalities of the red cells, white cells, or platelets (see this chapter)
10. Immunologic disorder: abnormal blood tests characteristic of SLE (see this chapter)
11. Antinuclear antibodies

A child is considered to have definite SLE if he or she has any four of the eleven criteria.

Although the onset of SLE occurs between the ages of twelve and twenty-five years in most patients, I have seen SLE in children as young as three years of age. In a pediatric rheumatology practice, it is not unusual to see SLE starting at the age of eight years. The incidence of SLE varies by sex and race. However, no one has ever sampled a completely homogeneous population to determine the precise number of children with SLE by race. I have previously published data from a large group of children I followed with SLE. Based on that experience, I estimated that among 100,000 female children of each race between the ages of nine and nineteen years, there would be 31 Asian girls with SLE, 20 African American girls, 13 Hispanic girls, and 4 Caucasian girls with SLE. I would also expect there to be one or two boys with SLE for every 100,000 male children.

Although chronic "failure to thrive" is the most common presentation in children, SLE can also begin in many other ways. Chronic swelling of the hands and feet, easy bruising, joint pains, abnormal urine tests, easy sunburn (photosensitivity), seizures, altered personality and depression, and even altered school performance all may be initial findings of children with SLE. However, it is important to remember that these are nonspecific symptoms that may occur in many different illnesses.

Some children with SLE reach my office after a long history of being evaluated for problems such as anemia, fatigue, fever, and weight loss without explanation. Less often the onset of SLE is sudden and dramatic, with bleeding from the lungs, kidney problems, or multiple-organ involvement. Again, it is important to remember that SLE is not the only disease that may cause these findings. Even when a positive ANA is present, SLE may not be the correct diagnosis. This is why it is very important that all such children be evaluated by a physician experienced with SLE.

Once the diagnosis of SLE is suspected, proper evaluation begins with testing for ANA. If the ANA test is negative, it is extremely unlikely that the child has SLE. (A variety of other rheumatic diseases may mimic the symptoms of SLE.) If the test for ANA is positive, further evaluation should include complete routine testing, such as a complete blood count (CBC), metabolic profile, clotting studies, urine analysis, and testing for Ro, La, Sm, RNP, and anti-DNA antibodies (see Chapter 24). Measurements of complement levels C3 and C4 should be performed. It is also useful to screen these children for thyroid function abnormalities, antithyroid antibodies, anticardiolipin antibodies, and rheumatoid factor. Sometimes it is clear that a child has SLE at the completion of these studies. In other cases, there are several abnormalities but not enough to make a definite diagnosis of SLE.

One of my patients is a young woman who was complaining of aches and pains when she was fifteen years old. There were no significant findings on examination, but her pediatrician was quite surprised when she tested positive for ANA. She was referred for evaluation, but her aches and pains had resolved by the time she came for her appointment. Her examination was entirely normal, but on repeat testing she remained ANA-positive and was also positive for Sm antibody. The remaining tests were normal. I did not make a diagnosis of SLE, but I continued to examine and test her periodically. She remained well until four years later, when she called to tell me she had developed a rash and joint pain. On examination, she had arthritis and a facial rash with an ulcer on the roof of her mouth. Blood tests again revealed a strongly positive ANA and Sm antibodies, but now anti-DNA (deoxyribonucleic acid) antibodies and decreased serum complement levels C3 and C4 as well. She had developed definite SLE, but we caught it very early. She was begun on low-dose prednisone and is doing fine years later.

The diagnosis of definite SLE requires that the child fulfill four of the eleven American College of Rheumatology criteria for the diagnosis of definite lupus. However, there are many children with SLE who initially fulfill fewer than four criteria. *If children have several findings that suggest SLE but do not fulfill criteria for a definite diagnosis of SLE, they should be monitored carefully.* It really does not matter whether they are said to have SLE, possible SLE, or probable SLE. The key to proper care for these children is to treat appropriately whatever problems they are having. If this is done, it will not matter if the ultimate diagnosis is SLE or another condition. They will have been receiving appropriate care either way. I sometimes see children with only three criteria who have been told because they do not have definite SLE, they do not need to be treated. This is incorrect.

Children with uncertain symptoms and relatives who have SLE are often of great concern to their families. Up to one-third of the relatives of a patient with SLE will be ANA-positive but have no disease. However, relatives of someone with SLE are at greater risk of developing SLE than the normal population. On one occasion I examined all the relatives of more than ninety children with SLE. When I tested everyone, I found there were thirty ANA-positive sisters among the relatives. Two had unrecognized SLE and were treated. I personally examined the remaining twenty-eight repeatedly for several years. No one developed disease during the first two years of follow-up. However, several developed definite SLE between three and five years after I first evaluated them. This group was clearly at increased risk relative to the normal population, but most of the twenty-eight ANA-positive sisters did not develop SLE.

Children who have nonspecific symptoms and a positive ANA require routine follow-up to look for evidence of disease. Their physicians must maintain an awareness of the possibility of SLE. Simply dismissing these children as not having criteria for definite SLE and never needing to be seen again is incorrect. Some physicians simply instruct the parents to bring the child back if more problems develop. I prefer to be proactive and periodically look for problems. This often allows me to begin therapy before the problems become more serious. It is well known that children with

SLE may develop kidney disease and damage to other organs without initially complaining of pain or discomfort. It is important to detect these problems as early as possible and to minimize the damage to vital organs.

CLINICAL MANIFESTATIONS OF SLE

The patterns of disease involvement with SLE range from children with fever, rash, aches, and pains but no serious organ damage to children with no complaints of fever or rash who are found to have serious kidney or blood (hematologic) involvement on a routine screening test. Serious internal organ involvement most often takes the form of kidney involvement, but the brain, heart, lungs, and other internal organs also may be seriously affected.

Many children with SLE have a mild version that is easily treated by an experienced physician, but other children have more severe problems and have serious internal organ involvement. As much as possible, it is important to recognize which children have mild disease and which children have severe disease. This cannot be done with absolute certainty. There are children who start out with mild disease and get worse over time. There are also some children who start out extremely ill, respond well to therapy, and do fine. The challenge for physicians and families caring for children with SLE is to find the proper balance between the side effects of the medication and the risks of damage from the disease (see the section on treatment below). When they can be recognized, children with severe disease should be treated aggressively *before* there is a lot of organ damage, not after. "Let's wait until we are sure the house is burning down before we call the fire department" is not a good approach.

Kidney involvement

Kidney (renal) involvement is one of the most worrisome aspects of SLE. However, there are varying degrees of kidney involvement, from the very mild to the very severe. Approximately two-thirds of children with SLE will have at least mild kidney involvement at the time they are diagnosed. Most but not all children with significant kidney involvement have evident abnormalities on a urine analysis when they are first brought to the doctor. In some cases, the presence of blood or protein in the urine was detected on a routine exam and lead to the diagnosis of SLE. Other children are brought to the doctor because of swelling of their feet and were found to have protein in the urine as the result of SLE. Red blood cells in the urine, white blood cells in the urine, casts (plugs of red or white blood cells), and protein in the urine all may be manifestations of SLE (note again that there are many other possible causes of these problems).

In a child with obvious SLE, the physicians may elect to treat with corticosteroids and do a kidney biopsy only if the child does not respond to this treatment. Other physicians will biopsy every child with SLE, while some biopsy every child with SLE who has abnormal urine tests. There is no single correct answer. If your child has had a kidney biopsy, there are several important things for you to know. The pathologist will look at the kidney biopsy and report the type of kidney involvement. Normally, this is done according to the World Health Organization (WHO) classification (see box). A class I or class II biopsy is not a cause for major concern. A class III, IV, or V biopsy is worrisome. In addition to telling you the WHO classification, the biopsy report should contain immunofluorescence results. This means that they have looked at the kidney biopsy to determine whether immunoglobulin or complement is being deposited in the kidney. The immunoglobulin may be reported to be in the glomerulus (the filtering portion of the kidney) or in the tubules (this is the part of the kidney that controls the flow of minerals such as sodium and potassium into the urine).

World Health Organization classification of renal biopsy pathology in lupus

- Class I: normal kidney
- Class II: mild glomerulitis
- Class III: focal segmental glomerulonephritis
- Class IV: diffuse proliferative glomerulonephritis (DPGN)
- Class V: membranous glomerulonephritis

If the immunofluorescence studies show a lot of immunoglobulin or complement in the glomeruli, this is worrisome. This is especially important if the biopsy is reported as WHO class III. Class III is focal segmental glomerulonephritis, which means that most of the glomeruli seen under the microscope are normal but that there are some (less than half) that show evidence of inflammation. This has long been thought to be a less serious degree of kidney involvement that does not require the same aggressive treatment as WHO class IV. However, that assumes that the damage has stopped. All too often, children with class III on their initial kidney biopsy go on to have class IV disease over time. In

WHO class IV (diffuse proliferative glomerulonephritis), greater than half the glomeruli are damaged. Everyone agrees that children with class IV are at significant risk of serious kidney damage and, ultimately, kidney failure. As a result, these children must be treated aggressively. Most physicians now look carefully at any biopsy interpreted as class III and treat the child aggressively if the immunofluorescence is strongly positive, since this suggests the disease is likely to become worse over time.

If your child has class IV renal disease, he or she needs to be treated aggressively. Some children with class IV do well, but others do not. If you are told that your child has a class IV biopsy, you need to know the "activity" and "chronicity" scores. Activity is a measure of the amount of cellular inflammation in the kidney. The pathologist looks at the glomeruli and determines how inflamed they are and whether there are large collections of inflammatory cells (these are often referred to as crescents). The presence of crescents means there is very severe, very active inflammation in the kidney. This is worrisome. A high **activity index** means there is a lot of damage going on right now. At the same time the pathologist will report a chronicity index. This is a very important number as well. The **chronicity index** is an estimate of the amount of scarring in the kidney. When a glomerulus is destroyed, it is referred to as sclerosed. Under the microscope, the pathologist can still see where the glomerulus was, but it is not working anymore. The greater the percentage of sclerosed glomeruli, and the greater the damage to other structures in the kidney, the higher the chronicity index.

If the chronicity index is very high, it does not make sense to treat the child aggressively. Badly scarred kidneys are not going to recover, no matter how hard you try. These children will ultimately need renal dialysis and kidney transplantation. The key to a successful outcome is to catch the involvement early and prevent the chronicity index from going up over time. *Although many different treatments have been recommended for children with lupus kidney involvement, only the systematic use of intravenous cyclophosphamide has been shown to prevent progression of the chronicity index over time.* Thus, it is very important that all children with a worrisome class III biopsy and all children with a class IV biopsy receive appropriate treatment. Some physicians do favor other therapies, but only intravenous cyclophosphamide has been proven to work in published studies.

WHO class V kidney biopsies are a special case. These biopsies show membranous nephritis. Membranous glomerulonephritis has a characteristic "wire loop" lesion on the kidney biopsy. It is associated with the loss of protein from the kidneys, causing significant proteinuria (protein in the urine). If the body loses too much protein in the urine, it leads to swelling of the legs and feet. This is a serious problem for several reasons. When the blood flows through the body, it is carrying both oxygen and many nutrients to the tissues. These nutrients are held in the blood by osmotic pressure (this is a balance between the level of molecules inside the blood vessel and the level of molecules in the tissues outside the blood vessel). When the osmotic pressure is proper, nutrients are allowed to seep out into the tissues where they are needed. If the kidneys are losing too much protein, there are not enough protein molecules in the blood to maintain the proper osmotic pressure. As a result, the water molecules in the blood leak out into the tissues, causing swelling.

One of the most important jobs of the kidney's filters (the glomeruli) is to keep the protein in the blood while taking unneeded water out. If the glomeruli are not working properly, they let protein escape into the urine. When too much protein escapes, the body cannot compensate by making more. The level of protein (albumin) in the blood drops and the osmotic pressure drops. When that happens, things start leaking out all over the body. Excessive water accumulates in the feet when the patient is sitting or standing up or around the buttocks if he or she is lying down. In an effort to correct the problem, the body starts making more of things that do not leak easily. Normally this takes the form of cholesterol. Children with nephrotic syndrome may have cholesterol levels in the 600 or 700 mg/dl range. This partially helps to fix the problem of water leaking out of the blood vessels, but these very high cholesterol levels often lead to early heart disease.

In addition to the problems resulting from excessive water leakage and high cholesterol levels, the prolonged proteinuria in children with class IV or V disease is damaging to the glomeruli. As a result, if children with proteinuria are not properly treated, the glomeruli will eventually fail. This can be partially prevented by the use of ACE inhibitors (a class of drugs used to treat high blood pressure). When enough glomeruli have failed, the kidneys are no longer effective and the child is in renal failure, which must be treated with kidney dialysis. Many doctors will treat children with class V disease with cyclophosphamide. It works, but not as well as it does for class IV disease. However, we do not have anything that is clearly better. Children with what is called mixed class IV and class V disease should be treated aggressively with intravenous cyclophosphamide.

All children with serious kidney involvement due to SLE need to be treated aggressively. All too often I see children who have been followed for "mild" kidney involvement for a long period of time. The treating physician did not become concerned until the serum creatinine level began to go over 2.0 gm/dl. Unfortunately, many of these children are found to have serious damage when a new renal biopsy is done. Things may not have looked bad on the first renal biopsy or maybe things were never bad enough "initially" to do a renal biopsy. The disease was allowed to smolder. The new biopsy shows a lot of scarring and a high chronicity index. It is now too late to do anything to prevent the kidneys from ultimately failing. These children need to have kidney transplants and will be on antirejection medicine for the rest of their lives. Many people tell me they are fearful of the side effects of being treated with intravenous cyclophosphamide to control SLE. However, the side effects of intravenous cyclophosphamide are far less than the side effects of chronic renal dialysis or the lifetime of immunosuppression required following kidney transplantation.

Brain and nervous system involvement

Children with SLE may exhibit a wide variety of brain abnormalities. Seizures, strokes, and other serious abnormalities are obvious but relatively infrequent. However, subtle problems due to brain involvement in children with SLE vary from difficulty with fine motor skills and poor penmanship to suddenly worsening grades and severe depression. These subtle problems are common. There are many psychological effects of being chronically ill. And there are also many psychological effects of having to take a lot of medicine, visit the doctor all the time, and have lots of blood tests performed.

I often listen to doctors arguing over whether a child's poor school performance and behavior problems are due to SLE, their medicines, or the situation. They want to decide that the answer is all one or all the other. In real life it is like arguing about the word "cat." Is "cat" a small furry animal because of the "c," the "a," or the "t"? After all, if I change the "c" to "b" it's "bat." But if I change the "t" to "p" it's "cap," but changing the "a" to "o" makes "cot." Well, this is ridiculous! All three letters go together in a specific order to make "cat" and they cannot be separated or assigned individual responsibility. They are acting together. In real life, the disease, the medications, and the situation all act together as well. It is never all one or the other. *If a child is not acting right, do not look for a single answer; assume that the disease, the medicines, and the situation all need to be evaluated and corrected as much as possible.*

Involvement of the brain in children with SLE has three primary forms. Some children have clotting disorders that lead to strokes that result in brain damage. Other children suffer brain damage because their lupus results in chronic inflammation of the blood vessels in the brain, and the inflammation of the blood vessels damages the surrounding brain tissue. A third group of children have brain problems because they have taken too much corticosteroid over the years. Each of these types of damage has its own peculiarities, but all three may occur in the same child at the same time.

A number of tests are used to evaluate a child with SLE who is showing neurologic abnormalities. An MRI will show structural changes in the brain. It will also show increased water content that can occur with inflammation, bleeding, or other problems. A CAT scan will show structural problems and may also demonstrate bleeding, among other problems. When these tests are normal, some physicians will recommend a lumbar puncture (spinal tap). This test will provide fluid to be analyzed in the laboratory for the presence of sugar, protein, cells, or immunoglobulins. All of these may be abnormal if SLE is affecting the brain. They also may all be normal. The most important reason to look at the spinal fluid in this situation is to make sure there is no infection or other unsuspected problem. Nuclear isotope brain scans called SPECT scans are utilized by some centers to evaluate brain function, but are generally considered unreliable in the setting of SLE.

Brain damage due to strokes is usually very dramatic. It can result in sudden inability to use a hand, leg, or whole side of the body. Sometimes the stroke may affect a speech center, making it impossible for the child to talk, or the balance centers, making the child unable to walk normally. Whenever there is a sudden change in the ability of a child with SLE to function normally, the brain should be carefully evaluated.

One of my patients was a teenage boy with SLE who loved to participate in sports. His disease was under good control and he was doing everything right. One day, the doctors on the ward at the hospital called to tell me that he was there. No one had called me initially because he had hit his head on the goalpost playing football and he had a simple concussion. When I went to see him, he could not move his head without the whole world spinning and was not talking. The neurologists saw him and said he must have hit his head hard to cause the concussion. We waited for him to get better, but things did not improve. When an MRI was done, it showed he had inflammation and damage in the part of the brain that controls balance. Once we treated the problem, he was able to tell us that while on the football field, he suddenly could not walk and fell down. He never hit his head on the goalpost. People assumed that was what happened when they found him on the field. The whole problem was a stroke from his SLE. The wrong story caused a two-day delay in proper treatment.

Brain damage due to inflammation of the blood vessels by SLE is often much more subtle. Margaret, whose story opens this chapter, became withdrawn and did poorly in school because she was suffering from brain involvement. Careful studies have shown that many children with SLE do not do as well as they should in school. In addition, they frequently use "bad" judgment. People often assume they are just bad kids. Many years ago I cared for Susan, a teenage girl who was sent to me because of SLE. The physician who sent Susan told me that she was trouble. She had been arrested for joyriding and hung out with the wrong crowd. She had a reputation for being nasty to her doctors, talking back, and often refusing to take her medications.

In addition to her other problems, Susan had developed ballism. Patients with ballism have trouble controlling their movements. This is the result of irritation of the part of the brain that controls motor coordination. When the ballism was active, Susan could not control the movements of her left arm. It would wave around wildly. When she took enough corticosteroids this was well controlled, but during "uncooperative" periods, Susan would not take her medicine. When the left arm began to wave around and she could not control it, Susan was always very annoyed. She would come to the hospital for medication. I would give her a high dose of corticosteroids in the hospital and the arm would come under control. We went through several episodes like this before I realized that at the end of each treatment for her ballism, Susan was polite and acted very respectful. Her misbehavior and refusal to take medications were also the result of her brain being involved by SLE, just like the ballism. When I put Susan on intravenous cyclophosphamide and got her SLE under long-term good control, she turned out to be a nice person all the time.

Heart involvement

Mild heart involvement is common in children with SLE but does not usually become significant. What this means is that careful studies looking for evidence of heart involvement often find changes, but they are rarely things that bring the child to the doctor. Involvement of the pericardium (the fibrous sack containing the heart) may cause chest pain. Your doctor will refer to this as pericarditis. This chest pain may be worse with deep breaths or made worse by changing position (such as leaning forward). This can be detected easily if an echocardiogram is performed. Children with chest pain must also be evaluated for pulmonary emboli (see below). Small amounts of thickening of the pericardium are often found in children with SLE who do not report chest pain, but if a child reports chest pain and there is thickening of the pericardium, a nonsteroidal anti-inflammatory drug (NSAID) may help. Another common problem is an increase in the amount of fluid around the heart. Since this fluid increase is also the result of inflammation of the pericardial sack, it is also termed pericarditis.

When the inflammation of the pericardium causes thickening, pain is the most common symptom, but it is rare for it to interfere with the function of the heart. The pain is thought to be due to the heart rubbing against the thickened pericardium. When the inflammation leads to increased fluid, there is no pain. Increased fluid in the sack around the heart is called a pericardial effusion. It should be suspected if the heart looks too large on a routine chest X ray. Normally, there is only a small amount of fluid around the heart and the tissues slowly absorb it as more is made. If there is a lot of fluid around the heart, it will ultimately interfere with the strength of the heartbeat and produce shortness of breath, swollen feet, and other signs of poor heart output (heart failure). This is easily diagnosed with an echocardiogram.

It is rare for the heart muscle to become significantly inflamed in children with SLE. If the heart muscle becomes inflamed, it is termed myocarditis. If myocarditis is present, there may be chest pain and there will be an increase in the level of creatinine phosphokinase (CPK), an enzyme that is found in heart muscle. This enzyme is found in other muscles as well and may be increased in many conditions. The laboratory can fractionate the CPK to tell whether it is coming from the heart, other muscles, brain, or elsewhere. Myocarditis may cause abnormalities in the heart rhythm that will show up on an electrocardiogram (EKG). It may also interfere with the ability of the heart to pump blood and produce signs and symptoms of poor heart output. Like the other heart findings, it is best evaluated by a cardiologist by means of an EKG and echocardiogram.

Buildup of abnormal material on the surface of the heart valves is another common cause of problems in children with SLE. There are four valves in the heart that control the flow of blood from one chamber to another. These valves are supposed to open fully to allow the blood to move forward freely but to close securely to prevent blood from flowing backward when the heart beats (contracts). Children with SLE often develop accumulations of fibrous material on the surface of the valves (the explanation is unclear). This is termed **Libman-Sacks endocarditis** and the accumulated fibrous material is referred to as "vegetation."

Libman-Sacks endocarditis is a worrisome problem for two reasons. First, the vegetations may become big enough to interfere with the proper opening and closing of the valve. When the valves do not open and close properly, the heart has to work harder, either pushing the blood past an incompletely open valve or making up for blood that flowed backward due to a valve that leaked, or both. If the heart cannot compensate for these problems, the result is heart failure with all of the associated symptoms.

The second reason Libman-Sacks endocarditis is a problem is that the vegetations on the valves provide a place for bacteria to grow. We all commonly get bacteria in our blood after brushing our teeth, getting dental work done, and when we have mild infections. Usually our bodies simply eliminate these bacteria without problems. However, if bacteria get into the vegetations on the heart valves of a child with SLE, they may start growing there. This can be extremely serious. As the bacteria multiply, they may spread through the bloodstream to any part of the body.

The bacteria growing in vegetations may also disrupt the vegetations and the valves themselves. This may cause problems by worsening the valve's function and thus heart function or by causing pieces of the vegetation to break off. If a piece of vegetation lands in the brain, it can cause a stroke. If it lands elsewhere, it can plug up the blood flow and cause major damage to the tissue where it landed. This breaking off into the bloodstream is called embolization, and the pieces that break off are called emboli. If the pieces that break off are carrying bacteria, they can cause an infection wherever they land. This is termed **septic embolization**. To minimize the risk of developing infected heart valves, children and adults with any type of heart valve involvement must take antibiotics before they go to the dentist. This is called SBE (subacute bacterial endocarditis) prophylaxis. Some doctors give antibiotics before dental visits to all the children they treat with serious SLE, even if they do not have definite heart valve involvement.

Heart valve involvement is usually detected by an echocardiogram. This will show how well the heart is beating, the motion of the valves, and any significant vegetation. The echocardiogram machines have become increasingly sophisticated and can see smaller and smaller abnormalities. However, in a suspicious situation, if the regular echocardiogram does not show vegetations, the physician may need to do a transesophageal echocardiogram (TE echo). This involves swallowing a transducer so that the physicians can look at the heart from another direction. It's hardly comfortable but it does give a much better picture.

Treatment of heart involvement varies with the type and severity of the involvement. Mild pericarditis may be treated with NSAIDs. More severe pericarditis is often treated with corticosteroids. In rare cases, this does not work or the problem recurs frequently or is very severe. When that happens, it may be necessary for a surgeon to open up the pericardium. If it is too tight, this will relieve the pressure. If it is full of fluid, this will allow the fluid to escape into the chest where other cells can absorb it and the pressure on the heart will be relieved. In general, this type of surgery has to be done only once and will permanently solve the problem.

The treatment of Libman-Sacks endocarditis is much more of a problem. If the vegetations on the valves are small, the doctors may choose to leave them alone. If they are breaking off and causing problems, the child may have to be given blood thinners (anticoagulants). If the vegetations are infected, a long-term course of antibiotics is required. If too much damage has occurred, it may be necessary to do open-heart surgery and replace the valve. Fortunately, with modern aggressive therapy this problem is becoming rare. I see it most often in children who were not diagnosed for a long time after their disease began and in children who were not adequately treated.

Another problem for children with SLE is the development of **arteriosclerosis**. Arteriosclerosis is the hardening of the arteries that occurs normally as people get older. In its severe forms, it causes narrowing of the coronary arteries, which leads to heart attacks, or myocardial infarctions. Chronic use of corticosteroids promotes the development of arteriosclerosis, so children who have received a lot of corticosteroids may develop arteriosclerosis in their teens or twenties. High cholesterol levels (like those seen in children leaking protein from the kidneys) also promote arteriosclerosis. Inflammation in the blood vessels promotes arteriosclerosis, too. Some children with SLE have all of these factors. As a result, some children with lupus that has been treated with moderate doses of corticosteroids for many years will have myocardial infarctions in their twenties or thirties. This is one of the strongest arguments for using strong immunosuppressive drugs early in SLE to bring it under control and minimize the amount of corticosteroids that the child takes over time.

Lung involvement in SLE

Lung involvement in children with SLE may take several different forms. Most children with SLE never experience lung symptoms. However, weakening of the diaphragm (the muscle that moves the lungs) is a common problem in children with SLE. This makes it more difficult for children with SLE to take a really deep breath and harder for them to cough deeply. This poor air movement combined with medications that interfere with the immune response makes children with SLE more vulnerable to **pneumonia**, or lung infections. In children with SLE, pneumonia needs to be treated aggressively.

Some children with SLE are found to have areas of inflammation in the lungs that are diagnosed as **fibrosis**, which is stiffening of the air cells (alveoli) in the lungs because of inflammation in the surrounding tissues. Small areas of fibrosis are not important and usually disappear with treatment of the SLE. Occasionally, children develop more severe pulmonary fibrosis, which may interfere with the ability of the lungs to move air in and out. If this progresses over time, it can be quite serious. In rare cases, children with areas of lung involvement may form pockets of nonfunctional air cells, or "blebs." If an area of fibrosis or a bleb breaks, air can leak out of the lungs and into the chest cavity. This is called a **pneumothorax**. When this happens, the child will experience severe chest pain and difficulty breathing. He or she needs to go to the hospital by ambulance immediately. Fortunately, this problem is uncommon.

Blood clots (**pulmonary emboli**) may occur in the lungs of children with SLE. The symptoms in children are the sudden onset of chest pain and shortness of breath. Although children with clotting problems and anticardiolipin antibodies are at greater risk of developing pulmonary emboli (see hematologic abnormalities below in this chapter), children without these findings may also have this problem. Any child with the sudden onset of pain and shortness of breath or severe chest pain must be promptly evaluated by an experienced physician. Blood clots may be diagnosed on the basis of X rays, CAT scans, MRIs, or ventilation perfusion (VQ) scans. Some newer tests such as D-dimer assays to detect blood clotting are also being evaluated. Children with blood clots will have to be treated with anticoagulants by an experienced physician.

Some children with SLE develop **serositis**, which is inflammation of the cells that line the inside of the chest or abdominal cavity (see the section on the gastrointestinal system below). When this occurs in the chest, it causes pain and difficulty in breathing. The symptoms are very similar to those of pericarditis and the two can be reliably distinguished only by carefully evaluating the pericardium on echocardiogram. The symptoms may also mimic those of a pulmonary embolus. Children with chronic chest pain will need to be carefully evaluated.

Pulmonary hemorrhage is a very serious complication of SLE. It is the result of chronic irritation of the blood vessels in the lungs. For oxygen to be moved from the air breathed into the lungs to the blood vessels in the lungs, the blood vessels must be very close to the surface. This oxygen exchange occurs in the alveoli. If the blood vessels are very irritated by inflammation, they may begin leaking blood into the alveoli. This prevents the proper exchange of oxygen. Poor heart function will make this worse, because it results in increased blood pressure in the lungs (pulmonary hypertension). Increased pressure leads to increased bleeding.

If the blood vessels in the alveoli begin to break down and blood begins to flow into the lungs, it is termed pulmonary hemorrhage. The body can handle a very little bit of bleeding, but significant bleeding may fill the lungs with blood, making it impossible for air to get in. If a child is coughing up blood, he or she should be taken to the physician immediately. Often coughing up a little bit of blood is not a sign of serious trouble, but it is better to make sure. A little blood can come from irritation in the airway or from blood swallowed because of a cut in the nose or mouth. If a child really is bleeding inside the lung, there is no way to put your finger on it to stop it. In the hospital, with a large intensive care unit and lots of hard work and good luck, we can often fix this, but it may be a fatal complication. If a child is getting short of breath and acting as if he or she is not getting enough oxygen, go to a hospital immediately. Worry about why later.

Hematologic involvement

Hematologic involvement refers to involvement of the blood-making system in the bone marrow or a problem in the mechanism of blood clotting. The most common hematologic involvement is anemia, or too few red blood cells. A little bit of anemia is common in children who are chronically ill for any reason. Children with SLE may also have anemia because of excessive bleeding. This can be bleeding from an ulcer, from the kidneys, from heavy menses, or bleeding from many other sources. Whenever there is a problem with the number of a type of cell that comes from the bone marrow, the physicians have to ask whether too few cells are being made or whether the cells are being used up too fast. In children with SLE, both answers may apply.

The anemia of chronic disease comes from poor uptake and use of iron; as a result, too few red blood cells are being made. However, if a child is bleeding, he or she will be anemic because the blood is being lost. Some children with SLE develop **hemolytic anemia**, a condition in which the body is destroying its own red blood cells because they have abnormal antibodies on their surface. Anemia of chronic disease results in a low hemoglobin and a low reticulocyte count. (Reticulocytes are newly made red cells.) Bleeding will result in a high reticulocyte count if the body has enough iron stores. If there is bleeding, the doctor should be able to find where it is occurring. Hemolytic anemia is suggested by finding low hemoglobin with a very high reticulocyte count without bleeding. It can be confirmed by special tests to detect antibodies on the red blood cells.

The condition of having too few white blood cells is called **leukopenia**. This is never thought to be the result of bleeding. It may result from the cells being used up very quickly in trying to fight an infection. It can also be the result of the cells being destroyed. In children with SLE, this happens because of antibodies in the blood called anti–white cell antibodies. Another possibility is that not enough white cells are being made in the bone marrow. This may be due to drugs, infections, or SLE.

Severe leukopenia is worrisome because there may be too few of the cells needed to fight infection. Levels under 1,000 white cells/mm^3 are worrisome. If the level is too low, the doctor may wish to give drugs to stimulate white cell growth. Any child with a low white blood cell count and a fever should be promptly checked by the doctor for evidence of infection. Children who develop large scabs on their lips without having been injured may be getting an infection from the normal bacteria in the mouth. This is often a sign of a dangerously low white blood cell count.

The third major type of cell made in the bone marrow that circulates in the blood is the platelet. Platelets are the sticky plugs that float around in the blood and immediately adhere to any damaged surface to start formation of a clot and limit bleeding. If the number drops too low, the child will start to bruise easily. With very low numbers, the child may start to bruise without doing anything. Lots of children bruise easily, but if your child has SLE and is starting to bruise too easily, make sure the doctor knows. If you look inside your child's mouth with a flashlight and see bruises on the inside of the cheeks, next to the teeth, that may mean the platelet count is very low. Call the doctor and insist on being seen immediately.

All of the hematologic abnormalities that occur in children with SLE need to be carefully investigated. Increasing the dose of corticosteroids treats most of them satisfactorily. If the problems are persistent or recurrent, there are other therapies. Surprisingly, cyclophosphamide has proven useful for these conditions, even though it may make the blood cell counts decrease after it is given. However, in these situations it has to be given with great care and only by someone with extensive experience. A variety of newer therapies are being used for these problems when they don't respond appropriately to corticosteroids.

Involvement of the clotting system

The clotting system is one of the miracles of the human body. Blood must be allowed to flow freely and easily throughout the body, yet any leakage must be promptly stopped. For this to happen, the clotting system must be carefully balanced to prevent clots from forming when they should not occur, while all the pieces are immediately in place to form a clot if necessary. It is best to think of all these pieces floating around in the blood like pieces of a puzzle. They will not all fit together unless the last critical piece is there. When a blood vessel is damaged, the last critical piece is exposed and all the puzzle pieces snap into place, forming a clot.

The most common example of a clotting disorder is **hemophilia**. Children who have hemophilia are missing one of the pieces of the puzzle. Some children with SLE bleed too much, and girls with SLE are sometimes recognized because of very excessive bleeding with their periods (**menorrhagia**). The bleeding in children with SLE is not like the bleeding in a child with hemophilia. If a child has hemophilia, you can mix his or her blood with a normal person's in a test tube and the blood clots normally. This is because the child with hemophilia is missing a factor that the normal blood supplies. However, when you add normal blood to the blood of a child who is bleeding too much because of SLE, often the blood still will not clot. This led to the concept of the lupus anticoagulant (an anticoagulant is something that prevents clotting). Most often children with SLE are not missing a factor. Instead, there is something in the SLE patient's blood that prevents clotting.

After much careful study, it has become clear that there is no single lupus anticoagulant. Instead, children with SLE may make a variety of antibodies that can be thought of as attaching to the puzzle pieces and getting in the way of their snapping together to form a clot. These antibodies often react with a class of molecules called phospholipids or cardiolipins, hence the terms antiphospholipid antibodies (APL) and anticardiolipin antibodies (ACL). These terms are almost, but not exactly, the same thing. The antibodies that interfere with clotting in different children with SLE may be very different from each other. In addition, over time they may change slightly. This is important because people with these antibodies sometimes bleed too much, but sometimes they clot too easily. If you think of the antibodies as sticking to the puzzle pieces, it's easier to understand. Some antibodies get in the way and prevent the pieces from fitting together properly (i.e., prevent clot formation), but other antibodies stick to the pieces in ways that make it easier for the pieces to attach to each other and form a clot when they should not.

Children with anticardiolipin or antiphospholipid antibodies need to be monitored for problems both from clotting and from not clotting. They may even have both problems at the same time. The doctors must try to prevent abnormal clots and to correct any abnormal bleeding. The key to this is stopping the body from making the antibodies that are sticking to the clotting molecules. Corticosteroids can do this and so can other immunosuppressive drugs.

There is a lot of controversy over what to do with children who have ACL or APL antibodies. If a child has had a clot, he or she has to be treated with anticoagulants. However, many children test positive for ACL or APL but have never had a problem. It might seem obvious to treat them with anticoagulants, but then if they get cut or fall they may bleed too much. It does not seem worth the risk for a child who has never had a problem. Some physicians feel it is best to just watch; others believe you should treat with a baby aspirin every day to try to decrease the risk. This seems safe, but so far it has not been proven to be effective. There is no certain answer. I treat my children with SLE who have ACL or APL with a baby aspirin every day if they have never had an abnormal blood clot. Children who have had problems with blood clots must be treated with anticoagulants (e.g., heparin and warfarin).

Gastrointestinal system involvement

The gastrointestinal (GI) system consists of several different parts. These are (1) the stomach and the intestines, which are responsible for the digestion of food, (2) the liver, which is responsible for storing digested food molecules, using most to synthesize substances needed by the body while removing inappropriate substances that get digested, and (3) the gallbladder and pancreas, which are responsible for making chemicals needed to aid in the process of digestion. All of these organs may be involved in children with SLE.

Irritation of the GI system occurs frequently in children with SLE. It may play a large role in the initial malaise that many children with SLE experience. The resulting pain and loss of appetite often lead to depression and weight loss. These are common problems in the period before diagnosis (note that this can happen in many other conditions, as well). The most common GI complaint of children with SLE is **nonspecific stomachache** (abdominal pain). This can be located almost anywhere in the abdomen. It may be associated with eating, or it may not. Often the first thought of the family and physician is that it is the result of irritation from the medications the child is taking. If it persists, everyone becomes worried about ulcers. One of the interesting things about caring for children with SLE is that stomach ulcers are rarely the explanation for abdominal pain. Although many of the medications used to treat SLE can cause ulcers, children with SLE do not often get ulcers. The time when ulcers do occur is usually in the setting of very severe active disease. (When a child is very sick in the intensive care unit, the stomach's protective barrier seems to fail and "stress ulcers" are common.)

The typical stomach irritation associated with medications is **gastritis**. Whenever a child with SLE is complaining of abdominal pain, there is a desire to stop the medicines (note that this is not possible for steroids, which cannot be stopped abruptly; see Chapter 22) and see whether the pain goes away. However, if the pain sounds like typical stomach irritation (gastritis) and all the medicines are important, it is often better to treat the irritation with medicines to prevent acid secretion or coat the stomach (e.g., using a beta-2 acid blocker or sucralfate). If these steps do not work, talk to your doctor about stopping the medicine, if possible, and see whether the pain goes away. If it does, restart the medicine. If the pain promptly comes back, that's a strong indication that the medicine is the cause. You and your doctor will then have to see whether there is an alternative medication that may be used.

Chronic abdominal pain in a child with SLE that is not resolved by changing medications needs to be carefully investigated. Some children have sensitive stomachs, but more serious problems can also begin with these complaints. One of the key aspects of SLE is inflammation of the blood vessels. If the blood vessels lining the intestines are inflamed, it may cause vague nonspecific pain. In some children this results in damage to the intestinal tract. This may take the form of **pneumatosis cystoides intestinalis** (gas-filled cysts in the wall of the bowel) or small areas of bowel that are infarcted because they do not receive enough blood. Both of these problems are difficult to diagnose on routine examination and may start with only vague abdominal complaints. Fortunately, they are rare in children whose SLE is well controlled. However, they must be looked for in children whose complaints continue. An experienced physician will know how to evaluate your child for these conditions.

Another cause of chronic pain in children with SLE is **serositis**, inflammation of the lining of the lungs or abdomen (serosa). The function of this lining is to keep everything moist and to remove any foreign material. If SLE causes the serosa to be irritated (presumably because of immune complexes deposited on it), the serosa will respond by releasing inflammatory cells and inflammatory chemicals into the abdomen. In mild cases this causes diffuse pain. In severe cases the pain may be quite marked and associated with "rebound tenderness." If a child has rebound tenderness, he or she looks very unhappy when you push down on the abdomen and feels much worse if you quickly let go. Any child with this problem needs to be evaluated promptly by a physician, as it is an indication of serious irritation in the abdomen. There are many possible causes, including infections. If, after careful investigation, SLE is determined to be the cause, it may need to be treated with more corticosteroids.

Irritation of the pancreas is another cause of chronic abdominal pain in children with SLE. When the pancreas is irritated, it will leak digestive enzymes called amylase and lipase. Normally, these go into the intestine and help to digest food. When they leak into the abdomen they cause pain and discomfort, a condition called **pancreatitis**. The levels of amylase and lipase can be measured in the blood and will be elevated if the child has pancreatitis. Sometimes the pancreas is irritated by inflammation due to SLE. Other times it is irritated by medications (e.g., corticosteroids) used to treat SLE. Your doctor will have to be very careful in analyzing this; one condition requires more medicine, the other less.

Other organs in the GI tract that may be irritated are the liver and the gallbladder. Gallbladder disease is particularly common in children with hemolytic anemia. This is easily detected on abdominal ultrasound. Usually, it can be followed conservatively, but if the gallbladder is very involved or has a lot of stones, it may need to be removed. Children with liver involvement often have an enlarged liver that can be felt on careful examination and may be tender. Elevation of the liver enzymes on the blood tests will confirm this (see Chapter 24).

The spleen is another organ in the abdomen that may also be enlarged in children with SLE. It is not really part of the GI tract; it is part of the immune system. An enlarged spleen may cause pain on the left side of the abdomen. The key for children with SLE and abdominal pain from both a parents' and physician's point of view is to thoroughly investigate pain that is severe or does not respond to the initial changes in the medication regimen. In some children the initial tests will be normal, but repeat testing a few weeks later will show problems. Children with continuing abdominal pain without adequate explanation should be carefully examined by a physician experienced in the care of children with SLE. The physician may require blood tests, X rays, abdominal ultrasound, and either an MRI or a CAT scan of the abdomen to look for explanations.

CHILDREN WITH SLE AND JOINT PROBLEMS

Although the family may not be aware of it, arthritis is often present when a child with SLE first comes to the doctor. It is usually very responsive to treatment with steroids or NSAIDs. As a result, arthritis is rarely a significant long-term problem. The exception is an unusual condition termed **Jaccoud's arthropathy**: a painless swelling, primarily in the fingers and wrists, which develops slowly during the course of SLE. It does not usually cause damage to the bones, but it may be painful and interfere with use of the hands. The explanation for this problem is unclear. Unfortunately, it does not respond well to medication.

Other bone and joint problems may develop during the treatment of children with SLE. The most common, worrisome problem is avascular necrosis (crumbling) of bone. Although the mechanism by which this occurs is not fully understood, it appears to be the result of decreased blood flow to the ends of the bones. This can occur in children who do not have SLE. It can happen to children with SLE who are not being treated with steroids, and it can happen to people being treated with steroids who do not have SLE. However, it is most common in children with SLE who are being treated with corticosteroids. The problem often begins with vague complaints of pain in the involved bone without any findings on examination.

Early in the development of avascular necrosis, the X rays will be normal. Sometimes avascular necrosis is suspected on bone scans because there is decreased uptake of the Tc99 by the involved bone (see Chapter 24). MRI is the most sensitive test for this condition. It will detect this condition very early. Sometimes children with a suggestion of avascular necrosis on MRI go on to recover. We do not know whether this means that the MRI was a false reading or whether early avascular necrosis is able to be reversed. However, if a child has definite avascular necrosis on MRI, it does not go away.

Unfortunately, the normal course of avascular necrosis is for the bone to crumble slowly under the continued stress of bearing weight. If this happens, it will be necessary for the joint to be replaced (see Chapter 25). In children with SLE, the hip is the joint most commonly affected, but shoulders, elbows, knees, ankles, and other joints all may be involved. The identical problem may occur in children with juvenile arthritis or JRA who have been treated with corticosteroids. There is no safe dose of corticosteroids with regard to this problem. Avascular necrosis has occurred in children who never got any corticosteroids. However, the more corticosteroids the child takes and the longer he or she takes them, the greater the risk. Children taking any significant amount of corticosteroids for more six months have a steadily increasing risk of developing avascular necrosis. In addition, a child who has had avascular necrosis in one joint is at greater risk of developing it in another joint. Reducing the risk of avascular necrosis is one of the reasons physicians try so hard to minimize the dose of corticosteroids for children with SLE.

LABORATORY TESTING AND TYPICAL PATTERNS OF DISEASE IN CHILDREN WITH SLE

Whenever physicians take care of large numbers of children with SLE, they are struck by the great variability of this illness. Approximately one-third of children have mild disease that never really causes major problems; many children have moderate disease that may be severe at times, but responds well to treatment. Many fewer children have obvious severe SLE right from the start. However, doctors in different locations describe seeing different percentages of children with severe disease. Different patterns of abnormalities may help to distinguish children with severe disease from the others.

Virtually all of the children with SLE are ANA-positive. However, many children test positive for ANA, but do not have SLE (see Chapter 24). Since ANA is clearly not the whole answer, physicians started to examine ANA more carefully to see whether different types of ANA were more strongly associated with SLE and with differing severity of SLE. Physicians soon recognized that there were different patterns of ANA (again, Chapter 24 discusses this in greater detail). Although a child with any ANA pattern could have problems, children with a "rim pattern" (seen under the microscope) were much more likely to be very sick.

Further study led to the recognition that children with rim-pattern ANA often have anti-DNA antibodies. Antibodies to DNA tend to be associated with more severe SLE and are infrequently found in children who do not have SLE. At one time they were thought to correlate with a greater frequency of renal disease, but this is now in doubt. With greater understanding and better testing we now know that antibodies to double-stranded (ds) DNA are the important ones. Antibodies to single-stranded or crude DNA extracts can be found in many different conditions and are not very meaningful. However, a child may be very sick with SLE and not have antibodies to dsDNA.

Further evaluation of patients with SLE led to the discovery of extractable nuclear antigens (ENA). These are Ro, La, Sm, and RNP (see Chapter 24). A lot of time and effort have gone into determining the importance of antibodies to these antigens. They do seem to be associated with different patterns of disease, but again there is not enough certainty to make definitive predictions. The clearest associations are with Ro and Sm. Often Ro antibodies are found in children with more rash, more than average complaints of arthritis, and relatively less kidney disease. A high titer of Ro and low or absent Sm have been described as typical of mixed connective tissue disease (MCTD; see Chapter 12). Over the years a variety of studies have suggested that adults with SLE who are Ro-positive have milder disease, but it is a generalization that does not always hold true. Ro antibodies are also associated with neonatal SLE and congenital heart block, discussed at the end of this chapter.

The other antibody that seems to be important is Sm. This antibody is not found in everyone with SLE. If it is present, it is associated with a greater frequency of severe disease. However, just as the association of Ro with mild disease is only approximate, so is the association of Sm with severe disease. Indeed, some children have antibodies to both Ro and Sm. The long and the short of this for a parent is simple. Do not get too concerned about which antibodies your child does or does not have. Make sure you have a good doctor and that the doctor is taking good care of your child's problems. Children with worrisome antibodies may do well, and children with protective antibodies may get in big trouble.

The key laboratory findings in evaluating a child with SLE are generally similar to those of children with other chronic illnesses. If a child is doing well, he or she should have a good hemoglobin level, a normal erythrocyte sedimentation rate (ESR), and a normal urine analysis. If all of these results are good, it is highly probable the child is doing well (though neurologic problems may still occur). The additional laboratory tests that are useful in evaluating a child with SLE are the serum complement levels C3 and C4.

ANA levels and anti-DNA levels rise and fall in children with SLE without a reliable association with disease activity. Sometimes it helps to think of the 10 percent analogy. If the ANA goes up, that's a 10 percent risk. If the ESR goes up, that's a 10 percent risk. If the hemoglobin falls, that's a 10 percent risk. If the anti-DNA goes up, that's a 10 percent risk, and so on. Any one test changing does not mean too much, but if they all start going the wrong way, be sure to pay attention.

The complement system plays an important role in attacking infectious agents. In the course of doing their job, the different components of the complement system are used up. Although the body is constantly making more, a drop in the level of the complement components in the blood suggests very active usage. This is true in children with SLE, as well. We know that much of the damage in SLE is brought about by the activation of complement following the deposition of immune complexes in the tissues. As a general rule, lower complement levels in the blood suggest a greater amount of ongoing damage. This is an imperfect system because doctors recognize that the levels in the blood are determined as much by how fast more is being made as by how fast it is being used up. There are very sophisticated tests to measure what are called complement breakdown products, but these tests are not routinely done.

All the laboratory findings in children with SLE are individual pieces of the puzzle. C3 and C4 are easily measured and the results are well standardized. In caring for a child with SLE, if the doctor looks carefully at all of his results and at the child, he or she will have a good idea of what is going on. Some children have chronically low C3 levels but do very well. Other children have normal C3 levels but develop more problems. While physicians would be unwise to disregard C3 levels, they are not the whole answer.

Another way to think about the evaluation of laboratory parameters in children with SLE is to understand that there are two types of tests. The routine tests that evaluate your hemoglobin, your kidney function, your liver function, and so on tell the doctor what is happening to those organs right now. Tests such as the ANA titer, the anti-DNA level, and the C3 and C4 levels, are more useful as predictors of the future. Nothing is a perfect predictor.

> Imagine if you are driving down the highway late at night. There is very little traffic and perhaps you are exceeding the speed limit. At the side of the road you see a large sign that says, "Warning construction ahead." There might be a big construction project, where workers might be there late at night, and you might have to suddenly come to a stop. On the other hand, workers might be there only during the day, and there may be no problem or only a need to change lanes. There's no way to be sure. However, a wise person would let up on the gas pedal, look around carefully, and be sure to keep his or her attention focused on the road until he or she was sure what was happening. That's how both parents and doctors should respond to changes in these predictive laboratory values. There might not be trouble, but everyone should be paying careful attention.

DRUG-INDUCED SLE

Drug-induced SLE refers to the development of a positive ANA and SLE-like symptoms in association with certain drugs. Among the drugs that can do this are commonly used drugs such as tetracyclines, including doxycycline, used in the treatment of teenagers with acne. However, this can also occur with many of the drugs used to treat children with seizures and some of the antibiotics, including isoniazid, which is used to treat tuberculosis. A wide variety of drugs have been suspected of causing drug-induced SLE in the past. For some drugs, the association with drug-induced SLE is well known, but for many others it is only suspected. The fact that a drug has been associated with drug-induced SLE does not mean that it should not be used. This is a rare complication. However, when evaluating a child with the new onset of SLE-like symptoms, these drugs should always be considered as a possible cause.

Children with drug-induced SLE can be significantly ill with fever, rash, and inflammation around the lungs or in the abdomen. However, a key to the diagnosis of drug-induced SLE is that it all goes away quickly if the drug is discontinued. If symptoms of SLE begin after a child has started on a drug but do not go away when the drug is stopped, it is not drug-induced SLE, even if it is a drug that is known to cause drug-induced SLE. This bothers me a little, too, but that's the official position of the American College of Rheumatology.

I am often asked whether a child who has SLE can use a drug that is known to cause drug-induced SLE. There was a lot of concern about this at one time. Some of the most important drugs for treating hypertension (a common SLE complication) in the past were also known to cause drug-induced SLE. Nevertheless, physicians often found it necessary to use them. There is no evidence they caused additional problems. Using drugs known to be associated with drug-induced SLE in a child with SLE does not seem to cause trouble. But everyone should pay attention to the possibility of side effects arising over time.

OTHER COMPLICATIONS OF SLE

Complications of SLE in childhood may be complications of the disease, of the therapy, or both. It is very important to understand that half of the children diagnosed with SLE in the 1950s (before the routine use of corticosteroids) were dead within two years. Although in part this was because only severe cases were properly diagnosed, it remains true that untreated SLE may be a rapidly fatal disease. Everyone must be concerned about possible side effects of treatment. However, it is obviously foolish to die from the disease because you were afraid you might get a side effect of the medications.

Severe complications of SLE, such as pulmonary hemorrhage, renal failure, and strokes, have all become less frequent with proper therapy. Infections remain a major concern for children with SLE, and children with SLE are subject to all the usual infections of childhood. In addition, children with active SLE often have poorly functioning white blood cells and reduced levels of complement. Since these are key elements in the defense against infection, children with active SLE are much more vulnerable to infection than normal children.

Another problem that leads to an increased frequency of infections is that children with active SLE often have a spleen that is not functioning well. Removing bacteria and other infectious agents from the blood is a major function of the spleen. Children who do not have a spleen (because of surgical removal due to injury, etc.) are well known to have more frequent **pneumococcal infections**. Systemic pneumococcal infections and pneumococcal pneumonia also occur more often in children with SLE. **Meningococcal meningitis** is another infection that occurs more often than expected in children with SLE.

Normally, the spleen, white blood cells, and complement play an important role in preventing infections. One important key to recognizing that the spleen is not functioning well in a child with SLE is the presence of Howell Jolly bodies on the complete blood count. These bodies are leftover nuclear material in red blood cells. A normally functioning spleen removes this material, and normal children do not have Howell Jolly bodies. If they are reported as being seen on the CBC smear, it means the spleen is not doing its job. Any patient with Howell Jolly bodies is at increased risk for infection. (Note: If someone has had his spleen removed, he will always have Howell Jolly bodies and will always be at increased risk of infection, but the physician should know this.) Finding Howell Jolly bodies is very important in someone whose spleen has not been removed. In these children it is a warning that they are at greater risk of infection than the doctor might have initially suspected. If a child with SLE is brought to my office or the emergency room with a significant fever and he or she has Howell Jolly bodies, I will most often admit that child to the hospital for observation even if he or she doesn't look very sick.

Parents are the most important line of defense against severe infection in children with SLE. You cannot lock your children in the closet to prevent them from ever being exposed to infections. You have to let them lead normal lives. However, do not let your child with SLE visit someone you know is sick. More important, if your child with SLE looks sick to you, insist that the doctor see him. A normal child who looks sick in the evening might safely wait until morning. In children with active SLE, the normal defenses are not working. If they look sick, it may not be safe to wait until morning.

When considering the possibility of infection, parents and physicians must remember that both active disease and the medications used to treat SLE decrease the child's ability to fight infection. Any child on a significant dose of corticosteroids or any amount of immunosuppressive drugs such as methotrexate, cyclophosphamide, or azathioprine, is at increased risk of infection. If the child looks sick, have her checked carefully. Too many trips to the doctor's office or emergency department may provoke complaints from the doctors and may be inconvenient, but that's far easier to live with than knowing you didn't act when you should have. Children with SLE can rapidly develop overwhelming infections requiring urgent care.

In some cases a child with SLE will be brought to the hospital looking extremely ill. It may not be clear to the physicians whether the problem is an infection or a flare-up of the SLE. Physicians who do not have a lot of experience with SLE will be very confused. For an infection they will want to use an antibiotic, but for a flare-up of the SLE they will want to use more corticosteroids. Often they are afraid more corticosteroids might make the infection worse. *The correct answer is to give both antibiotics and corticosteroids in this situation*. Often the infection makes the SLE flare up and this interferes with the ability of the white cells to fight infection. Other times the child came down with an infection because the SLE was flaring and again the white cells weren't able to fight infection. In either situation, using both corticosteroids and antibiotics is the best solution.

COMPLICATIONS OF TREATMENT

Corticosteroids have been a key element in the treatment of SLE since their discovery in the 1950s. They are effective in treating and preventing many of the complications of untreated SLE. However, they increase the incidence of infection, weaken bones, cause stretch marks, promote diabetes, and hasten arteriosclerosis and heart disease (see Chapter 22 for more detail). For the approximately one-third of children with mild disease, it should be possible to keep the dosage of corticosteroids at an acceptable level, and the likelihood of significant toxicity should be minimal.

Unfortunately, the remaining two-thirds of children with SLE may face a recurrent need to raise the corticosteroid dosage to a more significant level. This brings with it an increased risk of corticosteroid-related toxicity. Surprisingly, this is a greater problem for children with moderate disease than for the children with severe disease. In experienced centers children with severe disease are rapidly recognized and advanced to more aggressive immunosuppressive therapy. This normally allows a dramatic reduction in the dosage of corticosteroids. As a result, corticosteroid-related complications are often less frequent in this group. After recognizing this, many physicians have begun to advocate advancing children with more difficult moderate SLE to immunosuppressive therapy early in their disease course in order to minimize corticosteroid-related toxicity (see the next section below).

TREATMENT OF SLE

The key to proper treatment of SLE involves balancing the risks of the disease against the risks of the treatment. SLE is extremely diverse and many children have only mild disease that is easily treated with limited doses of corticosteroids. Other children have severe life-threatening SLE that requires aggressive therapy. There are no absolute guidelines for recognizing when a child needs to be treated with immunosuppressive drugs. However, it is clear that prolonged treatment with even moderate doses of corticosteroids will lead to significant side effects. Immunosuppressive drugs often seem like "scary stuff" to parents and physicians who do not work with them all the time. Although the immunosuppressive drugs may be associated with serious side effects, those side effects are very rare when experienced physicians give the drugs.

Many parents worry that their child will get all the side effects of immunosuppressive drugs. Virtually every child who takes a significant amount of corticosteroids does get corticosteroid-related side effects. In contrast, serious side effects of immunosuppressive drugs are rare. I've seen far more children do poorly and suffer permanent damage (even death) because their families were afraid to treat their SLE aggressively than I have seen children with serious side effects of immunosuppressive drugs. That does not mean that every child should be on immunosuppressive drugs.

For children with rash, malaise, and arthritis, but no evidence of significant renal or other internal organ involvement, initial therapy should be with a low dose of corticosteroids. Often this is combined with an NSAID to provide some additional symptomatic relief. Over the longer term the antimalarial drug hydroxychloroquine (see Chapter 22) has been shown to be very beneficial for this group. At the time of diagnosis, some physicians follow a cookbook approach of 1 or 2 mg/kg/day of corticosteroids (prednisone or its equivalent), but this is often excessive for these children. The physician should monitor that the children feel better and their laboratory abnormalities improve over a period of four to six weeks. As soon as it is clear that this has happened, the physician should try to begin slowly reducing the corticosteroids.

Some physicians like to use a very high dose of corticosteroids at the beginning and then dramatically drop the dosage when things look better. This is like putting the immune system on a roller coaster ride. In a sick child a high dose of corticosteroids may be necessary, but then a slow gradual progressive reduction in the dosage is much better. Even when physicians go very slowly, it is impossible to predict how much the corticosteroid dosage can be decreased before there is new evidence of disease activity (e.g., increased ESR, decreased hemoglobin [Hb], or decreased C3 or C4; see Chapter 24). If it is possible to reduce the corticosteroids (prednisone or its equivalent) to 0.2 mg/kg/day or less without recurrent disease, the child should be carefully followed on a low dose of corticosteroids.

Many parents are anxious to have their child discontinue steroids, but completely stopping corticosteroids is rarely advisable for children with SLE. Many years ago a very experienced rheumatologist described that last little bit of corticosteroids as "cheap insurance." Every physician who takes care of many patients with SLE has seen someone who was doing wonderfully on just five milligrams of prednisone daily and who suddenly got very sick when they tried to discontinue it. It is not impossible to discontinue corticosteroids, but if you are doing well on a small dose, it is probably unwise to try to stop completely. Even when there has been no evidence of disease for more than six months, I do not think stopping completely is the best idea.

The children who do not have internal organ involvement but develop more symptoms when the dose of corticosteroids is reduced are a difficult problem. Hydroxychloroquine often helps to bring the disease under adequate control. Some physicians have tried using low-dose methotrexate in this group, but the results are highly variable. Without evidence of internal organ involvement physicians are hesitant to recommend more aggressive therapy, but that may leave a child on too much corticosteroids for too long. In my own experience, children in this group who do not tolerate appropriate reduction of their corticosteroids usually progress to have evidence of internal organ involvement over time. It is important for physicians to monitor them carefully. Frequently, the first signs of internal organ involvement are changes in the urine analysis. Often these changes are minimal at first and might be dismissed. However, over time, it becomes clear that there is significant renal or other internal organ involvement.

Children who have internal organ involvement need to be treated aggressively. Although doctors tend to agree about the importance of treating renal involvement, there is less uniform agreement about when to treat other organ involvement aggressively. For children with internal organ involvement, it is often not possible to reduce their corticosteroids to an acceptable level (again, I consider this to be 0.2 mg/kg/day of prednisone or its equivalent). A variety of "steroid sparing" regimens have been recommended. Mycophenolate mofetil is one of the most commonly recommended immunosuppressive medications at present (see Chapter 24). It is helpful for some children. Other physicians may recommend low-dose methotrexate or azathioprine. Each of these alternative regimens has its advocates. None of them is always effective.

Children with moderate internal organ involvement represent one of the greatest challenges for physicians who specialize in the care of children with SLE. They often do not appear sick enough to warrant significant immunosuppressive therapy, but over the years they receive too much corticosteroids for too long. In the end these children often have significant corticosteroid side effects, continued smoldering disease, and a generally unsatisfactory outcome.

It is hard for parents to accept a recommendation for aggressive treatment for children with continued moderate internal organ involvement, because the disease is not that bad. Even many physicians do not believe that these children should be treated aggressively. However, when you watch what happens to these children over a five- to ten-year period, it is very discouraging. Ten years later, if they have not been treated aggressively, these children often have both significant corticosteroid side effects and significant damage from the disease, with no end in sight.

The reasons cited by many physicians to not use cyclophosphamide include the risk of infection, the risk of sterility, and the risk of cancer later in life. However, chronic use of corticosteroids and azathioprine or methotrexate also carries significant risk of infection, sterility, and cancer later in life. Many physicians assume these risks are greater for the children receiving cyclophosphamide, but there is no clear data to support this (I've reviewed it very carefully). The physicians who are opposed to cyclophosphamide refer to data from children treated for cancer. Those children often received multiple drugs and irradiation. The radiation greatly increases the risk of cancer and sterility. We do not give radiation to children with SLE.

The most compelling reason to use cyclophosphamide for children with moderately severe SLE comes from our experience in using it for the children with severe disease. Five or six years after receiving cyclophosphamide, most of the children with severe SLE are taking less than 0.2 mg/kg/day (prednisone or its equivalent) of corticosteroids and have no signs of steroid side effects. They have discontinued cyclophosphamide and all the other drugs except for the low dose of prednisone. They feel well and often tell me, "I do not remember I have SLE except when I have to come see you." In contrast, the children whom we did not put on cyclophosphamide because their disease was not that bad are still taking too much prednisone, have multiple prednisone side effects including weight gain and bone damage, and still have active disease. The children who had more severe disease at the beginning and were treated aggressively are doing far better both mentally and physically.

A physician who tells you that cyclophosphamide might have fatal side effects and prednisone does not has never seen a child stop all his or her medications because he or she refused to go on "looking so ugly." Some children admit they are not taking the prednisone; others just stop taking it and may suddenly die. It is very important for the physicians and parents who deal with these children on a day-to-day basis to be very aware of the emotional toll of acne, obesity, and stretch marks related to chronic corticosteroid therapy. In addition, corticosteroids may have significant negative effects on bone structure and heart function. Recently, one of my patients, a young adult who had been treated at another institution with many years of azathioprine and steroids, looked like he was doing fine. For twelve years his steroids went up and down, but they were never at a really high dose (maximum 40 mg/day of prednisone). He had mild renal disease but always did acceptably with azathioprine and was never treated aggressively. However, he had a massive heart attack at the age of twenty-eight and needed coronary artery surgery. Prolonged use of corticosteroids was his only known risk factor for heart disease.

There is no perfect answer for children with SLE at the present time. Years of experience and seeing what happens to children over time have made me very aggressive in trying to prevent the side effects of long-term corticosteroid usage. Some physicians are hesitant to use cyclophosphamide for involvement of the central nervous system, lung involvement, or milder kidney involvement. However, in my personal experience, children who have disease in any internal organ system that is not well controlled by an acceptable dose of corticosteroids do best if aggressively treated. Not every physician agrees. The parents must always make the final decision. My goal is to make sure that you have enough information to clearly understand the risks and benefits of the alternatives. Cyclophosphamide does not fix every child every time. It does have potential side effects, but these are rare when it is administered by experienced physicians. Corticosteroids and azathioprine sound safer in the short term. I do not believe the results are as good in the long term.

For children with severe internal organ involvement, especially kidney involvement, the majority of physicians now agree that cyclophosphamide is the best answer. In carefully controlled studies it has been clearly demonstrated that cyclophosphamide prevents continued scarring of the kidney, while prednisone does not. No one has studied azathioprine in this regard. The academic answer is, "We know cyclophosphamide works. Why should we subject patients to a different therapy that might not work?" The systematic use of monthly intravenous cyclophosphamide for seven doses, followed by cyclophosphamide every three months for an additional two to two and a half years has been shown to produce the best long-term outcome for SLE patients with renal disease (adults and children). It does not work for every patient. For the relatively few who fail, there is no uniformly accepted therapy. If you are one of the few unfortunate families in this group, you should find the most experienced center you can. Each has its own regimen for such children. We treat many such children at the Hospital for Special Surgery in New York City.

ADJUNCTIVE THERAPIES FOR CHILDREN WITH SLE

NSAIDs are often helpful in controlling the minor aches and pains associated with SLE. Children with SLE usually tolerate these drugs without difficulty. Just like children with other forms of arthritis who are on these medications, the children with SLE should have their liver function and kidney function monitored. SLE may make the children more vulnerable to the effects of NSAIDs on liver or kidney function. There are also reports of NSAIDs causing unusual reactions such as aseptic meningitis in SLE patients. Your physician should consider all of these issues when prescribing these medications. If something unusual happens when a child with SLE starts an NSAID (or any other new drug), it should be stopped and the physician notified. While these reports are a cause for concern, most children with SLE take NSAIDs without significant problems.

Bolus solumedrol refers to the use of very large doses of corticosteroids to control severe manifestations of SLE. In general this is considered to be 30 mg/kg up to a maximum of 1 gram of methylprednisolone. This large dose can be very effective in controlling sudden severe flares of SLE. Some physicians are tempted to use this therapy over and over again. In certain situations such as severe renal disease, it is often advisable to combine cyclophosphamide with bolus solumedrol each month until the disease comes under better control. However, bolus solumedrol is not without side effects. I've seen children develop serious infections, serious irritation of the pancreas, and avascular necrosis of bone after these treatments. It is best to treat bolus solumedrol as a "fire extinguisher next to the stove." It's very handy to have in case of emergency, but if you find yourself using it over and over again, you'd better change the way you cook.

Mycophenolate mofetil and azathioprine are immunosuppressive drugs that work in a similar fashion. There is much more experience with azathioprine, but mycophenolate mofetil is believed to have similar effects and perhaps fewer side effects. These drugs do increase your risk of infection. In addition, there is good data that azathioprine increases the risk of cancer and causes sterility in some children. Mycophenolate will probably be found to have the same effects once it has been around long enough. It blocks the same pathways azathioprine does, just at a different point. Nonetheless, these drugs may be useful for children who cannot receive cyclophosphamide. I also use them in children who have received cyclophosphamide but who have some continuing or new disease activity that I do not want to treat with too much corticosteroid.

Methotrexate has been very useful in the treatment of arthritis. It is generally used in a low dosage (less than 25 mg/week). Low doses of oral methotrexate have also been used as a steroid-sparing agent in children with SLE. In general, the response has not been dramatic. Physicians using methotrexate must be sure that the children are taking folic acid. Children with SLE who have chronic anemia may be deficient in folic acid. Higher doses of methotrexate given intravenously as part of multiple drug regimens for cancer have many more side effects. However, for children with severe SLE who did not improve with cyclophosphamide alone, we have had success using high-dose intravenous methotrexate in combination with cyclophosphamide.

Cyclosporine is a strong immunosuppressive drug that often interferes with kidney function (Chapter 22). It is known to cause kidney problems, and this has kept most physicians from using it for the treatment of SLE. However, there are occasional reports of its successful use. It seems especially useful in children with membranous glomerulonephritis (class V kidney disease) and excessive loss of protein in the urine. Cyclosporine should be given only by physicians experienced in its use. Like all immunosuppressive drugs, it is associated with an increased risk of infection and an increased risk of cancer.

New biologic agents and other experimental therapies are being tested in SLE. Some centers are also testing the use of autologus bone marrow transplants or very high doses of cyclophosphamide that completely suppress the immune system. These therapies need to be tested to see whether they are useful for children with severe SLE. However, at present, their use is restricted to specialized centers and they are being used only for children who have failed normal therapy. Fortunately, such children are rare. We are very lucky at the Hospital for Special Surgery to have access to the combined resources and experience of our own staff, Sanford Weill Medical College of Cornell University, Memorial Sloan Kettering Cancer Center, and the Rockefeller University. With this combined expertise we have been successful in treating some of the most difficult cases.

PROGNOSIS

If you have just finished reading above about how the most difficult cases are treated, you are probably very worried about the long-term outcome for your child. The key is that with early and aggressive treatment the vast majority of children do just fine. There are children who die from SLE. However, the survival rate is above 90 percent at five years in every experienced center. In many centers the survival rate is much higher. *Obviously, five-year survival for a fourteen-, fifteen-, or sixteen-year-old child certainly is not good enough.* The main reason for advocating early aggressive therapy is that we want to accomplish excellent forty-, fifty-, and sixty-year survival. Proof? Not yet. Someone will have to follow these children for fifty years into the future to "prove" that we've done the right thing. But we cannot keep doing what we know does not work while we wait forty or fifty years to get proof of the right long-term answers. I will be very disappointed if we don't have completely different answers about how to best treat children with SLE long before fifty years from now. With current state-of-the-art therapy, the majority of children will do very well. *Children with severe disease should be referred to the most advanced centers where they have the greatest likelihood of a good outcome.*

ANTI-RO ANTIBODIES AND NEONATAL SLE

It was a surprising finding when it was recognized that babies born with a problem called neonatal heart block or complete congenital heart block often had mothers with SLE. This does not happen to most mothers with SLE, but it may happen if the mother tests positive for antibody to Ro. Most children with congenital heart block have healthy mothers who report no medical problems. But when doctors began testing them, it was found that almost all of the normal, healthy mothers who gave birth to children with congenital heart block tested positive for antibodies to Ro. A few of these mothers had unrecognized SLE when examined carefully, and some of these mothers have gone on to develop SLE years later, but so far not most. There is a registry collecting information on all these mothers and their children (see Appendix for resources).

At first doctors were very worried that women who had SLE and were Ro-positive would be at high risk of having children with congenital heart block. This seems not to be the case. Most Ro-positive mothers have normal children. Even Ro-positive mothers who have had one child with heart block most often have normal children the next time. If a woman who is known to be Ro-positive becomes pregnant, she should be monitored carefully.

Evidence of congenital heart block can be detected before birth, and experienced doctors should be standing by to take care of the children when they are born. Most often congenital heart block is not life-threatening and can be treated with a pacemaker when the child is old enough to need it. Rarely, children with heart block are extremely sick and may not survive. The problem is sufficiently uncommon that we encourage women with SLE and antibodies to Ro to go ahead and have children when they are ready. But we want them to be carefully monitored during pregnancy.

Other complications that may occur in children of mothers with SLE include low levels of platelets, white cells, or red cells. These are thought to be the result of antibodies that have been passed from the mother to the child. These antibodies are usually cleared out of the child's system in a few days, and the problems are rarely severe. Other children of mothers with SLE may develop a rash when they are first exposed to the light or develop mild inflammation of the liver. These are all well-recognized problems that normally resolve after a few days to a few weeks. Serious complications in the children of mothers with SLE are infrequent.

SHOULD A WOMAN WITH SLE HAVE CHILDREN?

We know that SLE occurs more frequently in people of different races. It also occurs more frequently among relatives of people with SLE. This is evidence that genetics plays a role in the development of SLE. However, the risk of a mother passing SLE on to her child is very small. Precise numbers are uncertain, but one in fifty is the best estimate. Thus, the child of a mother with SLE is more likely to get the disease than a random child, but not enough so to discourage mothers with SLE from having children. If you are a mother with SLE considering whether or not to have children, the major concern is your health, not the risk of the child having SLE.

12

Mixed Connective Tissue Disease (MCTD)

Children with mixed connective tissue disease (MCTD) are antinuclear antibody (ANA)-positive. At one time this disease was thought to be a milder version of SLE. To understand this disease, it is necessary to understand that it was defined "backwards." A physician named Gordon Sharp noted an unusual laboratory finding in some patients who were antinuclear antibody (ANA)-positive. When he went back and looked at the patients who had this finding, they were most often "atypical" SLE patients. These patients differed from typical SLE patients in having more arthritis, more rash, more lung disease, and less kidney disease. Since many of these patients were also positive for rheumatoid factor (see Chapter 24) and had more arthritis than typical SLE patients, they were thought of as having "mixed" disease. Thus, the name was chosen to reflect this. It took only a short time once the disease was described in adults to realize that there were children with the same pattern of findings.

The precise relationship of MCTD to SLE and the other rheumatic diseases remains unclear. There are only three diseases that commonly cause nail fold capillary abnormalities (see Fig. 21 in Chapter 14, p. 199). These are dermatomyositis (a disease with muscle inflammation; see Chapter 16), scleroderma (a disease with hardening of the skin and poor lung function; see Chapter 15), and MCTD. Indeed, it is now well known that some children with MCTD will go on to develop scleroderma, but most do not. Obviously, these diseases are somehow interrelated, but there is no clear explanation yet. At some future time we may understand how MCTD, SLE, dermatomyositis, and scleroderma are all related to each other. Although MCTD was originally described as a subtype of SLE, it is probably more closely related to scleroderma and dermatomyositis. Children with MCTD often have mild muscle inflammation and may develop poor lung function.

Children with MCTD typically are brought to doctors because of cold, blue hands (Raynaud's), joint pains, and a positive ANA. Children with MCTD often have elevated muscle enzymes and rashes over the outer surfaces of their knees and elbows (just like those seen in dermatomyositis), but they rarely are significantly weak. Often they have a mild to moderate amount of arthritis, but they may not have been complaining about it. Children with MCTD usually do not have serious kidney involvement, but they may have some and it may become serious.

DIFFERENTIAL DIAGNOSIS AND LABORATORY FINDINGS

For most diseases, these are two separate headings. However, the clinical manifestations of MCTD overlap with dermatomyositis, SLE, JRA, and early scleroderma. In addition, over time, children initially thought to have MCTD may evolve into a clear case of one or the other disease. As a result, physicians must rely more heavily on the laboratory findings to confirm this diagnosis. The source of much of the confusion in diagnosing MCTD results from the unclear nature of the disease itself. Indeed, it is quite possible that we will ultimately realize that at least two different diseases have been grouped together as MCTD.

A high-titer speckled-pattern ANA is characteristic of MCTD. When the ANA subtypes are checked (see Chapter 24), children with MCTD are usually Ro-positive, RNP-positive, and Sm-negative (some have low-titer Sm). Because these children are often RF-positive, they may be referred for JRA. Another finding is that these children may have very marked elevation of their quantitative immunoglobulins, especially IgG (again, see Chapter 24).

Most children with MCTD were once considered atypical cases of SLE. Children with MCTD are often mistakenly diagnosed with SLE because of the strongly positive ANA. Findings that help in making the distinction between SLE and MCTD include the speckled pattern of the ANA, a positive test for rheumatoid factor, and usually normal serum complement levels. Antibodies to double-stranded DNA (dsDNA) are sometimes found in children with MCTD.

As noted above, children with MCTD often have many findings that are also seen in dermatomyositis and in scleroderma. In more severe cases, children with MCTD often have Gottren's papules and nail fold capillary abnormalities. They may initially have been labeled with one of these diagnoses. Although children with MCTD have the elevated muscle enzymes and rash, they do not tend to evolve into dermatomyositis. However, MCTD may develop into scleroderma over a period of years. The presence of antibodies to Scl-70, or anticentromere antibodies, strongly suggests the diagnosis of scleroderma. These antibodies may not be present initially but may appear years later.

COMPLICATIONS

The complications of MCTD are highly dependent on the evolution of the disease. The arthritis, rash, malaise, and Raynaud's phenomenon are usually easily treated with NSAIDs, low-dose prednisone, a calcium-channel blocker for the Raynaud's, and hydroxychloroquine. Inadequately treated children may have recurrent problems with Raynaud's and may have distal fingertip ulcers and even infarct parts of digits in the cold. (A digit is infarcted if the blood supply is cut off.) Physicians must emphasize to families the importance of treating the Raynaud's and seeking care if a digit does not warm up appropriately with return to a warm environment. The elevated muscle enzymes and the markedly elevated IgG level will usually respond to a moderate or low dose of prednisone.

Children with fever and distress should be presumed to have poor spleen function and should be hospitalized and put on intravenous antibiotics until it is assured that they do not have an infection. If the laboratory reports Howell Jolly bodies on the peripheral smear, this is evidence that the spleen is not functioning properly and there is an increased risk of infection. Some children with MCTD have poor blood circulation in their hands and feet. If the circulation to a finger or toe has stopped and it is numb and discolored, this is also a reason for immediate hospitalization. In most cases a numb and discolored finger or toe (impending digital infarction) responds to intravenous bolus solumedrol. A variety of regimens may be considered if this is not effective in restoring circulation.

Some children with MCTD will develop obvious scleroderma over time. They should be treated appropriately for that diagnosis. Other children do not develop the typical skin changes of scleroderma but may develop shortness of breath and pulmonary function abnormalities. Pulmonary fibrosis may occur, and I have seen children who developed a pneumothorax as a result. In other children, pulmonary fibrosis may result in pulmonary hypertension with resultant cardiac problems and an increased risk of infection.

Sudden overwhelming infection remains the most commonly reported cause of death for children with MCTD. This may be related to a high frequency of problems with the spleen (functional asplenia), as discussed for children with SLE. Parents of children with MCTD should be prompt in seeking medical care at the first suspicion of a serious infection.

MEDICAL TREATMENT

The standard treatment for MCTD is a low dose of corticosteroids combined with hydroxychloroquine and a nonsteroidal anti-inflammatory (NSAID) for relief of the arthritis. The corticosteroid dosage should be adjusted as necessary to correct the elevated IgG level, the erythrocyte sedimentation rate, anemia, and clinical symptoms. Significant Raynaud's syndrome should be treated with an appropriate calcium-channel blocker. Although stronger agents are available if these do not provide relief, most children with MCTD will do well on this combination.

For some children with MCTD, it is not possible to reduce the corticosteroid dosage to a satisfactory level. Methotrexate seems to be an effective steroid-sparing agent for these children. Most often it is necessary to treat them with higher doses of methotrexate, as are used in dermatomyositis and scleroderma (i.e., up to 1 mg/kg/week, 50 mg maximum). The key to successful treatment of MCTD is early recognition of the children who are at high risk for progressive disease. This group must be treated vigorously with the goal of bringing the disease under control. Children treated aggressively generally do well.

Stronger immunosuppressive agents are rarely necessary for the treatment of children with MCTD, unless the condition is evolving toward scleroderma. For children who do not respond to or tolerate methotrexate, azathioprine or mycophenolate mofetil may be considered. In the small subset of children who develop nephrotic syndrome, treatment with intravenous cyclophosphamide may be necessary and is often helpful. Children who progress to scleroderma are difficult to treat and should be treated as appropriate for scleroderma (see Chapter 15).

PROGNOSIS

The long-term prognosis for children with MCTD depends on the evolution of the disease. Most children do well with the treatment I have described. Many children seem slowly to resolve their disease over time and are able to discontinue all medications. Most of my initial teenage patients are now young adults. Ten years after diagnosis, they are doing well on no medication and without significant problems. However, children who develop significant lung involvement or other evidence of progression toward scleroderma are much more worrisome. These children need to be treated aggressively, but even so the prognosis is guarded, as it is for all children with scleroderma.

13

Sjogren's Syndrome

Children with Dry Eyes and Dry Mouth

The combination of dry eyes and dry mouth may be the result of inflammation of the glands that produce tears and saliva (lacrimal glands produce tears; parotid and submandibular glands produce saliva). The parotid glands are the large glands at the side of the face, just over the corner of the jaw. Normally, you do not notice the parotid glands. They lie flat against the face. However, if they are swollen they stick out on both sides of the face, just above the jaw line.

Children with Sjogren's syndrome are often sent to the rheumatologist by a dentist who has noted that they have unusually severe cavities or by an ophthalmologist who has noted that their complaints of eye discomfort are due to chronically dry eyes and poor tear production. Most of these children are antinuclear antibody (ANA)-positive. The majority of children with Sjogren's syndrome test positive for antibodies to Ro (see below). Other children with Sjogren's syndrome are sent to the rheumatologist because of Raynaud's syndrome and a positive ANA or rheumatoid factor.

When they are evaluated, some of the children with Sjogren's syndrome clearly have SLE; these children are said to have secondary Sjogren's syndrome. Sjogren's syndrome is also a known complication of rheumatoid arthritis in adults, but it rarely occurs in children with juvenile arthritis. I have seen children with sarcoidosis who had Sjogren's syndrome and arthritis. Children who have dry eyes and dry mouth but lack other findings suggestive of connective tissue disease have primary Sjogren's syndrome. However, over time some children with what was thought to be primary Sjogren's syndrome ultimately develop more findings and are diagnosed with SLE. The only way to deal with this is to treat the Sjogren's appropriately (usually with hydroxychloroquine and low-dose steroids) and to monitor them carefully.

One source of confusion in caring for children with Sjogren's syndrome is the involvement of the acinar glands. The acinar glands include not only the salivary glands, but also the pancreas. All the acinar glands are part of the digestive process. The parotid and submandibular glands produce amylase just as the pancreas does, and if they are inflamed, the level of amylase in the blood will be elevated. Doctors often measure the amylase level if they suspect pancreatitis (see Chapter 24). However, in children with Sjogren's syndrome, an elevated amylase level may reflect inflammation of the parotid gland. The child may not have pancreatitis. Sometimes children with Sjogren's have simultaneous inflammation in the pancreas and the parotid glands. It is important to recognize that there are several possible explanations for the elevated amylase level, and the physician must evaluate the child carefully for each of them.

Some children who develop recurrent swelling of the parotid glands are diagnosed with **recurrent epidemic parotitis**. This used to be common before everyone was immunized against mumps (mumps virus infection often causes swelling of the parotid glands). However, in reality, many of these children have Sjogren's syndrome. Children with Sjogren's syndrome may also be referred because they have developed arthritis. I recently had a child referred to me for knee pain. The mother was quite surprised when I asked whether he had problems with sores in his mouth or difficulty swallowing. When she told me about the dry mouth and his being treated for three episodes of epidemic parotitis, we promptly did the appropriate tests and confirmed the diagnosis of Sjogren's.

Kidney involvement with Sjogren's syndrome may take the form of blood in the urine or protein in the urine (hematuria and proteinuria). There is also an association with a condition called **renal tubular acidosis**. This is a condition in which the kidney loses its ability to regulate the amount of acid in the urine and the children cannot maintain a proper acid base balance. Children with this condition should be under the care of an experienced nephrologist.

COMPLICATIONS

The most common complications of Sjogren's syndrome are a direct result of the dry eyes. Dry eyes are easily scratched and the scratches (corneal abrasions) are both painful and ultimately damaging to the lens of the eye. These children need frequent monitoring by an ophthalmologist. The dry mouth causes poor dental hygiene and a very high frequency of cavities. These complications can become quite serious, and it is important to make sure children use artificial tears and artificial saliva if they need them. Special toothpastes and medicines to increase saliva production also help.

Most of the other complications of Sjogren's syndrome respond well to treatment. The kidney involvement usually is responsive to appropriate treatment by nephrologists. Sometimes children with Sjogren's syndrome develop abdominal pain and a rash over the fronts of their legs. If they did not have the other findings, this would be considered **Henoch Schoenlein purpura**. It is thought to result from deposition of large immune complexes in the skin and intestines. Children with this complication may also develop a flare of their arthritis and other problems and should be evaluated carefully.

MEDICAL TREATMENT

Artificial tears and artificial saliva are very important parts of the treatment of children with Sjogren's syndrome. Some teenagers are reluctant to use them at school, for fear of seeming different. However, the dry eyes and dry mouth can do so much damage that it is very important to encourage routine use of artificial tears and saliva even during school hours. Hydroxychloroquine is often helpful in slowing the progression of the disease. Corticosteroids are useful if the symptoms are more severe or progress despite the use of hydroxychloroquine.

Children who develop ocular, dental, or renal problems need to be treated appropriately for these problems. In most cases, these problems are not difficult to treat. There is an association between Sjogren's syndrome and lymphomas and Waldenstrom's macroglobulinemia in adults. This is not generally true in childhood. Most children with primary Sjogren's syndrome do well.

PROGNOSIS

The long-term prognosis for children with primary Sjogren's syndrome is unclear. Some children develop other rheumatic diseases over time. In that case, the underlying rheumatic disease determines the prognosis. Failure to attend properly to recurrent ocular or dental problems may produce significant problems. Serious complications related to kidney disease and vasculitis are infrequent. Because Sjogren's syndrome is rare in childhood, there are no good reports describing the extended follow-up of children with this diagnosis.

14

Raynaud's Phenomenon

Maurice Raynaud (1834–1881) was a French medical student in the 1860s who was required to write a thesis to fulfill the requirements for graduation from medical school. He described the color changes he noticed in the hands of some women while standing outside in the cold waiting for the street car during the winter in Paris. **Raynaud's phenomenon** refers to the typical hand changes he described. **Raynaud's disease** (primary Raynaud's) refers to the typical hand changes occurring in the absence of any other rheumatic disease. **Raynaud's syndrome** (secondary Raynaud's) refers to the typical changes occurring in the setting of an underlying rheumatic disease.

Many people experience cold hands whenever it is cool outside. This is not Raynaud's phenomenon. Raynaud's phenomenon results from spasm of the blood vessels in response to something happening. The vessels may spasm as a result of exposure to the cold, embarrassment, or another stress. The fundamental abnormality is the hyperreactivity of the blood vessels. Raynaud's may be the result of being thin (it is common for tall, thin women to have Raynaud's phenomenon) or of the blood vessels being sensitized by immune complexes or by inflammatory mediators (see Chapter 24) because the individual has an underlying rheumatic disease.

To have true Raynaud's phenomenon, there must be a three-phase color change. Initially, the tips of one or more fingers turn white as the blood flow is cut off by spasm of the blood vessels. Once the spasm passes, there is increased reactive blood flow and the fingers turn red then slowly back to their normal state of bluish discoloration, with sluggish blood flow.

Cold red hands or cold blue hands without the spasmodic white phase, do not constitute Raynaud's phenomenon.

The importance of Raynaud's phenomenon lies in its association with a variety of rheumatic diseases. While Raynaud's is common in thin young women, it is often the first manifestation noticed in children with progressive systemic sclerosis (see Chapter 15 on scleroderma). Raynaud's is also found frequently in children with other vasculitic diseases, such as lupus, dermatomyositis, and anticardiolipin antibody syndrome. It may occur in children with many other rheumatic conditions.

Since most young women with Raynaud's phenomena are healthy, it is important to understand how to recognize children in whom Raynaud's is a warning of an underlying condition. There are a number of simple steps for doing this. Every child with Raynaud's should have routine testing done, but boys with Raynaud's are more worrisome than girls, and children less than twelve years of age are more worrisome than older children. Tall, thin girls with a family history of Raynaud's disease are less worrisome than those without a family history.

As in every evaluation, a good history, careful physical examination, and appropriate laboratory tests are the key. When evaluating a child with Raynaud's phenomenon, the physician wants to know when it happens, how often, how prolonged the attacks are, and what other symptoms may be present. Long-lasting episodes of Raynaud's, a high frequency of episodes, shortness of breath, chest pain when the Raynaud's occurs, and morning stiffness (particularly in the fingers) all increase the probability that an underlying disease is present. When examining the child the physician should look carefully for nail fold capillary abnormalities (see Fig. 21) or distal fingertip pitting (see below). Either of these findings substantially increases the probability of an underlying disease being present.

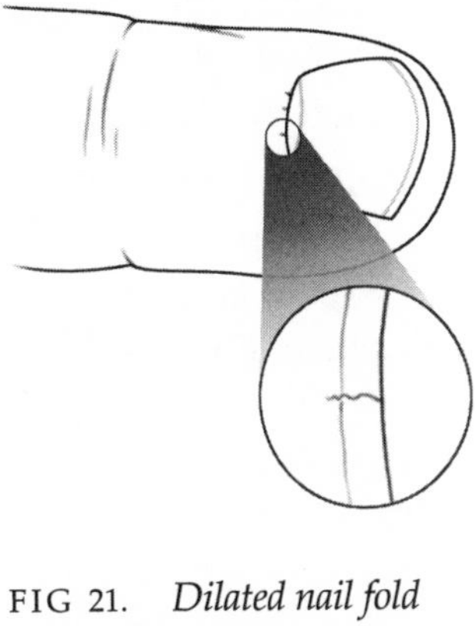

FIG 21. *Dilated nail fold capillaries may be easy to see with a small magnifying glass.*

Many physicians are concerned that they lack the proper equipment for nail fold capillary microscopy, but this can be easily done with an otoscope (the small hand-held magnifier used for looking in ears). In a normal individual, the nail fold capillaries cannot be seen, even with an otoscope. If red streaks are seen in the nail folds, it suggests the presence of nail fold capillary abnormalities and the child should be referred to an experienced physician for further evaluation. All ten fingers should be examined, as the presence of these abnormalities on any finger is significant.

Distal fingertip pitting is another important finding that is also easily detected on routine examination. These pits are little areas where the blood supply has been cut off and the skin and underlying tissues have atrophied. As a result, the areas often feel callused to the examiner. The child will describe decreased feeling in the fingertips, as one would expect from calluses. If you look carefully, you may be able to see the areas of thickened skin, often with little central depressions or scars. However, it is easiest to screen for these by feeling the tips of the fingers. The areas that are scarred feel like little bumps. They are harder than the normal skin. *The presence of either nail fold capillary abnormalities or distal fingertip lesions strongly suggests the presence of an underlying rheumatic disease.*

LABORATORY TESTING

Laboratory evaluation of a child with Raynaud's should include a complete blood count (CBC), erythrocyte sedimentation rate (ESR), antinuclear antibody (ANA), rheumatoid factor (RF), anticardiolipin antibodies, and thyroid function tests. If there are no suggestive findings on history or physical examination and all of these tests are normal, there is little likelihood of an underlying rheumatic disease. However, the presence of a positive ANA, positive RF, anticardiolipin antibodies, or an elevated ESR should all prompt more complete investigation, as should any suggestive findings on history or physical examination.

COMPLICATIONS

If a child is known to have an underlying rheumatic disease, the presence of Raynaud's phenomenon does not necessarily indicate more serious disease. However, there are several complications related to Raynaud's that must be considered. In more severe cases, children with Raynaud's may have problems not only in their fingers, but also in their toes, ear lobes, and tip of the nose. All of these areas should be protected if the child is to be subjected to significant cold exposure.

It is also important to recognize that children with increased vascular reactivity and Raynaud's phenomenon may have instability in other vascular beds. This is a rare complication, but I have cared for children with scleroderma who had chest pain and cardiac abnormalities due to documented constriction of their coronary arteries that occurred whenever their fingers blanched because of Raynaud's phenomenon. If the internal organs are being deprived of blood flow, the Raynaud's must be treated aggressively to prevent damage to these organs.

Any child who has distal fingertip pitting or a history of severe Raynaud's should not be unnecessarily exposed to cold stress. Digital gangrene with loss of parts of fingers or toes can occur. Whenever a child has prolonged loss of circulation to a finger or toe, he or she should be taken to a local emergency room. I tell my patients that if a finger is white and numb for more than ten minutes they should be inside making every effort to warm it up. If it is not clearly back to normal after half an hour, they should be on their way to medical help. High-dose intravenous corticosteroids and prostacycline inhibitors have both been used with good results in this setting.

MEDICAL TREATMENT

For children with Raynaud's phenomena without an associated disease, the most important aspect of treatment is common sense. The vast majority of children do well simply by dressing warmly and wearing gloves. If these measures are not enough, children may benefit from the use of calcium-channel blockers (Chapter 22). These drugs lower blood pressure by blocking blood vessel constriction. Hence, they serve to reduce the vasospasm that is the key to Raynaud's phenomenon. Most children tolerate the mild reduction in blood pressure associated with these drugs without difficulty, but some do get mild side effects. Many of my patients use these drugs only in the coldest weather. In addition to the calcium-channel blockers, it is possible to use drugs such as pentoxyfyline. This drug seems to reduce the incidence of Raynaud's, perhaps by making the red blood cell membrane more flexible so it is easier for the cells to get past the area of spasm. Some rheumatologists use aspirin and other agents with varying success.

For children with an underlying rheumatic disease, the key to relieving the Raynaud's phenomenon is primarily relief of the underlying condition. *In some children with an underlying rheumatic disease, Raynaud's may remain a problem when the majority of the symptoms have resolved. Symptomatic therapy with warm clothing and calcium-channel blockers may be helpful in these cases. Complete loss of blood flow for a prolonged period is extremely rare.* However, prolonged vasoconstriction can result in loss of the affected finger or toe. For this reason it is important that any child who has a cold white finger or toe that has not improved within a reasonable time period promptly seek appropriate medical care.

15

Scleroderma

Scleroderma is a broad term that simply means "hard skin." A variety of different diseases are grouped together under this diagnosis. The focal (or localized) forms of scleroderma are often mild and may not require any treatment. In contrast, **progressive systemic sclerosis** (also called **diffuse scleroderma**) is a life-threatening disease typically involving the heart, lungs, and other organs. Often when a family contacts me it is because they were told the child had scleroderma. They have no idea whether the child has a severe or mild form. Fortunately, the mild forms of scleroderma are far more common than the severe ones.

Because the different forms of scleroderma are so different from each other, it is necessary to discuss them separately. Typically, each of these conditions looks very different from the others, but children with confusing conditions that seem to overlap do exist.

LOCAL FORMS OF SCLERODERMA

Morphea

> Jill was an eight-year-old girl who developed a pink spot on her back. At first no one noticed, but it was obvious in the summer when she put her bathing suit on. It looked like a big pink circle with a whitish central area. Her mother thought first of Lyme disease, but two weeks of antibiotics had no effect. The lesion was treated with topical ointments for dry skin, then for ringworm, all without improvement. After six weeks Jill's mother took her to a dermatologist. He looked at the

Local or focal forms of scleroderma

Morphea
Linear scleroderma
Linear scleroderma en coup de sabre
Parry Romberg syndrome (the relationship of this syndrome to scleroderma is uncertain)
Sclerodermatomyositis
Other overlapping syndromes

Systemic forms of scleroderma

Progressive systemic sclerosis
CREST syndrome

Diseases that can evolve into scleroderma

Eosinophilic fasciitis
Mixed connective tissue disease (see Chapter 12)

Laboratory tests in scleroderma

Local or focal forms of scleroderma

- Antinuclear antibody (ANA) occasionally positive
- Rheumatoid factor (RF) usually negative
- Creatinine phosphokinase (CPK) mildly elevated in linear scleroderma and sclerodermatomyositis but not in morphea or linear scleroderma en coup de sabre
- Anticentromere antibody negative
- Anti-Scl-70 negative
- Other blood tests usually normal

Systemic forms of scleroderma

Progressive systemic sclerosis

- ANA often positive
- RF often positive
- Anti-Scl-70 sometimes positive (less frequent in childhood)

CREST syndrome

- ANA often positive
- RF sometimes positive
- Anticentromere antibody usually positive

Eosinophilic fasciitis

- ANA often positive
- Eosinophilia

Mixed connective tissue disease

- ANA positive
- RF most often positive; Anti-Scl-70 negative

lesion and did a biopsy. The report was "consistent with scleroderma." By the time I saw Jill the lesion had stopped growing and developed a thick white center that was firm to the touch. Jill never developed any other lesions. She was treated with over-the-counter topical agents to soften the skin. Over a period of several years the lesion softened. Now the lesion is evident only because she has an area of darker skin where it occurred. This skin is soft and feels normal. She's never had another problem related to morphea.

Morphea is the most common form of scleroderma in childhood. Morphea consists of areas of thickened skin commonly on the body (trunk), but sometimes on arms or legs. Families usually notice a patch of pink and irritated skin that looks like many common skin conditions. If the patch is due to morphea, it typically does not itch or hurt. Often the area of reddened skin does not attract any particular attention until it has persisted for several weeks. It will not improve with treatment for skin infections, but it might briefly look better if it is treated with corticosteroid creams.

Commonly, the family becomes concerned when either a second area of skin becomes involved or the area begins to enlarge. When areas of morphea are active, they slowly increase in size with the rim remaining pink, but the center turns whitish and becomes hard. Dermatologists usually make the diagnosis of morphea on the basis of either a skin biopsy or clinical experience.

Laboratory abnormalities are rare in children with morphea. Although some children have positive tests for ANA, tests for anti-dsDNA, RF, Scl-70, anticentromere antibody, and routine blood tests including complete blood count (CBC), erythrocyte sedimentation rate (ESR), and muscle enzymes should all be normal. If they are not, a full and complete evaluation by an experienced rheumatologist is in order.

Some lesions of morphea are very small (nickel- or dime-sized), while others can be several inches across. Over a period of years, they usually evolve from hard white areas to soft and darkened skin. (*Note:* In dark-skinned people the areas of morphea may remain lighter than the surrounding skin.) If the morphea is not interfering with function and there are only a few lesions, it may be best to treat it with topical creams such as vitamin E cream or cocoa butter. Many families feel these treatments make a difference. Chronic use of corticosteroid creams can damage the skin and should be avoided.

Medical treatment. Children with rapidly developing morphea lesions that are disfiguring may need aggressive therapy. In my experience, methotrexate therapy has been very successful in stopping the progression of morphea. Low doses of methotrexate given as pills are rarely effective, but moderate doses of methotrexate (1 mg/kg/week [maximum 50 mg]) given as subcutaneous injections are very effective. However, the lesions must be significant enough to warrant the risks, as well as the time, effort, and expense of therapy. Borderline cases may benefit from treatment with hydroxychloroquine (plaquenil; see Chapter 24).

Complications. Morphea has two main complications. First, the lesions are cosmetically unattractive. If they are in a place that is covered by clothing, the problem may be minimal. If the lesions are in a location that is easily seen by others, there will be a need to address the psychological issues associated with the invariable curious questions (see the section on dealing with friends and neighbors in Chapter 26). Second, the skin in the lesions will not heal well if it is cut or abraded. In rare cases, isolated lesions of morphea may be associated with mild arthritis or other rheumatic disease manifestations. These overlap conditions are of uncertain significance. However, any child with atypical lesions or unexpected problems should be carefully evaluated by an experienced rheumatologist. Most often nothing further is found.

Many parents worry that morphea lesions may be the first indications of systemic scleroderma. This is rarely, if ever, true. I have seen reports of children thought to have only morphea who later developed systemic disease. However, when you read the details, there was strong evidence suggesting systemic disease from the beginning (see the discussion below). Children with new onset morphea should be carefully evaluated by a physician who is experienced in dealing with children with scleroderma. An experienced physician may recognize indications that the child has a systemic disease. If there are no such indications, I recommend only periodic monitoring once the initial evaluation is complete.

Prognosis. The cause of morphea remains entirely unknown. Many ideas have been proposed over the years, but none has withstood the test of time. The key things for a family to know about morphea are detailed below.

- It usually goes away after a period of years and leaves only darkened skin behind.
- If there is a lot of it, or it is in places where it is disfiguring, morphea can be treated.

- The earlier in its evolution morphea is treated, the better the outcome.
- Children with morphea should be carefully evaluated for other evidence of rheumatic disease, but if nothing is found on careful examination at the beginning, the risk of other rheumatic diseases appearing later is small.

The long-term outlook for children with morphea is excellent. There should be no need for surgery or other aggressive interventions. Children with morphea should expect to grow up to lead normal, healthy, productive lives.

Linear scleroderma

Kathleen was a nine-year-old girl when her mother noted a patch of unusual skin on the top of her left foot. Over the next six months the area always looked irritated and red despite a number of treatments for athlete's foot and other minor conditions offered by her physician. No one was too concerned until new lesions appeared on Kathleen's calf. These were red at first and looked like an allergic reaction. Over time more lesions developed and they began to appear above the knee. Gradually, these lesions began to turn white, then darker and hardened.

When Kathleen was eleven, a neighbor pointed out to her mother that Kathleen was limping. When Kathleen was undressed in the doctor's office, there were mixed white, dark, and pink lesions all up and down her leg and even one on her stomach. The left leg was smaller than the right both in length and width. In addition, she could not straighten her left leg all the way. There was a tight band of skin behind the knee that prevented the leg from straightening.

By the time Kathleen came to my office, the linear scleroderma on her leg was well advanced and causing significant problems. It required a year of treatment with methotrexate injections and physical therapy before the skin was soft and she could fully straighten her leg. We did not discontinue the therapy until she had been stable for another year. Unfortunately, she lost a lot of muscle cells during the time before she was properly diagnosed and began treatment with methotrexate. As a result, the left leg is still thinner than the right. However, now she is able to function normally.

Linear scleroderma differs from morphea in that the areas of involved skin form linear bands instead of irregular ovals. These bands are often described as following the distribution of nerves (dermatomes), but this is not really true. Nonetheless, linear scleroderma usually does not cross from one side of the body to the other. The idea that irritation of the nerves led to the development of linear scleroderma received a lot of attention in the past. One group of researchers suggested linear scleroderma was the result of herpes zoster infection involving the nerves. Another group thought linear scleroderma was due to Lyme disease. These ideas have been disproved. The cause of linear scleroderma remains unknown.

A typical case of linear scleroderma is a child such as Kathleen (above) with a tight band of skin on the top of one foot extending up onto the leg. It may also begin on the hand and arm. These areas appear pinkish at first and don't hurt. Later they become pale and harden. A small area of involvement may be of little concern, but if a large area is involved, tightening of the skin may cause the leg (or arm, toes, etc.) to become bent.

We do not understand the patterns of linear scleroderma. Some children have one patch on one arm or leg. Others have several patches on one arm. Still others may have involvement of both the arm and the leg on one side, and the lesions may extend onto the trunk. Less frequently, both sides of the body are involved. Involvement of both sides of the body is unusual and should prompt careful investigation. However, involvement of an arm and leg on the same side is not uncommon.

Laboratory abnormalities in children with linear scleroderma are minimal. Although some children have positive tests for ANA, tests for anti-dsDNA, RF, Scl-70, anticentromere antibody, and routine blood tests including CBC and ESR all should be normal. Some children will have mildly elevated muscle enzymes. If a child has elevated muscle enzymes and the typical rash of dermatomyositis in conjunction with an area of linear scleroderma, the disease is termed **sclerodermatomyositis** (see below).

If the disease occurs while a child is still growing, it may interfere with the development of the underlying muscles, bones, and joints. This may result in an arm or leg that is much smaller than it should be and result in permanent disability. Because of this, areas of linear scleroderma that cross a joint (e.g., elbow, wrist, knee, ankle) require aggressive treatment. Although large-scale controlled studies are lacking, I have had excellent success in treating linear scleroderma with methotrexate. Over a six-month period, weekly methotrexate injections are associated with dramatic softening of the skin and reversal of contractures. Although this treatment cannot restore lost muscle or bone mass, it appears to stop the disease and allow further growth in young children. It should be started as soon as possible in children who are developing deformities.

scleroderma en coup de sabre should not extend below the eyelid. True Parry Romberg syndrome involves the entire side of the face. Some children fall in between.

Because there are children with varying degrees of involvement, there is no uniform agreement regarding where linear scleroderma en coup de sabre ends and Parry Romberg syndrome begins. If there is involvement of the tongue, it is Parry Romberg syndrome. I also believe all children with involvement of the brain underneath the lesions have Parry Romberg syndrome and not linear scleroderma en coup de sabre, but no one is sure. We are not even sure the diseases are truly different.

Laboratory abnormalities are minimal in children with both of these disorders. As with other forms of linear scleroderma, some children have positive tests for ANA, but tests for anti-dsDNA, RF, Scl-70, anticentromere antibody, and routine blood tests including CBC and ESR, should be normal. These children should not have abnormal muscle enzymes or muscle weakness.

Medical treatment and prognosis. Treatment and prognosis for this group of children remain uncertain. If the lesions are confined to the scalp and forehead, as in typical linear scleroderma en coup de sabre, they seem responsive to methotrexate. The long-term outlook for children with linear scleroderma en coup de sabre is generally excellent. In most cases the cosmetic deformity is minimal and can be well concealed by the hair.

Some children with linear scleroderma en coup de sabre have been described as having underlying neurologic involvement. Again, I believe this is more likely a manifestation of Parry Romberg syndrome, but the lines differentiating the two conditions are not clearly drawn. Children with linear scleroderma en coup de sabre may have some difficulties dealing with the impact of the cosmetic deformity. However, the prognosis for a normal and productive life is excellent.

Unfortunately, children with Parry Romberg syndrome and facial hemiatrophy are rarely recognized before the atrophy has become significant. In most cases, it does not appear appropriate to intervene medically at that point. However, in the hands of an experienced plastic surgeon that has worked with these children, cosmetic surgery is practical. There are multiple special considerations involved in this surgery and it should be only done by a team experienced in dealing with such children.

A significant percentage of children with Parry Romberg syndrome also have underlying central nervous system lesions. These may vary

Linear scleroderma en coup de sabre and
Parry Romberg syndrome

Linear scleroderma en coup de sabre is a particular form of linear scle roderma that may not truly be related to the other forms. "En coup d sabre" is a French phrase that was used to describe the injuries of foo soldiers struck on the head by the sword of a cavalry soldier riding horse. If the foot soldier survived his injury, there would be a scar anc thickened skin involving one side of the forehead and extending along the scalp toward the back. Children with linear scleroderma en coup de sabre have an area of thickened abnormal skin that resembles this scar, but they usually do not have significant underlying problems. However, the distinction between linear scleroderma en coup de sabre and Parry Romberg syndrome is unclear.

Parry Romberg syndrome is a gradually progressive facial hemiatrophy. In a full-fledged case, there is significant deformity, with one entire side of the face smaller than the other. This is in sharp contrast to typical linear scleroderma en coup de sabre, where the abnormality is confined to the forehead. While the changes of linear scleroderma en coup de sabre are usually confined to the skin, in Parry Romberg syndrome there is an increased frequency of underlying changes in the brain.

The difference between linear scleroderma en coup de sabre and Parry Romberg syndrome is best exemplified by involvement of the tongue in Parry Romberg syndrome. Not only is one side of the face smaller, but also one side of the tongue is smaller. Thus, Parry Romberg syndrome is clearly not a condition of the skin alone. However, both conditions may begin the same way and there are children who have areas of atrophic facial skin that do not clearly fit either category.

These illnesses typically begin in the first or second year of life. Most often the family will describe having noticed a pinkish lesion just to one side of the middle of the forehead. Since children in this age group fall frequently while learning to walk, most families assume the child simply banged his or her head. Over a few weeks the lesion does not go away as expected. Instead, the veins may become more noticeable in the pink area.

The lesion on the forehead is often present for months before the family begins to notice indentation of the bone under the pink skin. On careful examination, there may be a continuation of the abnormal skin underneath the hairline. In other children, the area of pink skin extends further down the face and along the side of the nose over time. Linear from benign nonspecific findings on MRI to vascular malformations or neurologic abnormalities. I evaluate all children who come to me with Parry Romberg syndrome with an MRI in order to see whether such abnormalities are present. Some children with Parry Romberg may have learning disabilities. Although some physicians dismiss this as a coincidence, I have seen it so many times that I believe the association is real.

Some children with Parry Romberg syndrome have developed inflammation of the optic nerve (the nerve in the back of the eye that provides vision). This is rare but requires immediate treatment if it occurs. I have also cared for children with linear scleroderma en coup de sabre who developed uveitis (ocular inflammation). *All children with these conditions should have periodic ophthalmologic evaluations.*

The combination of cosmetic and neurologic abnormalities in children with Parry Romberg syndrome makes the prognosis for these children more guarded. Most do well with corrective surgery, as needed, provided it is done by plastic surgeons experienced in dealing with this condition. A sympathetic family and physician are important. Special efforts must be made to help these children deal with the social stresses that result from their obviously abnormal appearance (see Chapter 26).

Sclerodermatomyositis

Sclerodermatomyositis is an overlap disorder that illustrates the foolishness of considering the rheumatic diseases to be completely separate entities. *Children with sclerodermatomyositis have a typical band of tight skin that appears to be linear scleroderma, but have muscle weakness, elevated muscle enzymes, and often a heliotropic rash* typical of dermatomyositis (see Chapter 16). The simultaneous occurrence of manifestations of two separate diseases in these children is unexplained. The muscle inflammation and heliotropic rash most often respond promptly to corticosteroid therapy and do not recur. The linear scleroderma lesion does not respond to corticosteroids, though it may become less pink in coloration. *PSS with elevated muscle enzymes is not sclerodermatomyositis.*

Laboratory abnormalities found in children with sclerodermatomyositis include positive tests for ANA. The routine blood tests may show a mild anemia, elevation of the ESR, and elevated muscle enzyme levels (CPK and aldolase; see Chapter 24). RF is rare and anti-Scl-70 is normally absent. Although diffuse sclerodermatous changes, rash, and elevated muscle enzymes may occur in mixed connective tissue disease, children with MCTD do not have linear bands of tight skin. Children with sclerodermatomyositis do not have the typical pattern of laboratory findings seen in children with MCTD and are most likely distinct.

Complications of sclerodermatomyositis are rare. Usually, the muscle inflammation and rash are easily treated with corticosteroids. The area of linear scleroderma is rarely large enough to cause concern. If it is crossing a joint or causing significant deformity, methotrexate therapy may be necessary. Many children have been treated with long-term hydroxychloroquine once corticosteroids were no longer necessary. Although a small percentage of children will develop further manifestations of rheumatic disease, in general the long-term prognosis is good.

Other overlapping conditions

As a physician caring for children with these diseases over a period of years, one cannot help being struck by the diversity of disease. Somehow all of these diseases that look so different in their typical forms are interrelated, but we clearly do not understand the connections. I have seen several children who simultaneously have skin lesions of morphea on their backs and abdomens, indentations typical of linear scleroderma en coup de sabre on their foreheads, ocular inflammation such as that seen in children with juvenile arthritis, and areas of linear scleroderma on their legs.

Other overlap conditions may also occur. The key element in caring for children who do not fit neatly into one category or another is to recognize each condition for what it is and treat each appropriately. At the same time, every atypical child must be carefully evaluated to make sure an alternative diagnosis has not been overlooked. Some of these children have been difficult to treat, and their long-term prognosis is uncertain. With the exception of neurologic and visual problems, none of the children in this section will have significant internal organ involvement.

SYSTEMIC FORMS OF SCLERODERMA

Progressive systemic sclerosis

The form of scleroderma called **progressive systemic sclerosis** (PSS), also referred to as **diffuse scleroderma**, is the most severe form of the disease with the subtle onset of skin tightening and, in many cases, shortness of breath. Children and families may be unaware of the disease until it has become well advanced. However, careful questioning may reveal that the disease had been developing for a long period. Because the onset of disease is slow and gradual, families often are unaware of the problem until a dramatic event occurs. Sometimes this is a cold, numb finger. Sometimes it is the inability to play favorite sports when the season starts. In other cases, the family suddenly realizes that the child cannot open jars or perform other minor chores that he or she used to do easily. These children have poor wound healing and may be brought to the physician because of painful sores that just do not heal. These commonly occur on the ankles, elbows, or fingers.

The most common early symptom of PSS is Raynaud's phenomenon. However, it is important to be aware that most people who have Raynaud's phenomenon do not develop rheumatic disease (see Chapter 14 above). Other common early symptoms of PSS are gradually increasing tightness of the skin and progressive stiffening of the fingers. Unfortunately, the disease often progresses so slowly that the child and family may be unaware of changes that are striking to the outside observer. With time, children may notice that it becomes more difficult to open their mouths fully to eat a large sandwich. Because they evolve slowly, none of these symptoms is likely to result in prompt referral to a rheumatologist. Typically, these children are ultimately brought to their physicians because of shortness of breath, difficulty swallowing, or weight loss.

An experienced physician easily diagnoses PSS when the skin involvement is prominent. The tight shiny skin is often accompanied by sores over the knuckles (Gottren's papules), abnormalities in the nail fold capillaries, and distal fingertip lesions (see Chapter 14 for a full discussion). This combination of findings is diagnostic of PSS. Less often children come to the doctor because of difficulty swallowing (involvement of the esophagus). They may have difficulty swallowing foods in large chunks or that have sharp edges, like potato chips.

Some children with scleroderma are first seen by their physicians because of chest pain. Most often they were at first dismissed, then sent to a cardiologist where the heart was found to be uninvolved and they were told the chest pain was due to heartburn. The distal esophagus is frequently involved in scleroderma, and the valve (sphincter) that keeps stomach acid out often fails to work properly. As a result, the chest pains are due to irritation of the distal esophagus by acid reflux. Occasionally, children present with chronic diarrhea and weight loss because the intestinal tract is affected by the scleroderma. In all of these cases, the key to the correct diagnosis is consideration of the possibility of scleroderma by a knowledgeable physician.

Other diseases may be associated with Raynaud's phenomenon or shortness of breath, but *the combination of shortness of breath and Raynaud's is highly suggestive of PSS or CREST syndrome* (see below). MCTD, dermatomyositis, systemic lupus erythematosus, and less frequently other rheumatic diseases may also have both symptoms. Parents often become concerned about the distinction between MCTD, PSS, and CREST syndrome. Typical cases of each can be easily differentiated. However, there is a broad spectrum of overlap among these diseases. While physicians have distinguished these diseases in textbooks, nature has not obliged. Over time, some children with obvious MCTD progress to having PSS.

The diagnosis of PSS is based on the characteristic findings on examination of the skin. In some cases, it is necessary to biopsy the skin for confirmation. However, the diagnosis is often obvious to an experienced physician. If confirmatory findings are present on physical examination and in the laboratory results, a skin biopsy may be avoided. The skin of children with scleroderma often heals poorly and the biopsy often leads to just one more scar.

There are several patterns of laboratory abnormality in children with scleroderma. No single test is abnormal in every child. Frequently, the routine tests (CBC, ESR, metabolic panel) are essentially normal. An increased number of eosinophils may be noted in the blood count. Very high levels of eosinophils may suggest **eosinophilic fasciitis** (see section below). Positive tests for ANA or RF are common but not necessary for the diagnosis. Muscle enzymes (CPK, aldolase) may be elevated. Antibodies to Scl-70 (antitopoisomerase antibodies) are less common in children with scleroderma than in adults but may occur. Anti-DNA antibodies are occasionally reported in low titer, but serum complement levels (C3, C4) should be normal.

With the exception of the finding of anti-Scl-70, it may be impossible to differentiate MCTD and PSS on a laboratory basis. Because some children with MCTD ultimately are diagnosed as having evolved into PSS, this may be a false distinction (see Chapter 12). CREST syndrome should be considered carefully in children with telangiectasias or high titers of anticentromere antibody (see section below).

Lung complications. The most severe complications associated with scleroderma result from involvement of the internal organs. Lung involvement that leads to progressive shortness of breath may be quite severe. Children with PSS should undergo periodic monitoring of their pulmonary function tests (PFTs; see Chapter 24). High-resolution CT scans of the chest are helpful to evaluate any child who has abnormal PFTs. Areas of fibrosis, or honeycomb, ground-glass appearance, indicate significant lung involvement. Over time, this involvement may lead to thickening and loss of elasticity in the lung tissue, much like what happens in the skin. These changes make it harder to move air in and out of the lungs and harder for oxygen to move into the blood.

Children with significant lung involvement should be aggressively treated. Over time, the difficulty of moving air in and out of the lungs places additional strain on the heart (it has to push harder to move the blood through the lungs because the lungs have become stiffer, and if the oxygen is not getting into the blood well, more blood will have to be pumped through the lungs to pick up the amount of oxygen needed by the tissues). The increased strain on the heart may result in enlargement of the right ventricle, leakage of the pulmonary valve, and increased pulmonary artery pressure. These are very worrisome findings: Untreated, severe lung involvement often leads to heart failure, pneumonia, or both.

Heart complications. Heart problems in children with scleroderma are usually the result of the extra stress put on the heart by the involvement of the lungs. However, some children develop involvement of the heart muscle known as **myocardial fibrosis**, which causes the heart to become stiff. It is as if extra fibrous tissue is forming in the heart, just as it does in the skin. When this happens, the heart cannot contract as well as it should. This can be detected by an echocardiogram. It is a very difficult problem to treat. Normally, heart failure is treated with agents such as digitalis that increase the strength of the heart's contractions. However, these agents may cause abnormalities of the heart rhythm. In children with scleroderma, treatment with these drugs may cause severe problems and I avoid them whenever possible. Children with significant cardiac compromise from scleroderma will need an experienced cardiologist to help in their care.

The outer covering of the heart (the pericardium) may also be involved in scleroderma. Most often this takes the form of thickening and irritation (**pericarditis**), sometimes with a buildup of fluid. If too much fluid is present, it becomes difficult for the heart to pump properly. This can be treated with medications, but if it is very severe, the fluid may need to be drained (pericardiocentesis).

Although children rarely have heart attacks (myocardial infarctions), the coronary arteries may become involved in children with scleroderma.

Gradual thickening of the coronary arteries is unlikely to cause problems until the children have become adults. However, some children develop overreactive blood vessels in the heart. This is essentially identical to what is happening in the blood vessels of the hands with Raynaud's phenomenon. Most often coronary artery involvement is discovered in children with scleroderma when they notice chest pain while they experience Raynaud's changes in their hands. The blood vessels in the heart are constricting at the same time as the blood vessels in the hands. This should be aggressively treated, as it may result in a heart attack.

Kidney complications. Involvement of the kidneys is another major concern for children with PSS. When an internal organ is involved in scleroderma, the blood vessels become thickened and narrowed. One of the normal functions of the kidney is to monitor the pressure in the blood vessels. If the blood vessels supplying the kidneys become thickened and narrowed, the pressure-monitoring cells (granular cells in the juxtaglomerular apparatus) respond to the drop in pressure reaching the kidney by releasing a compound called rennin. This causes the blood pressure to increase throughout the body. In children with scleroderma, the increased blood pressure leads to increased strain on the heart and other organs. Rarely, children develop an acute rise in blood pressure called **scleroderma renal crisis**. This is an acute life-threatening condition. Fortunately, a new class of agents for blood pressure control—the ACE inhibitors—is very effective in treating this problem.

Gastrointestinal complications. Children with scleroderma frequently have involvement of the gastrointestinal system. Tightness of the skin around the mouth can make it difficult to open the mouth widely enough to eat normal foods. The thickening of the esophagus (the swallowing tube that connects the mouth and the stomach) makes it difficult to swallow tough foods, such as meat. In addition, it is common for the valve at the bottom of the esophagus (esophageal sphincter) to lose its ability to close tightly. This results in acid washing up from the stomach (**gastroesophageal reflux**), causing severe irritation and often resulting in severe chest pain. Eventually, the gastroesophageal reflux may cause scarring of the esophagus, making it more difficult for food to pass through. Often the pain and discomfort caused by this combination of problems make the child not want to eat, and he or she will begin to lose weight.

Involvement of the intestines by scleroderma also takes the form of thickening of the tissues. This makes it difficult for the intestines to move food forward in the normal fashion. The result is poor absorption of nutrients and chronic bloating. Some patients have problems with constipation. Others have problems with diarrhea, and some have both problems. These digestive problems frequently worsen the child's weight loss. Liver involvement in children with scleroderma is rare. Some cases of **primary biliary cirrhosis** (an uncommon form of liver disease associated with scleroderma) have been reported.

Medical treatment. Proper treatment of childhood scleroderma remains controversial. However, it is generally agreed that treatment with D-penicillamine (which used to be the standard therapy) is ineffective. There is no clear agreement on the best treatment for mild cases. Some centers feel short courses of prednisone are helpful. I personally avoid them if possible.

The key to obtaining the best outcome for children with scleroderma is to prevent severe internal organ involvement. Since the disease is slowly and not always steadily progressive, it is difficult to perform scientifically accurate studies. Most centers will treat children with systemic scleroderma with mild agents such as hydroxychloroquine, unless there is severe internal organ involvement. If that is present, they will treat the children with intravenous cyclophosphamide.

My own preference is to treat every child with definite PSS with injections of methotrexate and oral cyclosporine. While this is not proven therapy, I have found it very successful in preventing progression of scleroderma. There have been studies in adults showing that low doses of methotrexate do not work. In my experience, the higher dose of 1 mg/kg is effective when given by injection every week.

Cyclosporin is another potent drug that provides additional benefit to these children. All of my PSS patients are treated with the combination of cyclosporine and high-dose methotrexate, and they do well. I do not wait for there to be severe problems; my goal is to prevent them. Families must be aware that not all physicians agree with this choice of therapy. Since no therapy for PSS has been proven effective, each center has its own preferences based on its own experience. This is very frustrating to parents. They want to know what the right answer is. It is difficult to explain that there is no right answer. Parents must choose a physician they trust and stick with a plan.

A variety of medications have been tried in adults with scleroderma. Thalidomide (a potent immunomodulator) and relaxin (a hormone that causes loosening of the skin) are both being actively investigated. The use of agents that block tumor necrosis factor alpha (TNF-α) is also being considered. See Chapter 22 for a fuller discussion of these medications.

An assortment of medications is used to address specific problems. For example, ACE inhibitors are used to treat increased blood pressure. Calcium-channel blockers are used to treat Raynaud's phenomenon. A variety of medications that block acid secretion are used to minimize damage to the esophagus. In addition, prostaglandins such as inhaled iloprost, a stable analog of epoprostenol, have been used to treat pulmonary fibrosis and the resultant increase in stiffness of the blood vessels in the lungs. There is no single best therapy, but it is important for parents to make sure that their children are being followed by physicians who are familiar with the most current recommendations.

Children with significant PSS should be cared for at major medical centers with experienced rheumatologists, pulmonologists, cardiologists, nephrologists, and specialists in intensive care—preferably with extensive pediatric experience. The primary goal of the pediatric rheumatologist must be to prevent progression of the disease and thereby prevent the child from needing the other specialists. However, often it is wise to have children with severe disease evaluated by all the members of the team. That way, the whole team will be ready to work together to correct serious problems, if they occur.

Prognosis. The prognosis for children with PSS is guarded. In the absence of significant internal organ involvement, children may live for decades. Some children with only skin involvement may find that their skin eventually softens and will do well. Children with significant heart, lung, kidney, or gastrointestinal involvement did poorly in the past. However, with more aggressive therapy the outlook is improving. There is reason to believe that continued aggressive treatment will allow children with PSS to lead successful lives.

CREST syndrome

CREST syndrome is a variation of systemic scleroderma that has several peculiar aspects. The name "CREST" comes from the findings of **calcinosis** (pieces of calcium under the skin), **Raynaud's phenomenon**, **esophageal problems**, **sclerodactyly** (tight skin on the fingers), and **telangiectasias** (small red spots due to abnormal blood vessels in the skin). The key findings that distinguish CREST from PSS are the presence of telangiectasias and anticentromere antibodies.

The general problems associated with CREST syndrome and their treatments do not differ from PSS. However, it is clear that these children are somehow different from the children with PSS. Often these children have less skin and kidney involvement, but more heart and lung involvement. Treatment is essentially the same for CREST and PSS. At one time, it was thought that the prognosis for CREST was better. In childhood this is uncertain.

EOSINOPHILIC FASCIITIS: A DISEASE THAT CAN EVOLVE INTO SCLERODERMA

Eosinophilic fasciitis is an unusual disorder characterized by the acute onset of pain and swelling in an extremity. It is named for the fact that in affected individuals, the connective tissue is inflamed (fasciitis) and there is an abundance of eosinophils (a white blood cell type associated with allergies and not commonly present in the fascia). Typically, the skin in the affected area is very red, tender, and swollen. This inflammation is followed by hardening of the skin and muscles in the area. Although the onset of eosinophilic fasciitis is commonly associated with extreme exercise or trauma, the cause is poorly understood. Evidence of inflammation, including an increased sedimentation rate and increased eosinophil count, are common. Internal organ involvement does not occur.

Some cases of **eosinophilic myalgia** syndrome were initially thought to be eosinophilic fasciitis. This is a syndrome with muscle pain and redness but not fasciitis. An epidemic of eosinophilic myalgia was apparently caused by contaminated L-tryptophan purchased in health food stores. Any child with eosinophilia and myalgias should be carefully questioned about their intake of vitamins, food supplements, and other agents. Most evidence points to a contaminated source of L-tryptophan as the cause of the problem, but these issues have never been fully resolved. I cared for one teenager with this syndrome who took lots of supplements but was sure none contained L-tryptophan. Since there is no real supervision of the manufacturers, one never knows for sure what is in supplements.

Eosinophilic fasciitis is usually very responsive to treatment with corticosteroids. However, the long-term course of the disease is highly varied. Sometimes the disease resolves entirely, but other cases persist with varying amounts of disease activity for years. A few children have ultimately developed PSS after initially being diagnosed with eosinophilic fasciitis. However, most cases have resolved completely over a period of months.

Children with eosinophilia and musculoskeletal complaints need to be evaluated very carefully. This combination of findings may occur in children with parasitic illnesses, eosinophilic vasculitis, and Churg Strauss disease. These diseases are uncommon but may be life-threatening if not properly recognized and treated. Children with these diseases may have rashes, but these diseases are not associated with hardening of the skin.

16

Dermatomyositis and Polymyositis

Hillary was a delightful four-year-old. She had a younger sister who was just beginning to walk when the family noticed that Hillary was asking to be carried and holding on much more often than she had previously. Her family thought this was a reaction to the increased attention given to her sister. But the next month she became increasingly "difficult." She often refused to walk and had tantrums if her family would not carry her. Hillary's bedroom was on the second floor. Although she would come downstairs in the morning, she insisted on being carried up to bed every night. One morning she wanted a doll from her bedroom but refused to go up the stairs to get it. The family could not understand why she was getting so lazy. Over the next few weeks they noted she was holding on to the stair rail with both hands when coming down the steps and seemed to be falling unexpectedly.

Concerned, the family brought her to the pediatrician. On examination she was weak and could hardly get up from a chair. She could not get up off the floor without assistance, and even when she was given help getting started, she needed to push herself up the front of her legs to rise to a standing position (this is called a positive Gower sign). Laboratory evaluation revealed an elevated erythrocyte sedimentation rate, elevated muscle enzymes, and elevated liver enzymes. She was referred for evaluation.

In the office Hillary could grab my fingers tightly with her hand but could not raise her arms over her head and could not lift her legs off the exam table. She had reddened and irritated elbows and knees. The family ascribed this to her frequent falling. She also had a pinkish rash over her eyelids that the family had not noticed. The diagnosis of dermatomyositis was made. She was begun on a low dose of corticosteroids, and within six months she had recovered completely.

Things you need to know

- Children with dermatomyositis do not have the increased risk of cancer described for adults with this disease.
- Polymyositis is rare in childhood. Any child with "dermatomyositis" without a rash—which is absent in cases of polymyositis—should be evaluated very carefully.
- Children with the characteristic rash of dermatomyositis and elevated muscle enzymes should be treated even if they are not weak. It does not make sense to wait for things to get worse.
- If a child with dermatomyositis develops a nasal voice or begins to cough when eating, it may signal involvement of the swallowing muscles. This places the child at high risk of aspiration and is an indication for immediate aggressive treatment.

DERMATOMYOSITIS

Dermatomyositis in childhood is characterized by proximal muscle weakness and rash. In most cases the disease begins slowly with the gradual onset of progressive weakness. However, a small percentage of cases begin with dramatic fever, rash, elevated muscle enzymes, and profound weakness. Dermatomyositis may begin in any age group, sometimes affecting very young children and at other times teenagers. The dermatomyositis that occurs in adults appears to be different from the disease in childhood. The key to the diagnosis is recognition of progressive muscle weakness involving the upper arms and upper legs to a much greater degree than the hands and feet (i.e., proximal muscle weakness). It is always associated with a rash, usually on the upper eyelids and over the elbows and knees.

There are a number of illnesses that may cause muscle weakness in children. In addition to dermatomyositis, the gradual onset of weakness in small children can come from botulinum spores (found in organic honey and possibly other unpasteurized or improperly processed foods), intrinsic muscle diseases, including muscular dystrophy, and a variety of metabolic diseases. The abrupt onset of muscle weakness may occur with viral infections, insecticides and other poisons, certain venomous snakebites, and some medications. During some flu epidemics many children will complain of pain in their calves and have elevated muscle enzyme levels. *The key finding that differentiates dermatomyositis from these conditions is selective proximal muscle weakness.* The children are weak everywhere, but the thighs and shoulders are much weaker than expected when compared with the hands and feet.

In children with dermatomyositis, hand and foot strength are relatively good (though they may be less than normal), while the ability to raise the hands over the head (e.g., when brushing the hair) and the ability to raise the legs (e.g., when going upstairs) are clearly reduced. An experienced physician can quickly recognize proximal muscle weakness. More important, any child of an appropriate age who cannot raise her arms over her head, get up easily from a chair, or get up off the floor without assistance should be evaluated by an experienced physician.

The diagnosis of dermatomyositis is made on the basis of the history and the physical examination findings plus appropriate blood tests. Either the creatinine phosphokinase (CPK) or the aldolase level will be abnormal in most children with dermatomyositis. These tests indicate muscle inflammation, but they can also be abnormal following viral infections or extensive physical activity (e.g., playing football, running track, lifting weights). Often these tests are not included in the routine metabolic panel and have to be specifically ordered by the physician. All of the "routine" tests, including the erythrocyte sedimentation rate, are occasionally normal, despite active dermatomyositis.

Absolute proof of dermatomyositis requires a muscle biopsy demonstrating the death of muscle cells with a characteristic pathologic pattern (perifascicular infiltration of inflammatory cells). The diagnosis can also be made if a electromyography (EMG) demonstrates a characteristic "spike and wave" pattern. The muscle biopsy and EMG must be done on the inflamed muscle. Since this is primarily a disease of the proximal muscles, doing the biopsy on a distal muscle is not helpful. In addition, not all proximal muscles may be equally involved. Biopsy of an uninvolved muscle may lead to a false negative pathology report.

Before a muscle biopsy is done it is often useful to obtain an MRI of the thighs. Inflamed muscles are swollen (edematous) and show up on the MRI because they have greater water content than uninflamed muscles. Thus, the MRI can show the surgeon which muscles are involved and where the biopsy is best done. However, once the MRI has demonstrated the inflamed muscles in a weak child, unless another cause of muscle inflammation is suspected, the muscle biopsy is academic. Many experienced physicians feel a muscle biopsy is unnecessary if the appropriate laboratory and physical examination findings are present. *Is a muscle biopsy necessary to make the diagnosis?* Most often I will not do a muscle biopsy. The characteristic history and examination findings with confirmatory laboratory tests are quite sufficient. If the MRI shows the inflamed muscles there can be little doubt of the diagnosis. Nonetheless, some families and physicians want the certainty that a biopsy provides. Unfortunately, children with dermatomyositis have poor skin healing. As a result the surgical site often breaks down and leaves a large scar where the biopsy was done.

The group of children who have a typical dermatomyositis-appearing rash with mildly elevated muscle enzymes but no evident weakness requires particular attention. These children clearly have the disease. Although I have heard physicians argue that they do not require treatment, the elevated muscle enzymes and rash are evidence of ongoing inflammation and damage. Rather than wait for things to get worse, I believe it is important to treat these children appropriately to bring the muscle inflammation under control. Often these children require only a short course of therapy and do well. This is a lot like putting out a small fire instead of standing around and waiting to see whether it turns into a bigger problem.

There are several subtypes of dermatomyositis that have been recognized by physicians. The most common form of dermatomyositis is typically referred to as **unicyclic**. This form of dermatomyositis most often occurs in small children, such as the girl described in the case history above. There is gradual onset of weakness and rash. On careful examination, these children do not have nail fold capillary abnormalities, poorly healing skin ulcers, or inflammation over the knuckles.

Children with **polycyclic** disease usually have the same initial symptoms as the children with unicyclic disease, but these children often do have nail fold capillary abnormalities, inflammation over their knuckles, and in some cases poorly healing skin ulcers. It is important to recognize that these children are different from the first group of children.

Treatment

Unicyclic dermatomyositis responds well to corticosteroids and typically disappears within six months of beginning treatment. Treatment beyond a modest to moderate dose of corticosteroids is rarely necessary. Long-term complications of this form of dermatomyositis (including calcifications) are very rare.

Treatment for children with polycyclic disease is more complex. They more often require moderate doses of corticosteroids and seem to relapse more often when the dosage is reduced. Methotrexate is often helpful for children with polycyclic disease, but these children may require therapy for six months or longer before they can be weaned off corticosteroids. Recurrences may occur, even years after the initial diagnosis. In some cases, children with polycyclic disease may require therapy with cyclosporine or, in rare cases, stronger immunosuppressive medications. Some physicians like to use intravenous gammaglobulin (IVIgG) in treating this group of children. I believe low-dose methotrexate is equally, if not more, effective, easier to administer, and far less costly. If they are aggressively treated, many of the children in this group do very well. Children with an extensive skin rash and skin ulcerations appear to have more severe disease and may follow a more protracted course.

Complications

Complications of properly treated unicyclic dermatomyositis are usually minor. There are two important types of complications that occur more frequently in children with polycyclic disease. Vasculitis (inflammation of the blood vessels) in the skin and muscles is characteristic of this form of the disease. Its presence is strongly suggested by the occurrence of nail fold capillary abnormalities and inflammation over the knuckles. In some children, there also may be vasculitis of the intestines that can produce severe abdominal pain and worrisome intestinal complications. Any child with dermatomyositis who has chronic or recurrent abdominal pain must be investigated very carefully. Vasculitis-related complications can also occur in other organ systems, including the central nervous system, lungs, and kidneys. Children with these complications are at significant risk and require aggressive therapy to minimize the chance of a poor outcome.

The second important type of complication that occurs more frequently in children with polycyclic disease is the development of **subcutaneous or intramuscular calcifications**. These calcifications appear as the muscle inflammation is disappearing and may be thought of as a scarring response. Unfortunately, they may cause major problems. The calcifications may become infected and there is a significant risk of severe infection. This most often occurs when the calcifications have formed over the elbows or other pressure points where they are constantly being irritated by pressure. They may spontaneously become swollen and tender, and then drain to the outside. The initial drainage most often is not infected, but once leakage to the outside occurs, there is a significant risk that the draining lesion will become infected.

Large calcifications within the musculature may be a source of ongoing muscular irritation and also may become infected. These calcifications can be seen easily on radiographs. Fine reticular calcification under the skin may also be seen on radiographs. There is little to be done for these complications. I have seen surgeons remove large calcifications, but this may be associated with poor wound healing and significant long-term problems. At one time, there were reports suggesting that these calcifications could be treated with warfarin, but this medicine has proven unsatisfactory. More recently, there have been reports describing substantial improvement of severe calcifications after treatment with bisphosphonates. The best therapy for calcifications is to prevent their occurrence by providing prompt diagnosis and treatment for children with dermatomyositis.

Children with polycyclic disease may have several recurrences of muscle inflammation over a period of two or three years. At the end of that period, they may be left with complications secondary to the development of calcifications or other internal organ involvement, but active muscle inflammation is less common. It is important to understand that individual muscle cells may undergo hypertrophy (grow larger) to increase strength, but we do not make new muscle cells. As a result, any muscle cells that die during the inflammatory phase of dermatomyositis are not replaced. While there are significant reserves, if too many are lost, a child will never be able to recover full strength. Again, prompt diagnosis and treatment are essential to the best outcome. Over time, many children with polycyclic disease slowly regain normal or near normal strength and are able to function well as adults. The calcifications may also disappear over a period of years, though not always and not all of them.

A third group of children with dermatomyositis has **chronic recurrent disease**. The relationship of this form of the disease to the other forms is unclear. Children with chronic recurrent dermatomyositis often appear more ill during the acute phase of their illness. Their muscle enzyme levels are often very high and do not seem to respond significantly to therapy. Vasculitis is a common component of this form of the disease. Children with chronic recurrent dermatomyositis frequently require treatment with corticosteroids and methotrexate, but may respond only incompletely. Fortunately, they are rarely as weak as their laboratory values would suggest. The long-term prognosis for this group is uncertain.

POLYMYOSITIS

> Sally was a six-year-old African American girl who was brought to me for a second opinion. Seven months previously, her mother had brought her to a local emergency room with cough, cold, and fever. Blood work was done and an X ray was taken. The child was sent home with cold medication. The next day, the emergency room physician called and insisted the child return to the hospital. Sally was hospitalized and begun on corticosteroids because her muscle enzymes were very elevated. After a week Sally was discharged and the corticosteroids were slowly withdrawn. Her mother had never noticed Sally to be weak and noted only the changes from being on steroids during the six months of therapy. At the end of six months, the corticosteroids were stopped completely. When the mother asked the doctors whether Sally was now well, she was told that nothing had changed. On evaluation, Sally was a delightful young lady with no muscle weakness. Laboratory testing, however, revealed a markedly elevated CPK with no additional findings. Sally has remained well for five years with no treatment, but her muscle enzymes remain elevated.

Polymyositis is extremely rare in childhood. The key factor differentiating it from dermatomyositis is the absence of rash. Children with polymyositis should have the same pattern of proximal muscle weakness as is seen in children with dermatomyositis. This is a rare condition and its natural history is unclear. We also are unsure of the significance of the muscle enzyme elevations in children, such as Sally, who have markedly elevated muscle enzymes without rash or evident weakness. Note that she was not being evaluated for weakness or pain; her elevated muscle enzymes were discovered "by accident." Her muscle enzymes did not normalize when she was initially treated, and since then she has done well without treatment. We do not know what the future holds for children such as this. None of those I have followed over the years has developed problems to date and I have followed some for more than seven years.

COMPLICATIONS OF DERMATOMYOSITIS AND POLYMYOSITIS

The common complications of dermatomyositis already have been discussed in the sections on unicyclic, polycyclic, and chronic recurrent disease above. In addition to these complications, there are rare complications related to **vasculitis of the central nervous system** (brain) in some cases of severe polycyclic disease. This can result in psychological disturbances, hallucinations, and even seizures. Children with these complications must be treated aggressively. The kidneys are also involved in some children with polycyclic or chronic recurrent disease. This may result in blood or protein in the urine (hematuria or proteinuria). Normally, this is not serious and does not lead to significant damage to the kidneys.

Lipodystrophy is a more unusual complication seen in some children with dermatomyositis. This condition is associated with widespread loss of subcutaneous fat. Some children have lesser areas of involvement, which is referred to as **localized** or **partial lipodystrophy**. Children with generalized lipodystrophy appear very thin. Characteristic of the loss of subcutaneous fat is the ability to easily see the blood vessels through the skin. Even in its partial form, this condition may be associated with abnormal lipid metabolism and diabetes with insulin resistance. Although some centers report this in as many as one-quarter of their patients, in most centers lipodystrophy is a rare complication. It may be seen in other rheumatic diseases, and its relationship to the diagnosis of dermatomyositis is unclear. Children with this condition will need to be under the care of a multidisciplinary team in an experienced center.

Medical treatment

The type of disease, the degree of weakness, and the nature of the complications determine the medical treatment of dermatomyositis. If a child is very weak, immediate intervention with high-dose intravenous steroids may be important. If a child has developed a nasal voice or has begun to cough when eating, immediate intervention is vital. These findings suggest weakness of the muscles needed for swallowing and thus indicate a risk of aspiration (food going into the lungs) that can be disastrous.

For children without evidence of vasculitis who are not profoundly weak, a low or moderate dose of corticosteroids is often sufficient. Some children with dermatomyositis have mild arthritis when they first come to a doctor's attention. This usually responds well to treatment with corticosteroids, but a brief course of nonsteroidal anti-inflammatory drugs (NSAIDs) may also be beneficial. Hydroxychloroquine (Plaquenil) is another drug that is often useful as a steroid-sparing agent in children with mild disease, especially where rash predominates.

Children with evidence of vasculitis (nail fold capillary abnormalities, poor wound healing, changes of the skin over the knuckles) often respond well to a moderate dose of corticosteroids. Typically, as the corticosteroids are withdrawn, these children develop recurrent problems. When this is the case, the addition of methotrexate is often beneficial. Alternative regimens include the use of cyclosporine, intravenous gammaglobulin, or—for severe methotrexate-resistant disease—cyclophosphamide. These agents are rarely necessary for unicyclic but may be necessary for more severe polycyclic dermatomyositis. Recently, preliminary reports have appeared describing the use of tumor necrosis factor alpha (TNF-α) blocking agents, such as etanercept and adalimumab, for the treatment of dermatomyositis (see Chapter 22).

Optimal therapy for chronic recurrent dermatomyositis and polymyositis in childhood remains unclear. These entities are not common. Most children are initially treated as if they had polycyclic disease, with subsequent therapy based on the severity of the symptoms and the experience of the physician. Children with characteristic rash and elevated muscle enzymes but not weakness do require treatment. We know they have ongoing inflammation, and there is no sense in waiting for enough muscle cells to die to make it obvious they are weak before we begin to treat them.

Over the long term, persistent weakness and secondary calcifications remain the most distressing problems for children with dermatomyositis. The weakness is the result of the death of muscle cells. Because we are unable to generate new muscle cells, the best therapy is prevention. Rapid diagnosis and appropriate treatment minimize the amount of muscle cell death. Since calcification in the skin and musculature is a healing response, early aggressive therapy is also the best means of preventing this problem. The role of bisphosphonates in the treatment of children with extreme cases of dystrophic calcification is under active investigation.

Physical therapy

Physical therapy to maintain range of motion and maximize the strength of the remaining musculature is a major component of care for children with dermatomyositis. During the period when there is active muscle inflammation, the therapists should concentrate on passive range of motion. Only after the muscle inflammation has been controlled should active exercises begin.

Surgical therapy

In general, surgical therapy is not a significant component of the care of children with dermatomyositis. Excision and drainage of infected calcifications may be necessary in some children. Poor wound healing limits the utility of surgical efforts to remove large calcifications. Children with inflammation of the vessels that supply blood to the intestines may require urgent surgical intervention.

Prognosis

The prognosis for most children with dermatomyositis is very good. Most children have unicyclic disease and do well. With early diagnosis and prompt therapy, most children with polycyclic disease also have a good outcome. An experienced medical team can usually handle recurrent infections of subcutaneous calcifications without major problems, provided the patient seeks care promptly. Most parents should regard dermatomyositis as a very treatable condition with an excellent prognosis.

Children with polycyclic disease associated with significant complications because of inflammation of the blood vessels supplying internal organs have a more guarded prognosis. This is also true for children who have lost substantial numbers of muscle cells or suffered significant intramuscular calcifications. These children should be referred to specialized centers where the best possible efforts can be made to avoid what is sometimes a very poor outcome. These cases are often the result of delayed diagnosis or inadequate therapy.

Recurrent lung infections resulting from excessive muscle loss leading to difficulty in coughing and maintaining respiration occur only in the most severe cases. Fortunately, such cases have become rare. It may not be possible to restore function to all of these children, and some of the most severe cases succumb to infections. However, with prompt diagnosis and treatment, the majority of children with dermatomyositis will do well.

17

Kawasaki Disease

Billy was a three-year-old boy who had always been in good health. Ten days before he was sent to my office, his mother noted that he appeared irritable. He had a low-grade fever and the next day he was taken to the pediatrician to be checked for an ear infection. The pediatrician noted that he had conjunctivitis (red, irritated eyes) and gave the mother drops. The pediatrician explained this was probably the result of a viral infection. Over the next two days Billy remained irritable. Although his eyes got better, his fever continued.

His mother noted a tender lump under his chin. She brought him back to the pediatrician. The pediatrician diagnosed cervical adenitis (an infection of a lymph gland in the neck area). Billy was started on antibiotics. He developed a rash the next day and the antibiotic was changed because he was possibly allergic. Three days later the mother returned to the pediatrician because Billy was not getting better. He still had fever; the tender lump under his chin was getting larger. Now his lips were dry and beginning to split. His tongue was red and irritated.

The pediatrician ordered laboratory tests and the white blood cell (WBC) count, erythrocyte sedimentation rate (ESR), and platelet count were all very high. Billy was sent to me and the diagnosis of Kawasaki disease was confirmed. He was treated with intravenous gammaglobulin (IVIgG) and his symptoms disappeared promptly. We monitored his heart and there was no sign of heart involvement. Billy recovered completely.

Things you need to know

- Kawasaki disease (KD) most often affects young children (mostly under the age of five years) and the diagnosis should be carefully questioned in anyone over the age of ten.

- *"Atypical" Kawasaki disease is almost always typical something else!*
- Children with Kawasaki disease who do not respond promptly to treatment with intravenous gammaglobulin should be carefully evaluated to be sure the diagnosis is correct, and corticosteroid treatment should be considered.
- It is not true that intravenous gammaglobulin is ineffective after the tenth day. Efficacy after the tenth day was never studied! The original study was set up to determine whether IVIgG was effective in preventing aneurysms. Since most aneurysms are thought to begin at or soon after day ten, earlier treatment gave IVIgG the best chance of blocking the aneurysms. Children seen after the tenth day were excluded from the study.
- If a child who is being evaluated for Kawasaki disease has a low platelet count, something is definitely wrong. KD does not cause low platelet counts.
- Kawasaki disease is not the only disease that causes coronary artery aneurysms or thickening of the coronary arteries on echocardiograms. These findings alone do not establish the diagnosis.
- Kawasaki disease is not the only condition that will cause peeling of the skin in the diaper area (perineum) or on the fingertips. Again, this finding does not establish the diagnosis.
- Anti-inflammatory therapy is important even after the IVIgG has been given. Children should be given one aspirin daily (baby aspirin for small children) to reduce the risk of heart problems, but traditional nonsteroidal anti-inflammatory drugs (NSAIDs), such as naproxen, are safer and easier to use as the main anti-inflammatory therapy. They can be given with the one aspirin daily. The NSAIDs should be continued until the erythrocyte sedimentation rate has been normal for several weeks. The duration of the aspirin therapy depends on the child's cardiac status.

Kawasaki disease usually begins in a young child as fever and irritability without apparent explanation. An ear infection may be suspected. Within the first few days, some children develop a swollen lymph node below the jaw. Usually, this is thought to be cervical adenitis and is treated with antibiotics. Young children with high fevers who do not develop a swollen lymph node are frequently begun on antibiotics for presumed ear infections. Some children already have a rash at this point, but often the child will develop a rash the next day that may be confused with an allergy to the antibiotic.

Physicians usually do not begin to think about KD until the child continues with fever and rash even after the antibiotics. In a typical case, the child will continue to look worse with inflammation of the eyes, which may look very bloodshot (nonpurulent conjunctivitis), and dry cracked red lips or an irritated tongue. These symptoms usually appear over the next few days of illness. Also about this time the hands and feet often become diffusely swollen. Laboratory tests indicate the white blood cell count is going up and so are the erythrocyte sedimentation rate and the platelet count, sometimes to very high levels. At this point your physician may recognize KD, or an infectious disease specialist may be called in to make the diagnosis of KD.

Early diagnosis of KD is difficult because many serious infections can look just like KD at the very beginning. The criteria require a fever for at least five days with no response to starting antibiotics. In careful studies, it has been noted that children with measles and severe streptococcal infections may fulfill the diagnostic criteria for KD. One interesting observation is the frequent occurrence of marked redness and swelling at the site of BCG vaccinations in children developing KD (note that bacillus calmete guerain [BCG] vaccinations are not commonly given in the United States).

Criteria for the diagnosis of Kawasaki Disease

Fever of at least five days' duration plus four or more of the following:

- Nonspecific rash, or polymorphic exanthem (any rash)
- Cracked (fissured), red lips or irritated tongue ("strawberry tongue")
- Diffuse swelling of the hands or feet with redness of the palms and soles
- Conjunctivitis, affecting both eyes without pus
- Swelling of the cervical nodes (nodes in the neck usually just under the chin)

ETIOLOGY

The cause of Kawasaki disease is not well understood. The disease tends to occur in epidemics, which suggests that it is an infection. However, infections usually spread among children in the same household. For KD it is rare (about 3%) to find a second child in the same household or a playmate with the disease. However, there is evidence that KD is spread by exposure to some type of agent. KD is more common in areas that have been recently flooded. It is also more common in households where the carpets have recently been shampooed. These observations suggest that dampness must play a role. Careful investigations of viruses, fungi, and bacteria have not been convincing. It is likely that KD is not a common result of an uncommon agent, but the uncommon result of a common agent. This would explain the disease's predilection for young children and occurrence in epidemics.

MEDICAL TREATMENT

Once the diagnosis of KD is established, the antibiotics can be stopped and appropriate anti-inflammatory therapy started. IVIgG is usually given right away because this often very quickly stops the inflammation associated with KD. The early administration of IVIgG (within ten days of the onset of symptoms) has been shown to reduce the risk of developing coronary artery aneurysms. If physicians are unsure of the diagnosis but want to treat with IVIgG, they should save a tube of blood for later serologic testing. IVIgG contains pooled antibodies from many different people. Once it has been given, serologic testing to look for other explanations for the child's illness will be unreliable for many weeks.

Some physicians mistakenly believe IVIgG should be given only during the first ten days of illness. This is wrong. Even if the disease has been going on for more than ten days, it is safe to give IVIgG, and the IVIgG is effective in treating the inflammation (see "Things You Need to Know" at the beginning of this chapter). The efficacy of IVIgG in preventing aneurysms when given after the tenth day has not been studied. However, it still does an excellent job of bringing the inflammation associated with KD under control.

Some children with KD have less common symptoms. One well-described pattern is the child with severe abdominal pain who has gallbladder involvement found on abdominal ultrasound. This responds to therapy for the KD and in most cases does not require special treatment. Severe headaches and neck pain are also well described but less common findings. Some children with KD develop **aseptic meningitis** ("aseptic" means not due to bacterial infection). If there is significant pain, a spinal tap may be necessary to make sure the child does not have bacterial meningitis. This is important because bacterial meningitis must be treated.

Arthritis with pain and swelling of the knees also occurs in some children with KD. Other uncommon but well-described findings include inflammation of the pancreas, the kidneys, and the urinary tract. All of these findings may confuse the physicians caring for the children, but in most cases if they are due to KD, they respond quickly to IVIgG therapy.

IVIgG treatment is followed quickly by an end to the fever and prompt improvement in other symptoms in children with typical KD. Occasionally, children require a second dose of IVIgG. *Any child who is not better after two doses of IVIgG should be carefully reevaluated.* I have seen children with polyarteritis nodosa, systemic onset JRA, and other rheumatic diseases and infections mistakenly diagnosed as having KD. They do not get better with IVIgG or improve only briefly.

At one time it was thought that treatment with corticosteroids might make a child with KD more likely to develop coronary artery aneurysms or make the aneurysms worse. This has now been disproven. If two doses of IVIgG have not made the child better, the diagnosis of KD should be reconsidered. In the absence of infection or other contraindication, corticosteroids may be given to children who have not responded to IVIgG. Although there are reported cases of children with KD improving significantly, then relapsing a few days later, this is rare. There are also reports of children having had KD twice, with months to years separating the episodes. These recurrences are very infrequent.

COMPLICATIONS

Once the diagnosis of KD has been properly established, the major concern is whether the child has any cardiac involvement. Early in the illness, a small number of children develop inflammation of the muscles of the heart (**pancarditis**). There are also children who develop coronary artery aneurysms very early in their disease. Children with very large coronary artery aneurysms (greater than 8 mm) early in KD have a high frequency of cardiac problems and should be cared for at an advanced center.

Fortunately, most children with KD have no aneurysms or only thickening of the coronary arteries on echocardiogram. This thickening is often not meaningful and can be seen in children who are sick with other conditions. Children without coronary artery aneurysms have an excellent prognosis. Although IVIgG decreases the frequency of coronary artery aneurysms, it does not always prevent them.

Children who do develop coronary artery aneurysms need careful follow up. There are two major concerns for children with coronary artery aneurysms. The first is that the aneurysm may become filled with clotted blood. This can cause a myocardial infarction by blocking the blood flow in the coronary artery. This complication may occur during the first weeks of illness. Fortunately, it is rare in children who are properly diagnosed and treated. The second major concern is that the area of the coronary artery damaged by the aneurysm may heal in a way that predisposes the child to heart problems years later. This is why it is important for children to have continued follow up by the cardiologist, even if they look perfect.

A small number of children with KD do develop aneurysms in other arteries of the body. These aneurysms may cause problems either during the initial illness or later. A variety of other unusual complications of KD have been described. Their relationship to the disease is uncertain. The long-term prognosis for most children who have been properly treated for KD is believed to be excellent.

DIFFERENTIAL DIAGNOSIS

The most important aspect of the diagnosis and treatment of KD is prompt recognition of the disease. At the same time, it is important to remember that there are a variety of illnesses that may produce a similar appearance. It is very important to be sure that the child is not suffering from a significant infection. Measles, streptococcal infections, drug reactions, and many forms of vasculitis may result in a clinical picture that satisfies the criteria for a diagnosis of KD. Hemolytic uremic syndrome has also been confused with KD.

There is a significant concern that children diagnosed with atypical KD in fact have another illness. Such children should be carefully evaluated. Coronary artery aneurysms may occur in children with a number of rheumatic diseases, including polyarteritis nodosa and Takayasu's arteritis. Further, thickening of the coronary arteries on echocardiogram is a nonspecific finding and should not be used to establish a diagnosis of KD. It may occur in many other conditions.

Mucocutaneous lymph node syndrome is simply an old name for KD. This is the name it was originally given by Dr. Kawasaki, who first recognized the syndrome among his patients in Japan. The name was changed to honor him years after his initial description of the disease. There is also an illness called **infantile polyarteritis nodosa**. The clinical symptoms of this disease are different from the normal symptoms of KD. However, when specialists compare the pathologic material from children who died of KD with material from children who died of infantile polyarteritis, it is not possible to distinguish the diseases. Most likely, infantile polyarteritis is KD. It is now rare for anyone to make the diagnosis of infantile polyarteritis.

Laboratory findings in KD typically include a dramatically rising white blood cell count, erythrocyte sedimentation rate, and platelet count. Failure of any of these indices to rise appropriately by the seventh day of illness should raise suspicion. A falling platelet count is never consistent with the diagnosis of KD unless there are severe complicating factors. Although small amounts of red and white blood cells may appear in the urine, significant kidney involvement is not a normal manifestation of KD. These findings should cast doubt on the diagnosis of KD and prompt a thorough reevaluation of the child.

18

Benign Hypermobile Joint Syndrome and Ehlers Danlos Syndrome

Benign hypermobile joint syndrome is not really a disease at all. Instead, *it is an inherited variation on normal*. Children with benign hypermobile joint syndrome are often referred to as double-jointed. Many children have loose joints or joints that pop out easily. The diagnosis of benign hypermobile joint syndrome requires that a child be able to do each of the following.

- Bend the fingers back over the wrist so that they are parallel with the forearm (i.e., they point straight backward)
- Easily bend the thumb back to touch the forearm
- Fully straighten (extend) the elbow all the way beyond straight (hyperextension)
- Fully straighten the knee beyond straight
- Bend the foot up to a greater degree than normal

The ability to bend joints to a greater than normal degree does not normally seem to be a handicap. Indeed, many young girls with benign hypermobile joint syndrome are extremely good gymnasts. They can do splits and other gymnastic activities that the other girls can only imagine doing. The problem becomes evident when they do too much gymnastics too early in life. Read Tania's story at the beginning of Chapter 5.

The role of the ligaments is to maintain the joints in proper position with respect to each other. If they are loose, they don't perform this function properly. Imagine that you have two sets of little wooden trains to play with. For one set the train cars are connected by metal hooks that hold each car firmly attached to the car in front. This train may not be able to turn sharply, but all of the cars will always remain in proper position. If you don't intentionally damage the set, the wooden train will stay in perfect condition. Now imagine another set with the train cars held to each other by rubber bands. These cars will be able to move about much more flexibly and the train will be able to make very sharp turns without difficulty. However, when you pull the train forward the second car may not begin to move right away. Instead it waits for the rubber band to become tight before moving. The same thing happens with each of the remaining cars. Once they all start to move the train will move well until the first car stops. Then the momentum of the second car is likely to cause it to crash into the back of the first car. Each of the remaining cars will also crash into the car in front of it. If you play with this train set very often, all of the cars will be damaged by the repeated crashes. Pretty soon it won't look nearly as good as the first train set.

In children with benign hypermobile joint syndrome, the ligaments are loose and the bones making up the joints are not held tightly in position. This allows the bones on each side of the joint to knock into each other repeatedly. Over time this leads to damage to the bones and joints that may become quite severe. You can't surgically fix the ligaments that are loose because the collagen they are made from is genetically weaker. The key is to recognize the syndrome and allow the children to reduce their activity and minimize the damage.

Most often the children I see with benign hypermobile joint syndrome are ten- or eleven-year-old girls who have been recognized to have a lot of talent in physical education class. They are taking extra gymnastics or ballet and are felt to have great potential. However, they are beginning to complain of pains in their knees or other joints after practice. This can result from overuse of normal joints, but the child with ligamentous laxity is likely to have both earlier problems and more severe problems. If the activity has been continued despite the pain, there may be joint swelling and pain on compression of the bones around the joint.

MEDICAL TREATMENT

The joint pains and irritation associated with benign hypermobile joint syndrome can be relieved with mild nonsteroidal anti-inflammatory drugs (NSAIDs), but the key to proper treatment is minimizing the activity until the body matures further.

PROGNOSIS

Most children with benign hypermobile joint syndrome do very well. They may need to work with a physical therapist to strengthen the muscles around the joint. Surgery is necessary only if severe joint damage has occurred. This is rarely the case. I occasionally see children who have had repeated surgery in an effort to stop the joint from popping out (recurrent subluxation). Because the ligaments are not made up of strong material, this surgery often fails repeatedly. It is best avoided if possible.

Significant complications of benign hypermobile joint syndrome are very rare. However, it is important to recognize that the same material that is used in making ligaments is used in making internal structures such as the ring (aortic root) where the aorta (the large main blood vessel that carries blood to the rest of the body) connects to the heart. If a child has very significant ligamentous laxity, he or she should have an echocardiogram done to look for any loosening of the aortic root. If this ring tears, it can cause a rip to form in the aorta and this can lead to sudden death if the aorta tears open. This probably does not happen to children with benign hypermobile joint syndrome, but some children with Ehlers Dahnlos syndrome are mistakenly thought to have only benign hypermobile joint syndrome.

At the present time, the relationship of Ehlers Danlos syndrome and benign hypermobile joint syndrome is complicated by a disagreement over nomenclature. Some physicians refer to benign hypermobile joint syndrome as Ehlers Danlos type V. This causes the children's parents to become very alarmed unnecessarily.

Classical Ehlers Danlos syndrome is a child who is tall (usually thin) with long arms, long legs, and long thin fingers (children with Marfan's syndrome may also have some of these characteristics). These children have a severe defect in their collagen and are easily recognized because it is easy to stretch their skin. If these children have a cut, it will heal poorly and the scars often become unusually large and thin ("cigarette paper" scars). By the time they are ten or eleven years old, these children have often had multiple orthopedic problems because of the loose ligaments. In contrast, a child with benign hypermobile joint syndrome may just be coming to medical attention at this age.

If you are evaluating a child for benign hypermobile joint syndrome, you should look carefully for any unusual scars. Ask the parents how well the child's skin heals. Any child with unusual scars, poor healing, or unusually loose joints should be referred to an experienced center where a complete evaluation for the possibility of Ehlers Danlos syndrome can be done. The evaluation of children in whom Ehlers Danlos syndrome is suspected should include an echocardiogram to evaluate the aortic root. This should be done when they are first brought to the physicians' attention, and periodically thereafter. However, it is unclear that children with simple benign hypermobile joint syndrome ever have these problems. If you are in doubt you should refer the child for further evaluation, but I would avoid scaring the parents by calling the problem Ehlers Danlos syndrome.

19

Fibromyalgia and Chronic Fatigue Syndrome

THINGS YOU NEED TO KNOW

The most important thing to remember in evaluating a child with fibromyalgia or chronic fatigue syndrome is to be sure the diagnosis is correct. Although these are complex syndromes that may be difficult to treat, many of the children who come to me who were originally diagnosed with these diseases had not gotten better because fibromyalgia or chronic fatigue were not the correct diagnosis. Every child with chronic pain and fatigue deserves a complete and thorough diagnostic evaluation. There should not be any significant laboratory abnormalities in children with either fibromyalgia or chronic fatigue.

Sue Ellen was a sixteen-year-old who complained of fatigue and weakness. She was unable to go to school because she could not get out of bed in the morning, complaining of hurting all over. Six months previously she had developed a severe viral infection with fever, rash, and diffuse aches and pains. Although the fever and rash had resolved within a week, she had never regained her strength. She had been seen by several physicians and had been treated for Lyme disease—despite negative blood tests—without response. A thorough physical examination and comprehensive testing found no abnormalities except for multiple trigger points (areas of the muscle that when compressed cause pain). It was carefully explained to Sue Ellen and her family that we would have to all work together to make her better. With the help of parents, family, and friends, a program of steadily increasing activities and school attendance was devised. She often became discouraged because she would try to do too much and exhausted herself. It took several months for Sue Ellen to resume her normal activities. However, once she realized that she was the most important member of the team working to make her better, she made steady progress to a full recovery.

Tracy was brought to me at the age of fourteen years, after being diagnosed with fibromyalgia by another physician. Tracy was obese and came from a troubled family. She was not very interested in physical activities and complained that she hurt all over and tired easily. Pressure over the expected trigger points for fibromyalgia produced complaints, but so did pressure in many other places. Laboratory evaluation indicated a mild elevation of the sedimentation rate and a positive antinuclear antibody (ANA) but nothing specific. Tracy was started on medication for fibromyalgia and followed carefully. After a few visits she came to trust me and openly asked for help with her depression. She was referred to a psychologist.

Over the next six months it was noted that Tracy was developing an increasing number of red spots on her hands and face. When examined, it was clear that these were telangiectasias. Testing for anticentromere antibody revealed that she was positive in extremely high titer, and we were able to begin appropriate treatment for her CREST syndrome. Had she simply been dismissed as another teenager with fibromyalgia, appropriate therapy for her CREST syndrome would have been significantly delayed and her prognosis worsened.

Mrs. Smith was the mother of a three-year-old girl who was referred to the neurology clinic because she was developing slowly ("developmental delay"). When the pediatricians evaluated Mrs. Smith's daughter, they found she did not reach the milestones of sitting independently, crawling, or walking by herself at appropriate ages. Even after she was able to do these activities, the little girl never wanted to play as much as her friends. She seemed very bright otherwise. She just "tired out" too easily. During the evaluation of her daughter it was noted that doctors had diagnosed Mrs. Smith with chronic fatigue syndrome. Mrs. Smith reported that all her life she had tired easily and never been good at getting everything done. Even as an adult she had been sent to a psychiatrist because she felt too worn out to get all her household chores done every day. Her doctors felt she was a typical case of chronic fatigue syndrome.

As the evaluation of Mrs. Smith's daughter progressed, it was evident that she was abnormally weak. A muscle biopsy was performed and it was found that the little girl had nemaline myopathy. This is an inherited condition that produced muscle weakness. Talking to Mrs.

Smith, the neurologist who cared for her daughter realized that Mrs. Smith had all the symptoms of nemaline myopathy as well. A muscle biopsy was performed and it was confirmed. Mrs. Smith's doctors had not realized that she had a genetic muscle abnormality. The diagnosis of chronic fatigue syndrome was wrong. Her case illustrates why it is important to make sure that a diagnosis of chronic fatigue syndrome is correct. However, it should be remembered that Mrs. Smith had been weak all her life. This is not the expected history in someone with chronic fatigue syndrome.

WHAT IS FIBROMYALGIA?

Children with **fibromyalgia** complain of widespread pain and fatigue that interfere with normal activities. Often they have missed many days of school because of difficulty getting up in the morning. With increasing school absences, these children have often been to a variety of physicians without a definitive diagnosis. The generally accepted criteria for a diagnosis of fibromyalgia require widespread pain (above and below the waist and on both the right and left sides) and the presence of at least eleven of eighteen defined "trigger points."

Many different causes of fibromyalgia have been proposed, but none is uniformly accepted. It often follows a severe viral infection or an injury. For the majority of children, it appears that the child never fully recovered from the injury or infection. Often the doctors have become frustrated because "it should have gotten better a long time ago." Because of the long-term nature of their complaints and their poor response to medications, children with fibromyalgia have one of the most challenging illnesses faced by physicians today.

Proposed explanations for the continuing pain and fatigue suffered by children with fibromyalgia emphasize increased sensitivity of the nervous system. This has been ascribed to damaged nerve conduction pathways, altered hormonal balance, persisting infectious agents, and many other possible causes. *None of the proposed explanations has provided the scientific basis for consistently useful therapy*. This has resulted in a large number of frustrated families and physicians.

The children and their families do not understand why the doctors cannot make them better. I often see children who have had a bad viral infection just like several of their friends, but unlike their friends, they just never recovered. They continue to complain that they are tired and do not feel well. Often they do not go to school or miss as many days of school as they attend. Whenever they try to do what doctors recommend to help them get better, it just makes them feel worse.

The first thing to do in such circumstances is a thorough historical, physical, and laboratory evaluation to find out whether something has been missed. Often this will yield an unsuspected clue and the child's regimen can be adjusted so that he or she recovers. However, in many cases, no explanation is found, but the child remains disabled.

CHRONIC FATIGUE SYNDROME

Chronic fatigue syndrome differs from fibromyalgia because the patients lack the typical trigger points associated with fibromyalgia. Like fibromyalgia, chronic fatigue syndrome is not associated with laboratory abnormalities, a known cause, or a known cure. Before accepting this label for their child, every family must be sure that a careful and complete medical evaluation has been done. Had Mrs. Smith's doctors listened to her history of lifelong weakness and carefully tested her strength, they would have suspected that she had a genetic disease.

Once the diagnosis of chronic fatigue syndrome has been established and other significant medical problems have been excluded, children with chronic fatigue syndrome should be rehabilitated just as I describe for fibromyalgia in the next section.

HOW TO TREAT FIBROMYALGIA AND CHRONIC FATIGUE SYNDROME

In the absence of a well-accepted scientific explanation for fibromyalgia, many physicians and families feel frustrated. They are waiting for someone to discover the cause and the cure. Unfortunately, they feel helpless because they do not know what to do. I point out to these families that simply tolerating the situation is unacceptable. Often, too much time and money have been wasted on promised "miracle cures," such as natural medicines, diets, or supplements. Instead, I ask the families to think of how they would respond if a truck had hit their child.

If you were walking in the crosswalk and got hit by a truck, you could easily suffer damage to the bones in both of your legs. This often requires operations to correct the fractures, and you are flat on your back in traction for many weeks. Then one day the orthopedist comes into the room, orders the traction removed, and announces that your bones have healed. The problem is that you do not just get up out of bed and walk away cured. While you have been flat on your back waiting for the bones to heal, you have suffered a major loss of muscle strength and endurance.

It is very difficult to start walking again. Even sitting over the side of the bed may make you dizzy. Relearning how to walk and rebuilding your strength and endurance is a slow and painful process. But there is no pill that makes it easy to do. In order to recover, people who have suffered major injuries go through a long and difficult period of gradual recovery of strength and range of motion. There is no magic. They have to do the work. The physicians and physical therapists can all provide guidance and encouragement, but only the patients can make themselves better. Emotionally, it's relatively easy if a truck hit you. There are lots of witnesses to what happened and no one is thinking this is your fault.

Children with fibromyalgia are suffering a similar degree of disability and have an equally difficult path to recovery. But it's much harder when no one understands what hit them. However, there is still only one person who can get these children going again, and that person is the patient him- or herself. There is no magic pill for fibromyalgia any more than there is a magic pill for being hit by a truck.

My own approach to caring for children with fibromyalgia is to emphasize rehabilitation and return to activities of daily living. If one views recovery from fibromyalgia as one would view recovery from a major physical injury, the appropriate steps become self-evident. At every step, the child, family, and physicians must recognize that there will not be a sudden, miraculous recovery. Progress is made through a rigorous program of slow and steadily increasing level of activities, just as if both legs had been broken. It is equally important for every member of the team to acknowledge the reality of the initial injury and the psychological difficulty of dealing with it, just as they would acknowledge the difficulty of recovering if the child had been hit by a truck.

The absence of a uniformly effective therapy for fibromyalgia places a significant burden on parents and physicians caring for these children. Several key points must be remembered.

- This is not a self-induced illness. The children definitely do want to get better.
- Children with this illness suffer from disordered sleep patterns.
- Opiate pain medications do not relieve any symptom other than pain. They frequently cause nausea, worsen sleep patterns, in-

crease ones' overall sense of ill health, and interfere with school attendance and normal life.

- Depression probably does not cause fibromyalgia, but fibromyalgia definitely does cause depression.

Children hit by trucks often recover faster than children with fibromyalgia because everyone understands their injury and everyone understands what has to be done to make them better. We need to treat children with fibromyalgia the same way.

Some children recover well with time, reassurance, medications, and support from their family and doctors. For more difficult cases, a hospital-based team approach is often beneficial. The team in a large children's rehabilitation center consists of nurses, social workers, psychologists, and pediatricians. Most often even children with difficult-to-treat fibromyalgia can be managed on an outpatient basis, but that does not eliminate the need for all the members of the team to participate in their care. Once the diagnosis of fibromyalgia has been confirmed, it is important for the family to meet with all the appropriate members of the team. Even while this is being done, the family can take the first steps toward recovery.

STEPS TO RECOVERY

Getting back on schedule

Anyone who has traveled overseas and suffered jet lag can immediately relate to the impact of disordered sleep patterns. Although a variety of remedies may be useful, the key to all of them is promptly to begin to set your body's wake/sleep cycle on the appropriate schedule for the time zone you are in. Similarly, families can start children back on a regular schedule of getting up at an appropriate time in the morning (the same time as if they were going off to school normally). This should be accompanied by a policy on lights, computers, televisions, video games, and so on that must be turned off at the appropriate time for a school night. *Do not expect instant success.* Inexperienced travelers often report two to three weeks of difficulty in adjusting to a new time zone. However, if you get up at the appropriate time in the morning, it becomes easier and easier to fall asleep at the appropriate time and sleep through the night.

Increasing physical activity

Even as the child is adjusting to getting up at the appropriate time each morning, it is important to begin a program of gradually increasing physical activity. For children in the rehabilitation center, this is done under the supervision of a physical therapist. For children being treated as outpatients, this may not be necessary if they are attending school. Children who are not attending school will need regularly scheduled physical therapy at least three days a week with parent-supervised physical activity on the other days. Too often families overreach in this initial physical therapy.

A child who has been incapacitated for a prolonged period will need to start exercising slowly. At first, three or four sessions of exercise lasting only fifteen minutes each may be all the child is capable of in a given day. Significant muscular discomfort normally accompanies the resumption of activities in someone who has been disabled for a prolonged period. This discomfort may be treated with nonsteroidal anti-inflammatory drugs (NSAIDs), topical creams for sore muscles, and massage. The key to the success of this program is that it be continued despite the muscle soreness and related complaints.

Physical and occupational therapy

Physical and occupational therapy play a vital role in the care of children with severe fibromyalgia. Just as children severely injured by a truck would never be expected to recover without physical therapy, a child with severe fibromyalgia should not be expected to do it on his or her own, either. The key is finding a therapist who understands that the injury in fibromyalgia is every bit as real as the injury to the child who was hit by a truck. The program of slowly increasing physical activities to improve strength and endurance must be tailored to the disability level of the child. However, it must have the ultimate goal of complete recovery. If a truck had hit the child, everyone would understand that complete recovery might require months of therapy and that even a year later the child might not be fully recovered. Fibromyalgia is no different.

Psychological and emotional support

During the initial weeks of establishing a program of normal wake/sleep hours and exercise, *it is normal for the child to increase his or her complaints and the parents to become discouraged.* Psychological and emotional support from the family and the psychologist treating the child is critical at this point. Antidepressant medications may be necessary for some children during this stage. Over a period of three months it should be possible to gradually increase the level of physical activity to the point where the child feels capable of returning to school. In a rehabilitation setting, this corresponds to three or more thirty-minute periods of sustained exercise each day.

It is normal for children to experience significant discomfort and resist the program of rehabilitation at several key points in time. Despite the best of intentions, at the beginning they will experience difficulty adjusting their sleep schedule and resuming physical activity. There is frequently another period of difficulty and resistance six to eight weeks into the program. At this point, children frequently decide, "This is not working and I'm tired of it." *Just as we would never allow a child to give up on recovering after being hit by a truck, we cannot let these children give up on recovering, either.* These periods of stress and frustration are a normal part of every recovery. Parents and even the children should be told to expect these periods in advance of their occurrence. Continuing physical, emotional, and psychological support is key to working through these episodes.

The major long-term disability associated with fibromyalgia results from the loss of strength and endurance and the accompanying loss of self-confidence and self-esteem that these children suffer. If a child was hit by a truck and had bad dreams or was afraid to return to school, no one would be embarrassed to ask for psychological help. Unfortunately, because we do not understand what happened to them, children with fibromyalgia often do not get the sympathetic support given to children with obvious injuries. From a psychological point of view, this makes the situation much worse for children with fibromyalgia. A sympathetic family, a sympathetic physician, and a sympathetic psychologist or psychiatrist are all very important.

Just as we would force a child who had an obvious physical injury to do the work necessary to recover, we must push the child with fibromyalgia to recover. Psychological support is critical for both the child and the family when the inevitable resistance occurs. There is no magic pill or diet. The physical and emotional pain of going a little bit farther every day and trying a little bit harder every day is often best dealt with by solid emotional support. A psychologist or psychiatrist can play a vital role in helping the child and family to deal with these issues.

Expect a relapse

Some children will relapse within four to six weeks of returning to school and having a full, normal schedule. The rehabilitation team routinely anticipates this setback. Children are so anxious to succeed that they often push themselves beyond their limits during their first days back.

Depending on the situation, the rehabilitation team may choose initially to have the child restart school on a part-time basis in order to avoid this problem. This is a decision that should be made by the entire team working together.

Periodic relapse or fear of relapse in association with viral infections and other stresses may occur. The key to successful management of these episodes is for the child and family to pull together and keep things on track. While it may be necessary to spend twenty-four to forty-eight hours in bed with "the flu," it is essential that children with a history of fibromyalgia promptly get themselves back on their feet and resume normal activity. The attitude of the rehabilitation team and family must be one of steady reassurance and support for the child.

Equally important in the care of children with fibromyalgia is recognition of the needs of the other family members (see Chapter 26). Children who are recovering from a severe illness are placed under significant additional stress when the stress of their illness is visibly upsetting other family members. Given the difficult nature of the gradual recovery process following any major injury, this additional stress may cause a significant psychological setback. This is why it is important that the entire family, including parents and siblings, be involved in the educational activities and psychological counseling that are part of the rehabilitation process. Too often other family members view the sensitivity of the child with fibromyalgia as manipulative behavior. These complex dynamics can be properly dealt with only if the entire family is willing to participate in the process.

Treatment in the home

Children with mild cases of fibromyalgia often do not require hospitalization. Their treatment should be based on the same principles as described above. It may be slower and more difficult because it is harder to provide a consistent wake and sleep schedule and physical therapy in the home environment. The key to success is willing participation by all family members. Everyone needs to help the affected child to recover. Often the school district has nurses and psychologists who can coordinate their efforts with the treating physician. Central to all of this is education of those caring for the child. Physicians, nurses, teachers, or others who convey a negative attitude toward children with fibromyalgia need to be properly educated.

Episodes of resentment and resistance are just as likely for children being treated at home as those treated in the hospital. Parents must be properly instructed both to expect these episodes and to deal with them in an understanding manner. However, understanding does not mean giving in. The program of exercises and activities necessary to regain strength and confidence can succeed only if it is carried out. Families that find themselves unable to handle the ups and downs of managing a child with fibromyalgia at home will need to consider inpatient therapy. With appropriate support from the physician and other care providers, most families can succeed.

Medical treatment

Medications are a key component of therapy for adults with fibromyalgia. They are less important in children. However, NSAIDs, including tramadol, may be helpful in controlling the aches and pains associated with activity. Amitriptyline is an antidepressant that has been found to have beneficial effects for children and adults with fibromyalgia. While some of the benefit may be from the antidepressant effect, amitriptyline appears to have additional effects that help fibromyalgia sufferers. Children who are greatly troubled by muscle spasm often benefit from the addition of cyclobenzaprine or a similar agent (all of these drugs are discussed in Chapter 22).

What I have described in this chapter is not a cure for fibromyalgia. None exists. Nor is there a cure for having been hit by a truck. Our goal must be to help children overcome the symptoms of fibromyalgia and regain useful lives. Children with fibromyalgia must be educated to understand their illness and how to cope with it. With the benefit of this knowledge, they can deal with recurrent symptoms that might occur and continue their lives in a normal fashion.

PROGNOSIS

The prognosis for children with fibromyalgia or chronic fatigue syndrome who get proper care is excellent. However, just as a child left to languish in bed after an injury would do poorly, so will a child with these illnesses. There is no reason that a child with fibromyalgia or chronic fatigue syndrome should not be able to be rehabilitated and to resume a fully productive life.

20

Reflex Sympathetic Dystrophy, Reflex Neurovascular Dystrophy, and Complex Regional Pain Syndromes

Fourteen-year-old Cindy was the ultimate figure skater. Her parents had met while skating in college. Briefly after college, her father had skated professionally, but shortly after graduating from college her mother stopped skating so they could start a family. Cindy's father was now a successful businessman, and Cindy's mother stayed home to promote Cindy's development as a figure skater. Cindy had been skating for as long as she could remember. But for the past six months Cindy had been unable to skate because of ankle pain. There was no doubt about how Cindy's ankle was injured. Hundreds of spectators witnessed her fall at the regional skating championships. X rays did not show a fracture but her orthopedist immediately placed her foot in a cast to rest the ankle and make sure it healed properly.

After three weeks of complete rest, the orthopedist expected Cindy to require only a few days of physical therapy before resuming full normal activity. However, when the cast was removed, Cindy continued to complain of pain and was unable to bear weight on her foot. Over the last few months every study has been performed to evaluate the ankle and find out why Cindy cannot walk or skate on it. Her blood work is normal, the MRI is normal, and X rays show only some mild osteoporosis (loss of bone density). Her bone scan shows patchy uptake that does not suggest a specific diagnosis. Since it has been six months from the time of her injury, Cindy's parents and the orthopedist are pulling their hair out.

Cindy's foot and ankle are steadily getting worse. The entire foot is purplish in color and cool to the touch. Cindy cannot put a shoe or sock on her foot and often complains that even the weight of a sheet on her foot causes severe pain. Figure skating and Cindy's entire future have been put on hold. How can she go on to become a professional figure skater and fulfill her dreams? Her parents are willing to try anything.

Reflex sympathetic dystrophy (RSD), reflex neurovascular dystrophy, and complex regional pain syndrome are all various names for the same condition. It is a cause of great frustration for parents and physicians, and it is far more common than you might think. RSD can involve the foot or hand. It rarely occurs in children under the age of ten, but may occur at any age thereafter. Because there is virtually always a well-documented history of injury, families and physicians are often distraught over their inability to fix the problem. The child who has suffered the injury is invariably described as "my best child," "the hardest worker," "truly dedicated," and so on.

The key to understanding RSD is to recognize that the problem is no longer a simple physical injury. Children with RSD are overachievers who have been put under too much pressure to perform. At first, parents often refuse to believe this. Like Cindy's parents, they know their child loves the activities she is involved in. The parents are sure they are not driving the child; the child is driving him- or herself to achieve. Any suggestion that there may be a psychological aspect to the problem is immediately rejected.

Frank was a twelve-year-old boy who loved to play tennis. He was referred to me because of pain in his hands with no obvious explanation. Could this be arthritis? The orthopedist had given up and the pediatrician knew that some recurrent athletic injuries were in fact arthritis. What did I think? On the first visit I took a detailed history from Frank and his mother. Frank's pain was only with activities. He did not complain of stiffness or pain at any other time. In fact, he could type and play computer games without difficulty. But he could not play tennis. Prior to seeing me Frank had had extensive X rays but no blood tests. I performed all the appropriate blood tests for arthritis, Lyme disease, and less common conditions and gave Frank a brief trial of nonsteroidal anti-inflammatory drugs (NSAIDs).

When Frank returned two weeks later, the blood tests were all normal, but there was no improvement. He still had to put the tennis racquet down as soon as he started to play. As I was questioning Frank, he and his mother began to argue. As I listened quietly they agreed to settle their argument "on the tennis court." It took only a few probing questions to determine that everyone in Frank's family was a big tennis player. Their usual way of settling disagreements was to play a tennis match. Winner of the tennis match was winner of the argument. Except, because of his hand pains, Frank could not play. With a little luck and careful questioning, the answer was obvious. After a few visits to the psychologist by Frank and his family to discuss normal adolescent issues related to growing up, Frank's hand pain disappeared.

Frank did not have RSD, according to the official definition. With some insight everyone could understand that the problem was a need for the family to discuss issues honestly, not solve disagreements by getting on the court. Frank was not yet old enough to defeat his parents at tennis. His hand pain saved him from the continued humiliation of losing every time.

It took many months before Cindy's family would agree to psychological intervention. When they finally did agree to seek help, Cindy's symptoms began to slowly disappear. Over a further six months of physical and psychological therapy, Cindy recovered completely. She did not go on to become a professional figure skater. One of the first things the psychologist discovered was that Cindy had dreams of being a fashion designer, not a figure skater. However, when all was said and done, the whole family could enjoy skating and everyone ultimately accepted that Cindy needed to grow up to be what Cindy wanted to be, not what her parents wanted her to be.

Extensive experience with children with RSD has allowed physicians to understand that it is invariably a "cry for help." The problem may be as obvious as Frank's or much more complex. The key to solving the problem is for everyone involved to realize after careful investigation that it is not simply a physical injury. Once this is done, the child and family can concentrate on solving the related issues and working with their physicians and psychologists to fully resolve the problem. Physical therapy is often still necessary because of the long period of disuse.

The first step in treating a child with RSD is to make sure the diagnosis is correct. As much as I have seen physicians fail to make this diagnosis, I have had children with undiagnosed arthritis referred as having RSD. The blood work is usually normal. In long-standing cases, X rays may show some mild osteoporosis due to disuse. An MRI may show some patchy marrow edema, and the bone scan may show increased uptake, decreased uptake, or patchy increased and decreased uptake.

On physical exam, the involved hand or foot is often markedly discolored. It may feel warm to the touch, but far more often it is cold. The child is often very tense when you examine the involved limb and may cry out with pain. However, it is often possible to distract or calmly to reassure the child and proceed to examine the limb fully. Often a child will cry out when I first take an involved foot in my hand, but then calm quickly as I rub the foot gently and continue to talk to him or her about a favorite activity. Most often, this will not work if there is a fracture, infection, tumor, or other significant injury.

Making the diagnosis of RSD is usually far easier than explaining the diagnosis to the family and getting them to accept the diagnosis. Affected children are almost invariably overachievers who are very anxious to please their parents. In many cases, the combination of an abnormal bone scan and the obvious initial injury make it very difficult for the parents to accept the idea that there is a psychological issue.

RSD is a true somatization disorder. This means that the child really feels the pain, and the pain is real. *The child is not making up a complaint of pain to manipulate the parents.* Since the child is in pain and the injured extremity is discolored, parents ask, "How can this be psychological?" It takes a lot of explaining to make the family realize that you do not think this is something the child is making up. RSD is not a voluntary illness. The children do not think to themselves, "If I say my foot hurts, I will not have to skate any more." *Whatever goes on in somatization disorders happens at a subconscious level that the child is no more aware of than the parents.*

TREATMENT

Once the diagnosis has been correctly made, physical therapy and psychological therapy become equally important. Physical therapy should concentrate on desensitization. The key is to persistently massage the tender extremity and gradually reassure the child that it is safe to put on a sock, to walk on the foot, or to use the hand. This is a process that may require weeks to months to accomplish. It should be accompanied by ongoing family psychological therapy to help the family and child understand the origins of the problem. (I have seen families refuse the psychological aspects of care and insist on only physical therapy. Although physical therapy may help even in the absence of psychological therapy, it fails to address the fact that this illness is a cry for help. In several cases, children whose parents refused psychological intervention when I diagnosed RSD recovered from their "injuries" but ultimately required psychiatric hospitalization.)

MEDICAL TREATMENT

Parents of children with RSD should be aware that pain specialists often believe that drug therapy is appropriate for these children. Corticosteroids, regional sympathetic blocks, and narcotic analgesics all may provide temporary relief but fail to address the primary underlying problem. In several studies of large groups of children, it has been shown that the long-term outcome is far better for children treated with physical and psychological therapy than for children treated with medications and injections.

21

Osteoporosis and Osteopenia

Charlotte was twenty-one years old when I first met her. She had been cared for by another rheumatologist for many years, but was referred to my hospital because of her need for joint replacement surgery. She was diagnosed with juvenile arthritis at the age of twelve years and treated with corticosteroids when her disease did not respond to NSAIDs. She felt much better with the corticosteroids and was able to attend school and go on to college. During the college years, Charlotte was away from home and managed her own medications. Although she was officially on a low dose of corticosteroids, Charlotte freely admitted that when she felt stiff or sore she would take extra. Charlotte completed college with honors and planned to go on to graduate school. However, she had fallen and broken her hip. X rays revealed that the hip had broken because her bones were so weak. Further evaluation revealed that she had weak bones throughout her body. Over the next few years she suffered multiple fractures with even the slightest injury. She continues with multiple operations, and because of her many problems she has never been able to attend graduate school.

Osteoporosis and osteopenia are conditions involving decreased bone mass and hence a decrease in the strength of the bones with an increased risk of fractures. A person has **osteopenia** if their bone mass is more than one standard deviation below the normal level and **osteoporosis** if their bone mass is more than two and a half standard deviations below the normal level. These definitions have been difficult to apply to children because the normal levels have not been well defined for children of different ages and races. However, precise medical definitions are not what parents should be concerned about. What it is important for parents to understand is that children who do not get enough calcium in their diet, children with chronic arthritis, children who take corticosteroids or certain other drugs (especially diuretics such as furosemide), and children with a variety of hormonal disorders are all at risk of decreased bone mass and easily broken bones.

Decreased bone mass in children is particularly disturbing because bone mass is normally increasing during childhood and then begins to decrease during adult life. If a child never reaches his or her expected peak bone mass level as a young adult, the risk of having significant problems later in life, as everyone's bone mass normally decreases, is much greater than normal. For parents, the first concern about osteoporosis or osteopenia may come when the doctor prescribes a medicine that is known to cause problems or when a doctor makes a casual comment when looking at the child's X rays. Sometimes the osteoporosis is not noticed until the child complains of back pain due to vertebral fractures that are the result of osteoporosis.

If your child is taking anticonvulsants (medicines for seizures), diuretics (medicine to help kidney function), or corticosteroids, you should be concerned about their effects on the child's bones. Children receiving drugs that are known to cause osteoporosis should be monitored carefully. If a child is discovered to have osteoporosis or osteopenia and is not known to have arthritis or be taking medicines that cause the problem, he or she should be carefully evaluated by an endocrinologist or other bone specialist to determine the cause. It is very rare for a child to have a low serum calcium level if he or she is consuming a normal diet. Most children with osteoporosis have normal serum calcium levels. *Young female athletes who train extensively while eating poorly are at particular risk for osteoporosis and stress fractures.* Teenagers should be specifically counseled that both alcohol and smoking increase the risk of osteoporosis.

Osteoporosis is best diagnosed and evaluated by physicians who are experienced in dealing with these problems. These may be orthopedists, endocrinologists, rheumatologists, or metabolic disease specialists. Although there are laboratory tests to help determine why a child has osteoporosis, *there are no laboratory tests that are regularly useful in detecting the problem.* While osteoporosis may be suspected on the basis of routine X rays, bone density studies should be done to confirm the diagnosis using DEXA (dual energy X-ray absorptiometry) or a similar technique. It is important to use a method of measuring bone density that will provide quantitative results so that changes in bone density can be followed over time.

COMPLICATIONS

The major complications of osteoporosis are fractures. These may be stress fractures in the limbs of athletes or vertebral fractures in children with chronic disease. Stress fractures become evident as pain at the site of the fracture. Vertebral fractures cause severe back pain. Occasionally, children are recognized to have osteoporosis only when they fracture an arm or leg after a minor fall. Because childhood is a time when bone mass is normally increasing, the most important complications of childhood osteoporosis may not occur until many years later. Everyone starts to lose bone mass gradually shortly before the age of thirty. Even if the loss of bone mass occurs at a normal rate, a person starting with a low bone mass because of childhood osteoporosis will reach a critical level much sooner than a normal individual.

For children with an underlying rheumatic disease, the key to the prevention of osteoporosis is control of the inflammatory process. However, while corticosteroids are effective anti-inflammatory agents, they promote osteoporosis. Their use should be restricted, but you do not want to risk serious damage from uncontrolled rheumatic disease because of the future risk of osteoporosis due to corticosteroids. *If a child or young adult requires corticosteroids, it is very important that he or she understands the importance of not taking extra when he or she feels bad.* The doctor may feel the need to increase the dose to improve disease control, but the doctor is also well aware of the need to reduce the dose as soon as possible. At one time it was thought that deflazacort might cause less bone loss than other corticosteroids, but this turned out not to be true when the dose was adjusted for equal anti-inflammatory effect.

MEDICAL TREATMENT

The most important element of treatment for childhood osteoporosis is prevention. Adequate calcium intake should be assured for every child. If extra calcium is given, it must be accompanied by vitamin D. While parents should assure that their children have adequate calcium and vitamin D in their diet, they must also avoid giving excessive amounts. *Excessive vitamin D consumption is dangerous and can be fatal.* Excessive intake of calcium should be avoided because it often causes constipation and stomach upset. This is not a situation where some is good so more must be better.

Attention to diet and appropriate supplementation should be adequate treatment for children with mild osteopenia. Children with fractures or DEXA-documented osteoporosis may require more aggressive therapy. However, appropriate treatment for children with osteoporosis remains controversial. Bisphosphorates such as Alendronate and other drugs used in adults may be required. They have been proven to reverse osteoporosis to some extent in children. However, their long-term safety for use in childhood is not established. Bisphosphonates are stored in the bones for many years. We do not know whether taking bisphosphonates earlier in life will cause problems for a woman if she becomes pregnant; this has limited our ability to use these drugs.

Calcitonin is an alternative therapy that deserves serious consideration. Calcitonin is a hormone that is normally made by the body to promote bone formation. Calcitonin isolated from fish is now available for prescription use. However, calcitonin is expensive and difficult to administer to children.

As noted above, the real key to successful treatment of osteoporosis is prevention. Monitoring the child's diet, avoiding smoking and alcohol ingestion, and whenever possible avoiding drugs that cause osteoporosis are easily taken steps that should minimize the frequency of osteoporosis in childhood. In contrast, all of the drug regimens used to treat osteoporosis are of uncertain benefit if the cause of the osteoporosis has not been addressed.

PROGNOSIS

The prognosis for a child with osteopenia is very good. Identification of any underlying problem, correction of the diet, and appropriate medical therapy should lead to improvement. The prognosis for children with osteoporosis is more guarded. Parents of children with osteoporosis must consider whether the children should be treated with bisphosphonates. At the time of this writing, the long term safety of bisphosphonates in children is unproven. There are also no clear data regarding their effect on future pregnancies. However, they have been shown to result in improved bone density. Children with severe osteoporosis should be referred to large centers with experienced staff where they may be offered the best possible therapy.

Part III

LIVING WITH A CHILD WHO HAS A CHRONIC CONDITION

22

Medications and Immunizations

Many books on health-related subjects start off with a long section on medications and how they work. The authors put the most important things, such as how and when to take your medication, monitoring, side effects, and when not to take your medications, at the end of the chapter. But many people never read to the end. They find the medicine they are interested in and skip everything else. I want you to understand why your child should take medicine (if they should) and how to be sure your child gets the best results. *So I've begun this chapter with the information that most authors put at the end. Do not skip it. Understanding your medications and taking them appropriately are vitally important in getting the best outcome.*

I do not discuss every possible medication in this chapter. I discuss the medications I commonly use. There are many choices and many individual styles. If your physician has recommended a medication not covered in this chapter, ask him or her for more information. At the right time and in the right place, there are a number of medications that I use that are not covered here. The omission of a medicine indicates only that it isn't something I use routinely or that I don't think of it as a rheumatic disease drug (e.g., I don't discuss antibiotics here).

GENERAL CONCEPTS

The physician strode confidently into the room and offered the child a cup of liquid to relieve his distress. "But wait," cried the parents, "does that have any possible side effects?" The physician paused thoughtfully for a minute and then began. "Well, if taken in excess, this can

> cause problems for anyone with heart or kidney disease. It may dramatically worsen both heart failure and kidney failure. It can cause problems with both nocturia and urinary urgency and frequency. If taken too rapidly, it may cause nausea. If too much is ingested and the body becomes overloaded, it may cause seizures. Excessive use is often associated with a bloated feeling, weight gain, and swollen feet. It should not be left on the skin for a prolonged period or it may result in maceration and skin breakdown. Further, you should always be careful where it comes from, because some sources are contaminated with bacteria or viruses capable of causing severe infections." With that the parents immediately jumped up and discarded the cup of water the doctor had brought because the child was thirsty.

No one likes to have to take his or her medicine and no one wants to take even the slightest risk of getting a side effect. Even most children who start off willing and excited about medications will become bored with taking them over time. Furthermore, most parents are not happy to give their children chronic medication. There is nothing wrong with feeling like you do not want to do it. *But children who do take their medicine routinely are the ones who get the best results, and that is what we want. The most important reason for writing this book is the realization that children often do poorly because their parents do not do what they are supposed to. This is because the parents do not understand why the doctors are telling them to do things* (see Fig. 22).

The key to getting the best results for your child is to select a physician you trust and then to follow his or her instructions. The doctor will tell you about possible side effects of medications and will monitor your child appropriately. This seems very simple, but there are two major sources of trouble. The first group of parents never wants to give the child medication but wants the problem to go away. *If only I could work miracles.* The second group realizes that their child is much better off when he or she takes the medicine, but they do not want to get the blood tests and come to the physician to be monitored.

Remember: Most medications for arthritis require a doctor's prescription. You cannot just go in and buy them. That means the doctor who prescribes the medication is taking responsibility for making sure that you are using the medicine properly and are being monitored. If you do not keep your appointments and you do not get the blood tests done, the physician cannot do his or her job. There is nothing more ironic to a physician than when the same parents who were very concerned about

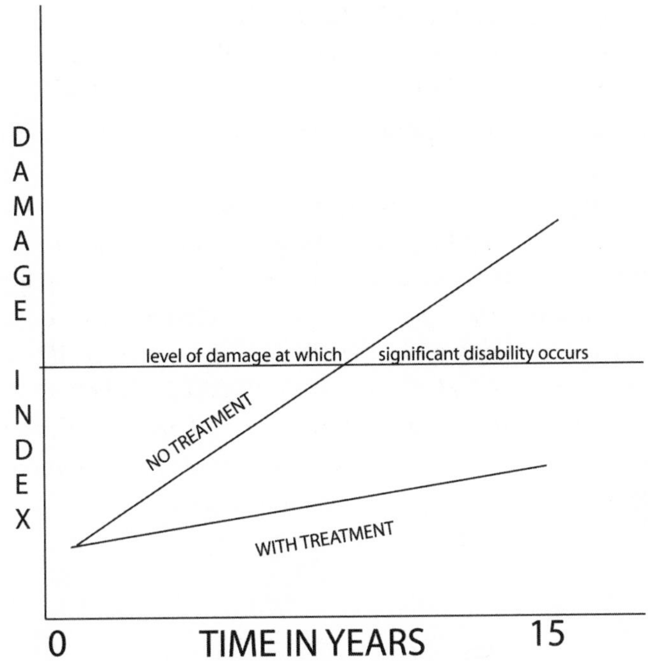

FIG 22. *Children who received treatment were able to continue functioning much longer after the children who did not receive treatment were significantly disabled, even though members of the treated group felt they never really "got better."*

side effects are the ones who keep forgetting to get the appropriate monitoring tests done.

When to withhold your child's medication. This is a subject that is frequently overlooked. If your child is sick with the flu or a virus and not keeping anything down, you do not want to give him or her nonsteroidal anti-inflammatory drugs (NSAIDs) or immunosuppressive medications. The only arthritis medication that is vital to take even when one feels sick is corticosteroids (see below). All the other medications should be avoided and you should call the doctor for instructions. Children who are not keeping anything down are at risk of getting dehydrated. They also are at risk of Reye's syndrome.

Reye's syndrome usually follows a viral infection with symptoms of nausea, vomiting, and sleepiness. This is an unusual condition of uncertain cause. What is clear is that aspirin and other drugs, including NSAIDs, may aggravate the condition. Untreated, it can produce multiple complications that may be life-threatening. NSAIDs should not be given to a child with nausea and vomiting who is at risk of becoming dehydrated. This includes aspirin and ibuprofen-containing products (e.g., Motrin and Advil).

It is also important not to give your child the medication if something goes wrong every time he or she takes it. If something unexpected is happening, it may be a side effect. The proper step is to stop giving the medication and call the doctor. If you keep giving the medication despite problems, you may make the whole situation worse. *If you stop the medication because you think it's causing a side effect or not helping, but do not tell the doctor, how is the doctor going to help you?* I always tell my patients that no medicine has ever been discovered that is the right medicine for every patient every time. If the one I'm giving you does not work for you, call me and I'll give you a different one.

GETTING YOUR CHILD TO TAKE THE MEDICATION

Getting your child to take his or her medication depends a lot on the age of the child. For babies, all you can do with pills is mash them up and hide them in applesauce or another favorite food and make sure it goes down. Liquid medications can often be put in with formula. A compounding pharmacist can make many medications that do not come in liquid form into liquids. You may have to ask around to find one, and your insurance company may not always pay the cost, but it may be worthwhile just to avoid the aggravation. Each medication is different, so check with your doctor.

For little children, it's best to make taking medication a positive experience. However, remember to keep the medication well out of reach. A small child who is rewarded for properly taking medication might take the whole bottle if he or she finds it. (Fortunately, the NSAIDs have a very good safety profile. You can take a lot without necessarily having bad effects, but do not take the chance!) Liquid medicines may be combined with something that the child likes (chocolate milk is popular).

For small children, pills can sometimes be chewed or swallowed. Otherwise, they can be combined with foods that cover the texture and taste, such as chunky peanut butter. Smashed pills can also be put in the middle of cookies such as Oreos. Some parents have found it useful to break pills into large pieces and slip them inside gelatinous candies (e.g., Gummi bears) that have been cut partially open with a sharp knife.

Some pills are coated to make them easier to take or to delay their absorption. The pharmacist may be concerned if you tell him you are crushing the pill since this interferes with the coating. It's true, but there may be no alternative. However, certain pills are designed to release a controlled amount of medicine over time. These should not be crushed. If you are going to crush a pill, make sure you have discussed this with the doctor first. In this age group, a compounding pharmacist can make a big difference by mixing the medication in liquid form and making the medicine a flavor the child likes.

For children over the age of six, education is important. They should understand when and why they take their medication, at least in broad general terms. Children over the age of twelve can usually be trusted to take their own medication, but there are always exceptions and you should base your judgment of this on your knowledge of your own child. Even if your child is a responsible teenager, you might ask yourself when the last time you had to refill the prescription was and how many pills are in the bottle. I've had disasters occur when children who were doing well for several years decided they really did not need their medicine anymore. By the time they realized they did need it and their parents and I discovered they were not taking it, it was too late to fix all the damage.

CHILDREN WHO FIGHT TAKING THEIR MEDICATION

There are a number of elements to consider in dealing with children who fight taking their medication. The easiest answer is to avoid getting into this situation. Finding a suitable compromise by making the medication into a liquid or offering ice cream, candy, and so on is usually preferable to an all-out battle. For children in the younger age groups, a reward system (or bribery) is often the easiest and most effective answer. As parents we all believe that we should not have to bribe our children to get them to do what they should be doing anyway. However, with over twenty-five years of experience in watching parents deal with their children, it's become clear that whether it's called a reward system or bribery, giving your children positive reinforcement for taking their medication works better than anything else. If you are concerned about the cost, remember how much more disease-related problems or psychotherapy would cost you.

If there are continuing problems in getting the child to take medication, it is important to deal with them openly. As children grow up they become increasingly frustrated by their lack of control over what happens to them. Often a struggle over taking medication is really a statement of, "I hate having my disease." If everyone can sit down and discuss what's going on, it may be possible to simply talk it out. If not, psychological intervention may be required. Often a child who completely refuses to take medication will respond quickly to being placed in a hospital environment where nurses instead of parents administer the medication. Awareness that the medication is a symbol of the disease and may become a focus of normal parent-child conflicts may help everyone bring the situation to a quick resolution.

WHAT IF THE MEDICINE IS NOT WORKING?

This question has no simple answer. It depends on the type of medication and the disease. You might be taking the wrong medicine. *Call your doctor. Make sure the name of the medication on the bottle is what it is supposed to be.* Not every doctor writes clearly and not every pharmacist reads carefully. All medications have a trade name and a generic name. Your doctor might have called the medication by its trade name and it may be labeled with the generic name. But if you are unsure, check. Today the trade and generic names of drugs can be found on the Internet in just a few minutes. If you don't have easy access to the Internet, take a few minutes to call your doctor's office and have someone check that your child is taking the correct medication.

If your child is taking the drug your physician recommended and it is not working, you might be expecting results too quickly. Some arthritis medicines do not make a big difference until they have been taken for several weeks. Other medicines may be very important, but instead of making the child feel better, they prevent him or her from getting worse. Be sure you talk to your doctor about your concerns. If you are not comfortable talking with your doctor or his office staff, you need to find a doctor you can be comfortable talking with.

Generic medications are another area of concern. Not all generic medications are equally effective. Some manufacturers make very good generics and save you money. Others, however, have less stringent quality controls. When you get a generic medicine from your pharmacist, you have to look carefully at the label to determine who made it. If you have been taking a generic made by one manufacturer without difficulty and then have problems, check to see whether the pharmacy gave you pills from another manufacturer. Even though the amount of drug in each pill may be the same, the coatings to prevent stomach problems, the ease with which the pill dissolves, and the filler material in the pill may all be entirely different. I have had patients suddenly get worse when they were changed to a generic. However, I also had a patient who suddenly "got worse" when careful investigation showed that he had been changed from the generic, to which he was accustomed, to the brand name pills.

PROPER MONITORING

I am forced to begin this section with a disclaimer. There is what a doctor must do to comply with the minimal requirements and there is what I believe a doctor should do to get the best possible results. What I am discussing here is what I believe should be done to get the best possible results. It does not reflect everyone's standard of practice.

Medicines tend to have two types of side effects. There are idiosyncratic reactions in which the patient responds in an unusual way. This is similar to an allergic reaction but not usually a true allergy. Some people are just unusually sensitive to certain medicines. Other side effects of medicines are related to the amount of the medicine, in terms of both the amount taken each dose and the total amount taken over time. These side effects require different types of monitoring.

For medicines such as NSAIDs, which are generally safe, I want children to be tested within two or three weeks of starting the medicine to look for any unusual reactions, six weeks after starting the medicine to look for any cumulative reactions, three months after starting the medicine, and then every three months thereafter. This is very conservative, careful monitoring, but as a result I have never had a serious medication side effect that did not resolve. There are many physicians who check much less frequently; usually there is no problem.

For medicines that are known to have an increased frequency or severity of side effects, such as methotrexate, I ask my patients to get their blood checked every week at the beginning, then every two weeks, and only when I am sure they are tolerating the medicine at full dose do I extend the frequency of blood tests to every month and eventually every three months. If parents add a new supplement to the child's diet, I start the monitoring tests over again. Some of the supplements increase the risk of side effects. *I recommend that children on supplements be monitored just as carefully as children on prescription medicines. There are numerous well-documented cases of children who became ill from dietary supplements.*

WHY TAKE MEDICINES IF THEY ARE POTENTIALLY DANGEROUS?

Imagine you are sitting in the library reading a book when six firemen come running in with axes and a fire hose, their boots clanking. "You cannot come in here with that hose!" the librarian shouts indignantly. "You're making too much noise, and my goodness, if you turn on that hose you'll get water everywhere and damage the books! It will take forever to clean up the mess." That's all true, you think. But then the fireman points to the smoke coming out of a vent on the sidewall and says, "Lady, if we do not start using this hose and get that fire under control, very soon there will not be any library or books to worry about."

Medications do have side effects and their use must be carefully monitored. That's why they are available only on prescription. However, if the majority of children did not do well, and the benefits did not far outweigh the risks, no physician would be recommending them.

Most medicines are not normally dangerous. Would you refuse to fly because you were told the pilot double-checked everything before he got on the plane? Pilots normally do that. Do you get off because the seats are equipped with seatbelts? It should reassure you that people are checking carefully and taking precautions, not make you more nervous. Careful people check everything not because they expect things to go wrong, but because they want to be sure that they do not. Even if you are only crossing the street, you are foolish to believe nothing could go wrong.

Some parents still want to know why they should give their children medicine. It is important to realize that very severe things can go wrong if the medicine is not taken. No sensible physician prescribes a medication unless he or she believes the potential benefits outweigh the potential risks. I often hear parents say, "It's only a sore knee" or similar things. But it's not. If children's problems are interfering with their abilities to keep up with their friends and do normal things, it's interfering with their concepts of who they are and their feelings of self-worth. Failure to take care of these problems may have disastrous consequences in both the short and long terms (see Fig. 22).

WHY DOES MY CHILD HAVE TO KEEP TAKING MEDICATION AND GOING TO THE DOCTOR EVEN AFTER HE OR SHE FEELS WELL?

> The old zookeeper smiled quietly to himself as he listened to the children talking. "Look at the big kitty cat, Mommy! Why do they keep him locked up in that cage? Can't they let the big kitty cat out, Mommy? Why don't they let us get closer? I want to pet him, Mommy!" The mother stopped to explain that the big kitty cat was a lion. A fierce animal that looked very calm and quiet when resting, but that could suddenly pounce on its prey with blinding speed and kill it mercilessly. The children were unconvinced. "It just looks like a big kitty cat to me, Mommy."

There are many times as a physician that I feel just like that mother in the zoo. Sometimes it's been several years since the child was brought to me with active disease that was causing serious problems. With the right medicines, hard work, and some good luck the child's disease has been brought under control. Other times it's just a few months after the disease has come under control and I'm just beginning to be fully confident that things are going to go well. But the parents who never missed an appointment while their child was sick now don't want to come back so often and don't want to keep giving the medicine. Like the children above, they see only a big kitty cat in the cage.

Many of the diseases I care for are chronic and recurrent. They can be controlled, but they can never be pronounced gone. When I have the disease under control the parents and their children would like to forget about it. They have forgotten that without the cage, the big kitty cat could again become a ferocious lion without warning. If you think this seems like a silly story, let me assure you that I've seen children suffer permanent damage because their parents thought the problem was gone and stopped the medicines. They stopped the medications because they ran out after forgetting to keep their appointments to have the blood work checked and the prescriptions renewed. After all, they did not see any problems, and they did not want to keep taking time off from work or dragging the child out of school to go to "unnecessary" doctors' appointments.

"DISEASE-MODIFYING" DRUGS?

In every discussion of drugs for children with chronic rheumatic disease, you will hear a discussion of disease-modifying versus nondisease-modifying drugs. Sometimes the disease-modifying drugs are referred to as DMARDs (disease-modifying antirheumatic drugs) or SAARDs (slow-acting antirheumatic drugs). This is a concept that requires further discussion. Ideally, there should be drugs that cure the rheumatic diseases. "Here, take these pills for ten days and the problem will be gone." Unfortunately, those pills do not exist. Instead, we have pills such as the NSAIDs (see below) that reduce inflammation and both decrease pain and increase function. We also have drugs such as the gold shots we used to use that seemed to "cure" some people. However, gold shots took a long time to make a difference and often had to be continued for many years.

With the development of newer drugs, there has been a lot of discussion about what constitutes a disease-modifying drug as opposed to what simply makes the patient feel better but does not fundamentally change the outcome of the disease. This is an important argument, but it has been misapplied and has caused a lot of trouble. The first thing to remember when dealing with children with arthritis is that we want the best possible outcome in terms of ability to function, not just day to day but in later adult life as well. If I decrease your pain and allow you to be more active and feel better about yourself, you will have a better outcome.

Some people are concerned that they may be giving their child a drug that has possible side effects but is not disease-modifying. Why bother? If the drug is not going to cure my child's disease, why can't I just have him deal with the pain so he does not have to risk the side effects of medicine?

Consider two construction workers who are working on a large project. I'll have them both come over to the examining area. I'll then take a brick that weighs exactly ten pounds and hold it exactly six feet over each one's right big toe—no shoes or socks. When I drop the brick on their toes they'll both scream in pain and will not be able to walk. I have dropped the same brick from the same height on both workers. Worker 1 is told he's a tough guy. He can rest or go home if he wants and come back when he feels he can work again—but he's not to take medications of any kind. Worker 2 is given NSAIDs that reduce the pain and inflammation. The NSAIDs do not change the fact that I dropped a brick on his toe. He, too, is told he can rest or go home, and to come back when he feels he can work again. Who is likely to be back on the job first, earning money again first, feeling better about himself first, and the more productive?

So taking NSAIDs may not change the fundamental nature of the disease, but it certainly will change the outcome by keeping the children in less pain, able to do more, and feeling better about themselves. The NSAIDs may not be disease-modifying, but they certainly modify the functional outcome, and that's what's most important.

For adults with rheumatoid arthritis there has been an extensive discussion of how to define "disease-modifying." To concentrate on objective measurements, the original plan was to concentrate on observing the changes in the bones on X rays. Actively inflamed synovium will begin to make holes in the surrounding bones. These holes are called erosions and can be seen on X ray. So for the original studies, two groups of patients on different medications were compared for the number of new erosions seen over a period of years. If patients on one drug developed fewer erosions, then the drug was disease-modifying. Most physicians now agree that this misses the point. What counts is whether you can go to work or school every day. That is determined more by how much pain and stiffness one has than by the number of erosions. However, it is important to keep up the search for a drug that truly cures the disease.

NONSTEROIDAL ANTI-INFLAMMATORY DRUGS

Nonsteroidal anti-inflammatory drugs (NSAIDs) are the mainstay of therapy for most children with rheumatic disease. All of them interfere to varying degrees with the cyclooxygenase pathway. This pathway is responsible for the production of prostaglandins, which are important inflammatory mediators (chemicals that cause fever, pain, and irritation). By blocking the production of these inflammatory mediators, NSAIDs serve to reduce the amount of pain, fever, and irritation that the child experiences.

Most of the NSAIDs interfere with cyclooxygenase-1 (COX-1) and cyclooxygenase-2 (COX-2). A few primarily interfere with COX-2, and I discuss them separately below. Choosing the proper NSAID for a given child involves balancing convenience, cost, effectiveness, and probability of side effects. All of the NSAIDs can irritate the stomach, irritate the liver, interfere with kidney function, or result in a rash. However, all of them can be used safely with appropriate monitoring.

Side effects of NSAIDs

Allergic reactions can occur with any medications. Few children are allergic to NSAIDs, but if there is a history of allergy to aspirin or similar medications, one should be cautious. Some children who are allergic to aspirin are allergic to all NSAIDs, but others are not. You will need to work carefully with your doctor to evaluate this problem if it occurs.

All NSAIDs may irritate the lining of the stomach. This may cause indigestion or loss of appetite. It is important to make sure the child takes the medicine on a full stomach. If the stomachaches are common or persistent, make sure your doctor is aware. He or she may choose to change the medication or add another medication to protect the stomach lining. Some children have developed ulcers while taking NSAIDs, but this is uncommon. Remember, if every NSAID causes a child to have stomachaches, perhaps something else is going on.

Bruising is a common side effect of all of the COX-1 NSAIDs. These drugs interfere with platelet stickiness and cause one to bleed or bruise more than one would otherwise. Frequent bruises over the shins are common for children on NSAIDs, but if they are significant, the physician should do blood tests to make sure there is not another explanation. It is also important to stop the NSAIDs before any elective surgery where there is a high risk of bleeding. Consult the physician doing the surgery. It may be necessary to stop the NSAIDs two weeks in advance.

Liver irritation may also occur with these medications. Most often the patient is not aware of the liver irritation, and it is detected only by blood work. With aspirin, liver irritation was very common and mild inflammation of the liver was tolerated. Given the variety of medications available today, we are less tolerant of liver irritation, but minimal amounts are acceptable.

The NSAIDs also affect the kidneys. They usually interfere with the rate at which the kidneys filter the blood, or the glomerular filtration rate. This means that the child will hold more water in the body. This causes a few pounds of weight gain and may be reflected in a drop in the hemoglobin value and slight rise in the BUN level. These are normal effects of the medications.

In some children using NSAIDs, the kidneys become irritated, resulting in a condition called **interstitial nephritis**. This is a more serious condition that requires stopping the NSAID. It may have to be treated with steroids and could result in permanent damage. Routine urine tests are part of monitoring for side effects of NSAIDs in order to detect any signs of this problem. It may not occur until many months or years after starting the medication. This is why the monitoring must continue.

An unusual skin rash called a **pseudoporphyria reaction** has been described in some children on NSAIDs. This skin rash appears when the child is out in the sun. At first, it just looks like a number of tiny blisters. However, the blisters leave a small scar when they heal. With continued medication and continued sun exposure, there will be more and more blisters and scars. The medication should be stopped and the sun avoided until the medicine is cleared from the body. This reaction has been noticed most often with naproxen, but that may be because so much naproxen is used. It has been reported with other NSAIDs, and all children on NSAIDs should be monitored for it.

Behavioral problems in children taking chronic medication can result from many different causes. In general, the NSAIDs do *not* cause misbehavior, changes in attitude, poor sleeping, difficulty studying, or similar side effects. However, very strong NSAIDs, such as indomethacin, are known to cause headaches, depression, and dizziness. If there is a significant behavioral problem in a child on an NSAID, I will observe at first and then stop or change the NSAID to see whether there is an improvement in the problem.

Other problems may occur. This list is not comprehensive. Almost anything can happen to someone and possibly be the result of an NSAID he or she was taking. In large studies to document the safety and efficacy of new medications, there are groups of patients taking placebo (sugar pills with no active ingredient). There are always patients taking the sugar pills who complain of headache, itching, sweating, constipation, diarrhea, difficulty concentrating, and so on. However, there are often a few more patients with these complaints in the group taking the real medication. If you are concerned that your child may be experiencing a side effect of medication, be sure to discuss it with your doctor.

Important things for parents to remember

I have prescribed NSAIDs for thousands of children without ever seeing a side effect that did not go away when the drug was stopped. In twenty-five years I have briefly stopped or changed the NSAIDs in many children with complaints of stomachache, but I have seen only three ulcers due to NSAIDs. I would never prescribe these drugs if I did not think the benefits far outweighed the risks. Nonetheless, I monitor very carefully with blood and urine tests (see the guidelines above). If a parent describes a change he or she thinks might be due to the NSAIDs and it continues, I always stop the NSAID to see whether it goes away, then carefully restart the NSAID to see whether it comes back. If it does come back, I stop the drug.

As a physician I want to give children with arthritis the NSAID that makes them better with the least likelihood of side effects and the greatest convenience. The probability of side effects is different for each of the NSAIDs. If there were one NSAID that was more likely to make children better and less likely to cause side effects, all of the others would be discarded. Instead, doctors must start with the easy ones and carefully move on to the stronger ones if the response to the easy ones is inadequate. The list of side effects is essentially the same for all the NSAIDs; it is the probability of the side effects that changes.

One of the most common problems is for children to be treated with only one NSAID and told there is no other choice. The physician may either stick with that NSAID, even though it is not working well, or recommend jumping to a second-line drug without trying any other NSAID. Despite their similar mechanisms of action, all NSAIDs are not the same. I often use the analogy of ice cream. All ice cream is ice cream. However, there are many different flavors, and some people love chocolate but hate strawberry, or the reverse. Furthermore, there are many different brands of ice cream and the chocolate flavor of one brand does not really taste exactly the same as the chocolate flavor of another brand. Some of the NSAIDs are far more effective for certain types of arthritis. Failure to recognize the different types of juvenile arthritis (see Chapter 7) means that many doctors have failed to recognize that different NSAIDs are better for different types of diseases.

Many physicians will not prescribe NSAIDs that have not been specifically tested and approved by the Food and Drug Administration (FDA) for use in childhood. However, the testing costs a lot of money and there are not that many children with arthritis. As a result, many excellent drugs have never been specifically approved for children. That does not mean that they cannot or should not be used by physicians who are experienced with them, do appropriate monitoring (see above), and are comfortable with their use. In some cases, newer drugs have been shown to be more effective and safer, but some physicians continue to use the less effective and more toxic drugs in children because no one has specifically told them the safer drug is approved for children. Changing to the appropriate NSAID can often make a dramatic difference for a child. However, it may take some trial and error. You cannot predict which NSAID will be most effective for a given child just by looking at him.

In the paragraphs that follow I discuss the NSAIDs that are commonly used and the ones I prefer to use. This is not a complete list of all NSAIDs or of every NSAID I ever use. I have found a variety of NSAIDs that I am comfortable using in children and feel are effective. I have not tried them all, and the absence of an NSAID from this list simply means I do not use it often. A few, like aspirin, are included because other physicians commonly use them, even though I rarely do. The FDA has not specifically approved all of these medications for use in children at this time. That means they cannot be advertised "for use by children"; however, it does not mean children cannot use them.

Aspirin

Aspirin was the original NSAID and was the mainstay of therapy when I began my career. Aspirin is a short name for acetylsalicylic acid (ASA). Salicylic acid is derived from plants and was a natural therapy in ancient times. In the eighteenth and nineteenth centuries, the active ingredient was isolated from the natural preparation. This allowed chemists to modify it to acetylsalicylic acid, which is the aspirin we use today. Aspirin is much easier on the stomach than salicylic acid was, but still not ideal. The main goal of pharmacists in developing all of the NSAIDs described below has been to increase the efficacy of the medication without increasing the toxicity of the medication.

On a worldwide basis aspirin remains one of the most widely used treatments for children with arthritis. However, its use in the United States is limited by the ready availability of other medications that are more convenient, equally effective, and less likely to cause side effects. Disadvantages of aspirin include the following.

- The dose needs to be given three or four times each day.
- It is available only as pills.
- Aspirin frequently upsets the stomach.

Although aspirin is available without a prescription, regular use must be monitored, just like the use of prescription NSAIDs, to minimize the risk of severe and even life-threatening side effects. Aspirin has all of the side effects described for NSAIDs, and in many instances they occur more frequently with the use of aspirin than with the prescription NSAIDs. A variety of alternate forms of salicylate are available, including choline salicylate (which comes in liquid form), but these are infrequently used. The modern NSAIDs are more effective, more convenient, and less irritating to the stomach. An additional concern in the use of aspirin is that it has been linked to Reye's syndrome (discussed above).

Naproxen and ibuprofen: propionic acid derivatives

Naproxen and ibuprofen are marketed under a variety of different names (Alleve, Naprosyn, Motrin, Advil, Nuprin, Buprofen, and more). Both are available in liquid form and are used extensively in the treatment of children with arthritis. Naproxen has an advantage in being given twice a day, while ibuprofen may need to be given as many as four times a day. Ibuprofen liquid and pills, and some forms of naproxen pills, are available without a prescription. The reason ibuprofen liquid, but not naproxen liquid, is available without prescription, is unclear. *Both of these drugs require monitoring, just like all the other NSAIDs, whether a doctor prescribes them or you buy them without a prescription.* Other than stomach upset, side effects of these medications are relatively infrequent. However, all of the side effects listed in the section on NSAID side effects may occur. These NSAIDs are effective for true pauciarticular onset JA and helpful in many other conditions. For many children with more difficult forms of JA, more potent NSAIDs may be necessary.

All of the following drugs require a prescription in the United States.

Nabumetone

Nabumetone (marketed as Relafen) is an NSAID that is useful for pediatric rheumatologists. It seems to be very effective for arthritis while rarely causing stomach irritation. It's easy for parents because it has to be given only once each day. Although it does not come as a liquid, it will dissolve in warm water without any apparent loss in efficacy. It can also be crushed. Since it has a long half-life (it stays in the body longer, which is why it needs to be given only once a day), it can easily be given after dinner for a peak effect the next morning, when it helps to reduce morning stiffness.

Diclofenac and tolmetin sodium (phenyl acetic and heteroaryl acetic acids)

Diclofenac and tolmetin sodium are marketed as Voltaren and Tolectin, respectively. They are effective for all onset types of JA and for spondyloarthropathies. Many children who are not doing well enough on naproxen or ibuprofen dramatically improve when switched to diclofenac. However, complaints of stomachache and increases in liver enzymes seem more common with these medications. Physicians prescribing them must monitor the children for these problems. In general, I prefer diclofenac to tolmetin because of fewer complaints of stomach irritation; also most preparations of diclofenac are enteric-coated (a special coating that slows the rate at which the pill dissolves so that most dissolves in the intestines) to protect the stomach. A compounding pharmacist can make diclofenac into a liquid for small children. The liquid cannot be enteric-coated, but that does not seem to cause problems.

Piroxicam (enolic acids)

Piroxicam (marketed as Feldene) is an NSAID that is very effective for many older children with spondyloarthropathies and the related types of arthritis. It has a very long half-life and slowly builds up to an effective level in the body. Often it takes two or three weeks to start having an effect. However, it is often very effective when other NSAIDs have not been sufficient. Gastrointestinal side effects and renal side effects may be more common with piroxicam than with other NSAIDs and do not always occur at the beginning of therapy. All NSAIDs require continued monitoring. I have seen interstitial nephritis as a complication of piroxicam more often than other NSAIDs, but it can occur with any NSAID.

Indomethacin (arylalkanoic acids, or indole acetic acids)

Indomethacin (marketed as Indocin) is generally agreed to be the most potent of the routinely used NSAIDs. It is an excellent inhibitor of inflammation. Indomethacin is also much more likely to cause side effects. In addition to the side effects listed for all NSAIDs, it is common for children on indomethacin to complain of headaches. However, many of the children old enough to talk about it say that the trade-off in improved relief of arthritis is worthwhile. The headaches can be treated with acetaminophen and do decrease over time. Some individuals become depressed when taking indomethacin, and the physician and family must watch out for this complication. In small children, it may cause inexplicable temper tantrums. Kidney and liver irritation are also well-recognized side effects.

Because indomethacin is very effective and is available as a liquid it has a valuable role in the care of children with arthritis. In children with systemic onset arthritis, it may relieve fever and other symptoms when no other NSAID is effective. Indomethacin is also very effective for some children with spondyloarthropathies who have not responded to other NSAIDs. However, it requires careful monitoring. If you were to look at the chemical structures of the different classes of NSAIDs, you would notice diclofenac and nabumetone are more closely chemically related to indomethacin than most others. They are not as strong as indomethacin, but significant side effects occur far less often.

Selective COX-2 inhibitors

Over the last few years, there has been a tremendous increase in interest in the NSAIDs that are selective COX-2 inhibitors. Many of the side effects of the NSAIDs are the result of their effects on COX-1. Drugs that affect only COX-2 should have fewer side effects as a result. In many ways this is true, but part of the efficacy of the normal NSAIDs comes from their effect on COX-1. I have had families whose children were doing very well on a regular NSAID come and request one of the selective COX-2 inhibitors after seeing all the advertisements. Frequently, the children have had increased problems with their arthritis when the medication was changed. If your child is doing well on an unselective NSAID, there is no good reason to change to a selective COX-2 inhibitor. These medications do not seem to be as strong as many of the other NSAIDs. However, if the unselective NSAIDs are causing a lot of stomach irritation, the selective COX-2 inhibitors may be a big improvement. *It should be noted that it is not impossible for the selective COX-2 inhibitors to cause stomach irritation or ulcers. They just cause these problems much less frequently.*

Celecoxib (Celebrex). Celecoxib (marketed as Celebrex) is a useful selective COX-2 inhibitor that provides a good level of relief for some children. Celecoxib is available as capsules that can be opened. The powder can be mixed with a variety of foods if necessary, but you should check with your physician and pharmacist before doing this. It has a reduced frequency of side effects, but this medication does contain sulfa and *children who are allergic to sulfa drugs may be allergic to celecoxib.*

Rofecoxib (Vioxx). Rofecoxib (marketed as Vioxx) is the second widely available selective COX-2 inhibitor. It has two advantages in pediatric rheumatology. It comes in a liquid form as well as pills, and it does not contain sulfa. A number of my patients with sensitive stomachs have done well on this medication.

Valdecoxib (Bextra). Valdecoxib (marketed as Bextra) is a newer selective COX-2 inhibitor. Some adolescent patients have found it effective when the others did not work adequately. However, it contains a sulfa-moiety and *could cause an allergic reaction in children who are allergic to sulfa drugs*. It does not come in liquid form.

For many people with mild arthritis, selective COX-2 inhibitors are adequate therapy. For children with more severe arthritis but who experience repeated stomach irritation with NSAIDs, it may be best to combine a selective COX-2 inhibitor with a second-line medication that is not a COX-1 inhibitor. The key is having a knowledgeable physician who has experience using these medications in varying combinations.

SUCRALFATE (CARAFATE)

This drug is not an anti-inflammatory. Rather, *it is a drug that was developed to minimize stomach irritation secondary to other medications.* It is frequently added by rheumatologists if a child complains of stomach irritation with their NSAIDs. Sucralfate is a surface active agent. I always visualize the old TV ads for another product that talked about a protective coating action and showed the product spreading to cover the inside of the stomach. That product didn't really do that, but sucralfate does. The drug coats the inside of the stomach but lets the medicine get absorbed into the body. It dramatically reduces irritation of the stomach. I'm not enough of a chemist to explain how that works, but it does.

The key thing to remember about sucralfate is that it takes time for the medication to dissolve in the stomach and spread over the surface to provide its protective action. You should not swallow sucralfate and your other medicines together. The sucralfate should go down at least a half an hour in advance of the other medicines. If you take your medicines with meals, it is recommended that you take the sucralfate, eat your meal, then take your other medications.

Side effects of sucralfate are rare. A few people have been allergic to it. Others have complained of bloating or constipation. Some of my patients say it makes them feel full. It is available in liquid form for small children.

SULFASALAZINE (AZULFIDINE)

Sulfasalazine is a drug that was developed in the 1930s, when there was still a strong consideration that rheumatoid arthritis was caused by an infection. A Swedish scientist chose to combine the salicylic acid from aspirin with sulfapyridine (one of the early antibiotics). When I began my career, this drug was used by gastroenterologists to treat children with inflammatory bowel disease but was considered ineffective for children with arthritis. I can still remember going to my mentor, Dr. Virgil Hanson, and asking about reports in the British literature that the drug was effective. He assured me that it did not work in his experience.

In the mid-1970s we were just beginning to realize that many different diseases were being described as JRA. It turns out that *sulfasalazine is very effective for spondyloarthropathies (enthesitis-associated arthritis),* which are common in Northern European and Asian populations, but less effective for other forms of arthritis in childhood. At that time, children with enthesitis-related arthritis were still diagnosed as having JRA. The British physicians were having good success using it on their Northern European population. However, in Los Angeles at that time very few of our patients were Northern European or Asian. As a result, sulfasalazine was rarely effective in Dr. Hanson's experience. *This illustrates why it is important to know exactly what condition you are talking about and not lump all children with arthritis together as JRA.*

Often children with enthesitis-related arthritis who have not responded to the other NSAIDs respond dramatically to this drug. The mechanism of action of sulfasalazine is unclear. In the body, the drug is broken down into the aspirin-like molecule and the antibiotic. However, neither alone seems to be as effective. Sulfasalazine can be used in addition to other NSAIDs, so it can be added to the regimen of a child who is not doing well enough without stopping the medications the child is already taking.

The major disadvantage of sulfasalazine is that *anyone who is allergic to sulfa drugs will be to be allergic to sulfasalazine.* These allergies often take the form of skin rashes that can be quite dramatic. Other common side effects include liver irritation, stomach upset, and decreased white blood cell count. Allergic reactions require stopping the drug; other problems might respond to changing the dose. Because of the allergic reactions, I usually start children on a small dose of sulfasalazine and monitor them carefully as I increase the dose.

For children who have shown significant active arthritis that responded well to sulfasalazine, I will continue the drug for years. Although there is no hard data, I have had a number of children who did well for years, stopped sulfasalazine, and then had problems again within a few months. These problems ultimately came back under control with sulfasalazine, but the children had suffered that much more joint damage in the interim.

Parents frequently ask me why they should use sulfasalazine if it often has side effects. The answer is that this drug is extremely effective for children who do not get the side effects. If a child does not have an allergic reaction to the drug, he or she can often tolerate it without difficulty for years (properly monitored). I have many patients who did not need to take potentially more toxic medications such as methotrexate because this drug was effective for them.

HYDROXYCHLOROQUINE (PLAQUENIL)

Hydroxychloroquine is an interesting drug that has been widely used in the treatment of rheumatic diseases since the 1950s. It is a derivative of quinine, which was originally used to fight malaria (you will hear doctors refer to hydroxychloroquine as an "antimalarial"). Quinine was first reported to be beneficial for patients with rheumatic disease in the 1890s. Hydroxychloroquine is a derivative that has fewer side effects. The precise mechanism of action of hydroxychloroquine remains unknown. The drug is very slow in its onset of action. You will not take one and feel better. Indeed, families often wonder whether their child just got better, rather than the improvement being the result of hydroxychloroquine. However, many controlled studies have shown that the group of patients receiving hydroxychloroquine did better than the group that did not.

Hydroxychloroquine has been found to be helpful in children with most forms of arthritis, systemic lupus erythematosus, dermatomyositis, and scleroderma in both its localized and systemic forms. It is probably helpful for many other conditions as well. At one time, it was thought that hydroxychloroquine was uniquely effective for skin manifestations of dermatomyositis and SLE, but it is not clear that this is true.

One of the most interesting things about hydroxychloroquine is that evidence suggests that it truly is a "disease-modifying" drug. That means that it can change the long-term outcome of the disease (see discussion above). Hydroxychloroquine is probably the safest of all the medications that are thought to be "disease-modifying." It is rarely associated with toxicity.

Unfortunately, if you look hydroxychloroquine up in the reference books, there is a discussion of possible blindness. No parents in their right mind would give their child a drug that was likely to make the child blind. It is important to know that this warning comes from a period in the late 1960s and early 1970s when the wrong dosage was used. Once the dosage was corrected, this problem essentially disappeared. Your physician will recommend an eye examination by an ophthalmologist before your child starts the drug and every six months while taking the drug. This is to check for any evidence of damage to the eye by the hydroxychloroquine.

Checking the child's eyes before starting the medication allows the physicians to detect any abnormality that might be present for another reason. If this was not noted before starting, and found while the child was taking hydroxychloroquine, it might be mistakenly thought to have come from the hydroxychloroquine. This would cause the physicians to stop the drug unnecessarily. In many years of prescribing hydroxychloroquine, I have had a small number of patients where the ophthalmologist thought there might be an early problem. I stopped the medication. I have never had a child or parent notice any vision-related problem due to hydroxychloroquine.

Since hydroxychloroquine appears to be safe and effective, but very slow-acting, children are often kept on it for years and years. Like all medications, hydroxychloroquine can be associated with a wide variety of minor complaints or abnormalities on blood tests and so needs to be monitored appropriately. Fortunately, these problems are very infrequent. Hydroxychloroquine is unique in that it is probably one of the worst-tasting pills. The modern preparation is coated so that it can be swallowed without being tasted, but if you have to crush or break the pill for your child, it tastes terrible. A compounding pharmacist can provide it in liquid form and add ingredients to hide the taste.

DOXYCYCLINE (VIBRAMYCIN)

Doxycycline is marketed under a wide variety of trade names around the world. It is a tetracycline antibiotic that has received a lot of publicity because it is used for Lyme disease. It is also useful for patients with arthritis. *The use of doxycycline and related tetracyclines in children is restricted by the fact that tetracyclines permanently stain growing bones and teeth.* Most physicians prefer not to use doxycycline before the age of twelve, though some physicians will use it earlier.

The discovery that doxycycline is effective for arthritis generated a lot of publicity. The physicians who initially proposed the use of doxycycline thought that it was effective in treating certain infections that caused arthritis. Instead, it has been shown that doxycycline works by blocking a group of enzymes called metalloproteinases. This effect is independent of its effect as an antibiotic. Chemists were able to synthesize a derivative of doxycycline that did not work as an antibiotic but still reduced arthritis.

In addition to staining teeth and bones in young children, doxycycline causes a number of children to complain of stomach upset and photosensitivity (they sunburn easily). These complaints limit its use. It is also used in the treatment of acne in teenagers and in the treatment of Lyme disease. Some caution using doxycycline for acne is necessary, because it has been associated with rare cases of drug-induced SLE.

There are a number of good controlled studies indicating that doxycycline is an effective adjunctive (extra) agent for patients with arthritis, but the vast majority of teenagers I give it to discontinue it because of chronic stomachaches. Patients also must be warned that they may be very sensitive to sunburning (photosensitive) when taking doxycycline. They should always use sunblock and be careful when exposed to the sun for prolonged periods. *Because it permanently stains developing bones and teeth, doxycycline should not be given to young children.*

IMMUNOSUPPRESSIVE DRUGS

If a child with arthritis has failed to respond to NSAIDs, hydroxychloroquine, and sulfasalazine, the family will have to consider immunosuppressive medications or one of the newer biologics discussed below (although the biologics are classified separately, they are in fact immunosuppressive). Fortunately, the majority of children with arthritis do not require immunosuppressive drugs. However, children with more severe arthritis will do much better if they are appropriately treated and their disease is brought under good control. Stronger immunosuppressive drugs are commonly used for children with illnesses such as systemic lupus erythematosus, dermatomyositis, scleroderma, polyarteritis nodosa, and Wegener's granulomatosis.

There are several important considerations in the use of immunosuppressive drugs for arthritis and related conditions. If you read about these drugs in books or elsewhere, you will discover they have all sorts of possible side effects. In the high dosages used for the treatment of children with cancer, these drugs have many major side effects. However, it is very important for parents to understand that although the drugs may be the same, in general, the dosage of the immunosuppressive drugs used in the treatment of children with arthritis is far lower.

As you read through the sections that follow, keep in mind that your doctors are trying to get the best possible outcome for your child. I have been caring for children with rheumatic diseases for over twenty-five years. The majority of the poor outcomes I have seen were the result of families refusing aggressive therapy for severe disease. If your doctor is recommending aggressive therapy, it is because the doctor believes it is more likely that your child will suffer permanent injury from the disease than the medication. With careful monitoring, poor outcomes due to medication are extremely rare. If planes routinely crashed, no one would fly. Thousands of planes fly every day. That does not mean we can ignore plane crashes; it means we should only fly after due consideration and with airlines we have confidence in.

Certain potential side effects have to be considered with every immunosuppressive medication. The two most important are the increased risk of infection and the possible increased risk of a malignancy (cancer) later in life. In all of the rheumatic diseases, the body is acting as if it is trying to control an infection. The inflammatory reactions that result involve the release of many damaging substances (cytokines and similar agents) that are intended to kill bacteria and viruses. In children with arthritis, the cells of the immune system are making and releasing these agents, and the joints and other tissues are being damaged. Immunosuppressive drugs block the production of these damaging substances, thus preventing the damage to the joints and other tissues.

Some immunosuppressive drugs (such as cyclosporine, tacrolimus, etanercept, infliximab, adalimumab, and thalidomide) work by directly blocking the messengers that stimulate production of the damaging substances. Other immunosuppressive drugs work by interfering with DNA synthesis and killing cells that are trying to divide. In children with arthritis, most of the cells trying to divide at any given time are the ones that are making the damaging substances. However, if a child on immunosuppressive drugs develops an infection, he or she does not have full use of these substances to fight off the infection. This is why careful monitoring and experience are so important.

In addition to preventing infections, the immune system is charged with monitoring the body for any cells that have reproduced themselves incorrectly (e.g., something goes wrong when the DNA is being copied). If the immune system finds a cell that is incorrectly made, it tries to destroy it. Some incorrectly made cells are the beginnings of cancer. Because the immunosuppressive drugs weaken the immune system, it might be easier for some of these cells to escape detection and become cancer. Moreover, the drugs that interfere with DNA synthesis may fail to kill a cell but may instead cause it to develop incorrectly.

So why would anybody ever take immunosuppressive drugs? Again, it's a matter of carefully balancing everything and realizing that almost every plane lands safely. Physicians reserve these drugs for children whom they expect will do poorly if they are not aggressively treated. Every immunosuppressive drug increases the risk of infection. Every immunosuppressive drug increases the risk of having cancer later in life. Every immunosuppressive drug may interfere with the ability to have children. *But at the dosages normally used for the treatment of children with arthritis, all of these problems are rare. Most often immunosuppressive drugs simply make you better.*

Prescribing medications is often like being the wise man in a mythical village. It is a wonderful place ruled by a good king. However, to keep evil at bay, the dragon must be fed fifty people each year. The king cannot make such a choice from his subjects. Instead, a hundred people are chosen by lot and assigned to stand in a house with no roof where the dragon comes to eat. The house has two rooms. One room has red walls and one room has blue walls.

Since you are a wise man, some of the people who must stand in the house come to you and ask what to do. Experience has taught you that the dragon prefers to eat people in the red room. However, the dragon is nearsighted. Every year he eats forty people from the red room, but misses ten times and eats ten people in the blue room. Your advice is always to stand in the blue room. Every year there will be someone in the red room who lived and someone in the blue room who did not. There is no foolproof advice. But the blue room is clearly the better choice, even if the advice seeker's best friend survived in the red room the year before.

Methotrexate

Methotrexate has significantly improved the outlook for many children with arthritis. Before methotrexate became widely used for arthritis in the 1980s, children who did not respond to NSAIDs were treated with "gold shots" (see below). If you were allergic to the gold shots or had a toxic reaction, there were very few choices left. Methotrexate is now one of the mainstays for the treatment of children with significant arthritis. As noted above, much of what you may read about negative effects of methotrexate is related to the doses used in the treatment of children with cancer. The doses for cancer therapy are frequently ten times higher and in some cases hundreds of times higher than the doses used to treat arthritis.

In the doses used in cancer therapy, methotrexate works by interfering with DNA synthesis and blocking the rapid reproduction of cells. However, in the dosage normally used for children with arthritis, methotrexate is believed to have a different mechanism of action. Nonetheless, it is very effective at reducing pain and swelling for children with most forms of arthritis. Careful studies in adults suggest that it may reduce the number of erosions and be a disease-modifying drug. It is certainly a drug that improves function and controls arthritis symptoms for most children who take it.

Most often methotrexate is given as pills that are taken just once each week. Some physicians start out at the full dose and monitor blood work after a few weeks. However, there are children who are unexpectedly sensitive to methotrexate. I prefer to start out with a small dose and monitor the blood tests every week until I am sure the child is tolerating the drug. Children on methotrexate should take folic acid. Use of folic acid has sharply reduced the frequency of side effects. There are many different stories about how the folic acid should be given. It doesn't matter how it is given as long as it is taken. My patients take 1 mg every day (even the day when they take the methotrexate) and do fine.

The onset of action of methotrexate is slow. It usually begins to show effects after a few weeks, but it may be six to twelve weeks before it is clearly having a significant effect on the arthritis. This is especially true if it is begun carefully, using a low dosage. For many children, methotrexate is a very effective drug and provides excellent control of the arthritis. The normal dosage range used for children with arthritis (5 to 10 $mg/M^2/week$) is far below the amount used by cancer specialists. For children with severe disease, there may be some benefit to increasing the dose significantly.

At higher doses, many physicians prefer to give methotrexate as an injection. This has the advantage of consistently delivering the same dose to the body. If a child is taking pills, he or she may not get the same effect every week because of differences in what was eaten the day the pills were taken and other factors that influence the absorption of the methotrexate from the stomach. In addition, methotrexate injected under the skin is absorbed and distributed through the circulation before it reaches the liver. Pills are digested and go into the portal circulation (the blood vessels draining the stomach and intestines) that goes directly to the liver. Since methotrexate is known to have a negative effect on the liver, at higher doses it is thought the shots are safer.

Many children who were having significant problems with arthritis do well after starting on methotrexate. Although there is no uniform agreement, most physicians will keep children on methotrexate until they have been well for at least six months. Some physicians then reduce the weekly dose, while others prefer to spread the dose out so that it is given every two weeks, then every three weeks, and so on, until it is slowly discontinued over a period of many months. Unfortunately, the arthritis flares in a substantial proportion of children as the methotrexate is withdrawn.

Common side effects of methotrexate include nausea, minor changes in the white blood cell or platelet count, and liver irritation. The nausea often responds to reassurance. However, methotrexate-induced nausea is not coming from stomach irritation; it is a "centrally acting agent." If the nausea is severe, it can be treated with ondansetron (Zofran), which is commonly used by those receiving cancer chemotherapy. Changes in the blood counts and liver enzymes are monitored through the blood work. Sores in the mouth or an irritated tongue are rare in children taking folic acid. Children with warts will often notice that their warts either return or get worse when the methotrexate reaches an effective level.

Children taking methotrexate also need to be careful about going out in the sun. Although most children have no problem, some children are very easily sunburned when they are on methotrexate. It is important to be sure that your child is not excessively photosensitive before spending a day in the sun when he or she is on methotrexate. Another side effect of methotrexate noted in adults is rapid appearance of rheumatoid nodules during methotrexate therapy. This is rare in children.

In addition to the side effects discussed for immunosuppressive drugs in general, methotrexate may have side effects that include problems with the blood cell counts or liver function. In rare cases, methotrexate can also cause kidney and lung problems. It should be very carefully monitored in children with preexisting liver, kidney, or lung conditions. Methotrexate is normally excreted by the kidneys, but it is not removed by dialysis. If your child has serious kidney problems, make sure your doctor is aware. If your child develops serious kidney problems, be sure the methotrexate is stopped or monitored very carefully.

When methotrexate first began to be used for patients with arthritis, many underwent periodic liver biopsies to assure they were not developing cirrhosis of the liver. However, these routine biopsies were not found to be helpful. Children with persistent or recurrent liver enzyme abnormalities should be taken off methotrexate. Failure to do so could result in long-term liver damage. However, this is rarely necessary.

Occasional mild abnormalities in the white blood cell count or liver enzymes may be the result of viral infections or other unrelated problems. These situations are best dealt with by withholding the methotrexate until the problem corrects itself, then restarting the methotrexate while monitoring carefully to make sure the problem does not return. *Everyone must remember that individuals using methotrexate must not drink alcoholic beverages.* The use of alcohol greatly increases the risk of liver damage. If your child drinks alcohol, make sure the doctor knows. If you can't trust them to stop drinking, don't let them take methotrexate.

Cyclosporine and tacrolimus

Cyclosporine (marketed as Neoral or Sandimmune) and tacrolimus (marketed as Prograf) are closely related immunosuppressive drugs that are primarily used to prevent organ transplant rejection. Cyclosporine was discovered first and is used more widely, but tacrolimus may be more potent and have fewer side effects. However, there is only limited experience with the use of tacrolimus for arthritis at present and I restrict the rest of this discussion to cyclosporine.

Cyclosporine works primarily by blocking synthesis of IL-2 (a messenger molecule) and preventing the recruitment of additional inflammatory cells to a site of inflammation. It also affects IL-3, IL-4, and IFN-gamma, which are messenger molecules (cytokines) that promote inflammation. Since cyclosporine has an independent mechanism of action, in most cases it can be added to the other medications a child is taking.

Cyclosporine may be very beneficial in children with enthesitis-associated arthritis, systemic onset arthritis, inflammatory bowel disease–associated arthritis, dermatomyositis, and other vasculitic illnesses. It is also useful for the treatment of ocular inflammation (uveitis). However, a child's response to cyclosporine is unpredictable. Some children who have not responded to other medications have dramatically improved with the addition of cyclosporine. At the same time, I have used it in other children, in seemingly identical situations, without benefit.

Cyclosporine is associated with a variety of side effects. It interferes with the immune system and has essentially the same risks as the other immunosuppressive drugs. In addition, the larger doses used to prevent organ transplant rejection are often associated with kidney damage (renal toxicity). At the low dosages used for children with arthritis, these side effects are uncommon. However, children on cyclosporine should have all the normal monitoring tests (see above) with extra attention to make sure the urine and blood pressure are checked routinely. Changes in the blood pressure or evidence of kidney irritation do occasionally occur at low doses, but with proper monitoring the drug can be discontinued as soon as they appear. In children who are carefully monitored, side effects are infrequent and generally resolve quickly with discontinuation of the drug.

Cyclosporine has several peculiarities. One is that it promotes hair growth—not just the hair on the top of the head, but hair everywhere on the body. This may become unsightly, but if the cyclosporine is correcting the disease, it is acceptable. *Cyclosporine is also unusual in that it binds very strongly to glass.* That means if you open the pills and put the medicine in a glass of water, the cyclosporine will bind to the glass and none will go into the child. Liquid cyclosporine is provided in a special container and must be administered directly to the child. You can't mix it in another container. Another peculiarity is that *children taking cyclosporine must avoid grapefruit juice.* There is a chemical in grapefruit juice that inactivates cyclosporine. Orange juice, grape juice, and other juices do not contain this chemical. If you are giving your child a lot of juices or juice-flavored drinks, check the label carefully.

Leflunomide (Arava)

Leflunomide (marketed as Arava) is another of the immunosuppressive drugs that works by interfering with DNA synthesis. However, at the very low doses used by rheumatologists, it is suspected that leflunomide has other anti-inflammatory effects as well. In adult studies, leflunomide has proven effective for rheumatoid arthritis. It is a new drug, and at present the studies in children have not been published. I have had good results in teenagers with polyarticular arthritis and enthesitis-associated arthritis who have not been able to tolerate other agents. Most physicians feel that leflunomide is appropriately used only after methotrexate and perhaps one of the biologics has been tried. However, this is a matter of individual judgment.

Leflunomide can be added to NSAIDs and other medications. It does not act at the same point as methotrexate, so the two drugs can be combined, but both may cause liver and blood cell abnormalities and their combined use requires careful monitoring. As with other immunosuppressive drugs, leflunomide has a slow onset of action but appears to be disease-modifying.

Leflunomide differs from most of the other immunosuppressive drugs by being highly concentrated in the enterohepatic circulation. What this means is that the drug is absorbed by the body, processed by the liver, and released from the liver into the intestine, but then reabsorbed into the body from the intestine. Instead of being removed from the body, as are most drugs, the active part of leflunomide stays in the body for a long period of time.

To take advantage of the fact that leflunomide is very slowly removed from the body, patients are given a big dose for the first few days, then a much smaller everyday dose. This is generally advantageous. However, if you need to get the drug out of the system (e.g., because of a side effect) the child must be given cholestyramine. This is an agent that binds to the leflunomide products in the intestine and prevents them from being reabsorbed. Once bound to cholestyramine, the active compounds are carried out of the body quickly.

Leflunomide requires careful monitoring of the child, just as in the case of any other immunosuppressive drug. It may cause problems with the liver, the blood-forming cells, or elsewhere. It also may increase the risk of infection, as do the other immunosuppressive drugs. Since it is a new agent, we still have a lot to learn about how well it is tolerated, which situations to use it in, and what problems may arise. Diarrhea seems to be an occasional mild side effect.

Mycophenolate mofetil (Cellcept)

Mycophenolate mofetil (marketed as Cellcept) is a newer immunosuppressive drug that inhibits DNA synthesis. It is primarily used for the treatment of organ transplant recipients but has been increasingly used in the treatment of children with SLE and other vasculitic diseases. It has also been used for the treatment of children with uveitis associated with JA and in adults with psoriatic arthritis. At present, the role of mycophenolate mofetil in the treatment of children with arthritis has not yet been defined. It is useful for some children with SLE (see Chapter 11).

Azathioprine (Imuran)

Azathioprine is one of the oldest of the immunosuppressive drugs. As do many of the others, it works because it inhibits DNA synthesis. There is extensive experience using azathioprine in the treatment of children with arthritis and the vasculitic diseases. In the past, it was the primary immunosuppressive therapy used for children who failed NSAIDs and gold shots. With the widespread use of methotrexate, there has been much less need for the use of azathioprine. It has all of the side effects of immunosuppressive drugs listed above. In addition, it is well known to sometimes cause liver irritation and problems with blood cell counts. It has also been associated with pancreatitis.

The proper role for azathioprine at present is unclear. It has been useful in children with severe polyarticular-onset and severe systemic onset JA. Newer agents, such as leflunomide and mycophenolate mofetil, were developed with the intent that they would be more effective and have fewer side effects. At present, we do not have enough experience with the newer drugs to make a definite statement about their relative safety or effectiveness. However, many physicians will try leflunomide or mycophenolate mofetil before azathioprine.

The biologics etanercept, infliximab, and adalimumab may greatly reduce the need for drugs such as azathioprine. However, on a worldwide basis, many physicians continue to use azathioprine because they have extensive experience with its use and it is far less expensive. Azathioprine has been used extensively in the treatment of children with vasculitic diseases.

Cyclophosphamide (Cytoxan)

Cyclophosphamide is the most potent of the commonly used immunosuppressive agents. *It is rarely used in the treatment of children with JA.* Its use in the treatment of SLE is discussed in detail in Chapter 11. Cyclophosphamide can be given as daily pills or as intravenous injections. The intravenous injections are given on a variety of schedules, but the most common is monthly for a period of months, followed by every three months until the course of therapy is completed. Except in special situations, *daily pills should be avoided*, as they have a much higher incidence of side effects than the intravenous injections.

Children receiving cyclophosphamide must be carefully monitored for evidence of bone marrow and bladder irritation. It is impractical to measure white blood cell counts and all other tests on a daily basis. If the medication is being given intravenously at intervals, all of the necessary tests can be done before each dose. Daily use of cyclophosphamide pills is associated with an increased risk of infection and a greatly increased risk of bladder damage. The damage to the bladder can lead to persistent bleeding and has been associated with the later development of bladder cancer in some patients.

Periodic intravenous injections of cyclophosphamide not only allow more careful monitoring, but they also allow the physicians to make sure the child is well hydrated to prevent cyclophosphamide breakdown products from being allowed to sit in the bladder for a long period. In addition, most physicians administer MESNA intravenously after the cyclophosphamide. MESNA is a compound that binds to the cyclophosphamide breakdown products and neutralizes them. This reduces the risk of bladder irritation.

Intravenous cyclophosphamide has been used for the treatment of children with systemic onset JA who failed all other therapies. Although there are several small reports in the literature describing success, it is not generally utilized. The treatment is difficult for the child and family. At best it made some children better. A number of years ago I tested it on a group of eight children with severe disease. After one year, all elected to discontinue treatment. They did not think it made enough difference. With the current availability of many new therapies, the role of cyclophosphamide in the treatment of children with arthritis is extremely limited. However, it remains a mainstay of therapy for children with vasculitic diseases, including SLE, dermatomyositis, and scleroderma.

Chlorambucil

Chlorambucil is a very potent immunosuppressive agent that does not have the bladder-irritating properties of cyclophosphamide. It has been used for systemic onset arthritis, vasculitic diseases, uveitis, and a variety of other life-threatening conditions. It is a very effective immunosuppressive drug. Chlorambucil does not have the problem of bladder irritation that cyclophosphamide has, but it does significantly impair the ability to deal with infections.

Chlorambucil is not widely used because it has been associated with the development of leukemia, sterility, and other complications far more often than the other immunosuppressive drugs discussed here. It should be considered only in the most difficult situations and used only by physicians with experience. Nonetheless, there are situations in which its use is appropriate.

GLUCOCORTICOIDS (STEROIDS, CORTICOSTEROIDS, PREDNISONE, METHYLPREDNISONE, DEXAMETHASONE, CORTISONE, HYDROCORTISONE)

The discovery of steroids was a major advance in the care of children and adults with rheumatic diseases. The beneficial effects of steroids result from their ability to block the effects of most inflammatory messengers (cytokines) and decrease the activity of the cells that promote inflammation. For children with severe diseases, the corticosteroids have vastly improved their quality of life. However, the excessive use of corticosteroids has many negative effects. Corticosteroids should be used only when necessary. Excessive and unnecessary use of corticosteroids may cause great harm.

Steroids are simultaneously a blessing and a curse for children with JA. With a large enough dose of corticosteroids, virtually all of the manifestations of JA will rapidly disappear. The discovery of these drugs at first was considered a miracle, but it rapidly became obvious that their continued usage caused an unacceptable level of side effects. When considering the use of these drugs, it is important to remember that they may be absolutely necessary and life-saving under certain circumstances but that prolonged use in significant dosage is inevitably associated with complications.

For children with JA, corticosteroids should be thought of as a fire extinguisher next to the stove. If everything is going up in flames, the fire extinguisher is very handy. On the other hand, it makes a mess of your kitchen that takes some time to clean up. Further, if you have repeated need for the fire extinguisher, you're doing something wrong. With the ready availability of biologics, oral steroids should be necessary only in the treatment of systemic onset JA, never pauciarticular onset JA, and rarely polyarticular onset JA. Corticosteroids are routinely used in the treatment of vasculitic diseases.

The adrenal gland in the body normally makes a certain amount of corticosteroids every day. If the adrenal gland fails, the result is a severe and life-threatening condition called **Addison's disease**. When your child takes extra corticosteroids every day, the body recognizes that there is no need for the adrenal gland to make more. If this continues for a long period, the adrenal gland may not be able to produce an adequate amount of corticosteroids. This is termed "adrenal suppression."

There are two important consequences of adrenal suppression. First, if corticosteroids have been given long enough to shut down the adrenal gland (weeks, not days), they cannot be stopped abruptly. Instead, they must be withdrawn slowly to give the adrenal gland time to resume normal function. Second, if your child is taking corticosteroids and becomes ill with nausea and vomiting, or if for any other reason your child cannot take the normal daily dose of corticosteroids, he or she needs to be given the dose by injection. This usually requires a visit to the doctor's office or the emergency room.

Even for children who have been able to discontinue corticosteroids, extra should be given if they need surgery or are under any form of significant physical stress, since their adrenal glands might not be able to produce the additional corticosteroids needed to deal with the stress. Make sure any doctor caring for your child knows that he or she is taking or has taken corticosteroids if this is the case. They will then know to take extra precautions, if necessary.

Glucocorticoid side effects

Cushing's syndrome
Fluid retention
Increased appetite
Weight gain
Truncal obesity (skinny arms and legs, but increased fat on back and stomach)
Moon facies (fat cheeks)
Stretch marks
Acne
Growth retardation
Bone-weakening calcium loss
Avascular necrosis
Muscle weakness
Poor sugar control (diabetes)
Cataracts
Increased intraocular pressure
Increased infections
Oral and vaginal thrush
Atherosclerosis
Hirsutism (extra hair growth)
Mood changes

Side effects of corticosteroids

The side effects of corticosteroids are very common. These are not unusual side effects; they are normal effects of taking extra corticosteroids (see box). In addition to the common side effects listed, corticosteroids also may cause high blood pressure, mood changes, inflammation of the pancreas, and pseudotumor cerebrae, which is increased pressure in the brain associated with severe headaches and visual problems.

So why take corticosteroids? The answer is that most children with JA should not be taking corticosteroids. However, children with diseases such as SLE and dermatomyositis often must take corticosteroids. For children with arthritis, corticosteroids should be reserved for those who cannot carry out their normal activities of daily living despite an adequate trial of other medications. Preferably, children who are having trouble should be placed on a disease-modifying drug before they get to the point where they cannot function well.

In some cases the disease is evolving rapidly or has a significant head start and the child requires corticosteroids. Even then, they should only be used for children with JA until one of the disease-modifying drugs can take over and the steroids can be withdrawn. In contrast, children with vasculitic illness often require chronic corticosteroid therapy. Most of the negative effects of corticosteroids are related to either the highest daily dose taken or the total amount taken over time, but side effects such as avascular necrosis of bone may occur after only the briefest exposure.

Many parents are very worried about the possible side effects of immunosuppressive drugs. It should be remembered that in the hands of experienced physicians, the severe side effects of immunosuppressive drugs are very rare. The negative effects of corticosteroids are very common. Before the widespread use of disease-modifying drugs, it was common to see a large number of obese children with bad hips sitting in wheelchairs waiting for the arthritis clinic to open. The corticosteroids made them obese and weakened their hips. By avoiding the excess use of corticosteroids, experienced pediatric rheumatologists have made such children rare in their clinics.

Despite their negative side effects, there are times when corticosteroids are important. For children with life-threatening vasculitic diseases, corticosteroids are often mandatory. Even so, the dosage should be minimized by the appropriate use of immunosuppressive drugs. This is discussed in greater detail in Chapters 10 to 16. For children with systemic onset JA with macrophage activation syndrome or other severe manifestations, corticosteroids are often mandatory. In the other forms of JA, corticosteroids can generally be avoided. However, if a child is unable to function adequately to attend school because of active arthritis, a short course of low-dose corticosteroids may be necessary.

A number of alternative regimens for the use of corticosteroids have been proposed. Many physicians have argued that given every other day, corticosteroids are less toxic. It is certainly true that 10 mg of prednisone every other day is less toxic than 10 mg every day. However, it is unclear that it is less toxic than 5 mg of prednisone every day, which may in fact be more effective. Some physicians claim that very high doses given every other day have few side effects. It is untrue.

In some situations, physicians use high doses of corticosteroids given intravenously. This is thought to have fewer side effects than high daily oral doses of corticosteroids. On a one-time basis this is probably true. However, this has not proven to be true when the high intravenous doses are given routinely. Many physicians were very excited when deflazacort became available. It was thought to be a corticosteroid that would "spare the bones." Unfortunately, on an equal-dose basis that is true, but if the dose is adjusted to get an equal therapeutic effect, there is an equal bone loss effect.

The widespread use of biologics, immunosuppressive drugs, and improved NSAIDs has led to a significant reduction in the use of corticosteroids in the treatment of JA. As further methods of treating JA are developed, the number of children suffering from significant corticosteroid toxicity should continue to fall. However, until we have a suitable replacement, it is important to have corticosteroids available for those times when an immediate and dramatic effect is necessary.

Intra-articular corticosteroids (aristospan, celestone, depo-medral)

These corticosteroid preparations are often used for intra-articular injections. That means that the drug is injected directly into the inflamed joint. For many years physicians were worried that this might weaken the joint. It is common to hear about athletes who have had multiple joint injections and had badly damaged joints in the end.

In the 1990s when MRI machines became widely available, a group of children who needed intra-articular steroid injections to treat arthritis in their knees were studied. This study took MRIs before injection, a few weeks after injection, and several months after injection. These serial MRIs demonstrated that the injections had a very positive effect on reducing the inflammation and promoting healing of the cartilage. When athletes do badly, it is because they resume harmful activities after their knees are injected. Children with arthritis who receive intra-articular injections are instructed to rest.

With the increased use of intra-articular corticosteroid injections, it has been easier to bring arthritis that is primarily affecting a single large joint under control. Intra-articular corticosteroid injections should be considered for a child with a single swollen joint who is not responding well to NSAIDs. Studies even suggest that the liberal use of intra-articular injections has reduced the frequency of leg-length discrepancy in children with "true" pauciarticular onset arthritis. Since the therapy is generally safe and effective (see below), it should probably be done sooner than later.

A number of physicians believe it is appropriate to anesthetize a child with three or four swollen joints and then inject each of the joints. It is my belief that if there are more than two swollen joints, it means that the disease is not under adequate control. These children should be given better systemic medication instead of multiple joint injections. The likelihood of long-term benefit from multiple joint injections in this setting is small, but this remains controversial. The children will definitely feel much better for a period of days after several joints are injected because the corticosteroids slowly leak out of the joints and have a systemic effect just as if they were taken by mouth. This effect is minimal if only a single joint is injected.

I normally do not anesthetize children for joint injections. Anesthesia carries its own set of medications and risks. However, it certainly can be done if the family requests it. Since I rarely do more than one joint, I find joint injections to be a quick and easy procedure. The joint to be injected is cleaned with surgical soap (betadine). Then a sterile cloth is placed around the spot to be injected. Numbing medicine can be injected around the area of the joint (this burns a little and I give children the choice of skipping it).

Once the area is properly cleaned, the physician simply slips the needle into the joint and injects the corticosteroids. For an experienced physician, this is usually very easy. Although children up to age twelve years or so will need to be helped to hold still when it hurts, most children tolerate this very well with positive reassurance from parents and the doctor. Do not say it will not hurt. That's not true. I always tell children it will hurt for a minute and challenge them to see if they can say "Ouch" louder than I can. In the distraction of listening to me say "Ouch," many of them forget to.

It is very difficult to predict for how long an intra-articular joint injection will provide relief. Sometimes there is only a single involved knee, and after it is injected the child never has trouble again. Other times the knee is injected and there is no apparent improvement. Most often joint injections provide two or three months of relief and allow other medications to take effect and control the disease. A frequent need for joint injections suggests that the child's disease is not being adequately controlled by the systemic medications.

There are very few risks associated with intra-articular joint injections. The greatest risk is that associated with anesthesia if children are anesthetized. Since I rarely inject multiple joints, I do not find anesthesia necessary except under unusual circumstances. Other risks associated with intra-articular joint injections include the risk of an infection as the result of being injected (I've never seen it), an unusual "crystal reaction" to the injected medication (I've never seen that, either), and damage to the skin around the injection site.

If corticosteroids leak into the skin and adjacent tissues during the injection, they cause loss of fat under the skin. This might sound like a good thing, but it is not. Consider the hands of a grandparent over the age of eighty. You can clearly see the veins and other tissues through the skin. This is because they have lost all of the subcutaneous fat. A similar thing happens if the corticosteroids leak under the skin. I often see children who come to me after being treated elsewhere who have pea-sized dimples at injection sites around their knees. These are not a big problem, but I have also seen larger areas of damaged skin that look like a bad scar. I can assume only that they are the result of poorly done joint injections.

Whenever a joint is injected, it is important for the physician to use a short-acting agent such as betamethasone if the area being injected is close to the surface (a tendon, a finger, or a wrist joint). Using a short-acting agent minimizes the risk of skin damage. Long-lasting agents such as triamcinolone hexacetonide should be reserved for large joints such as knees and hips.

There has been a lot of discussion about how much to limit activities after injecting a large joint. Our goal is to suppress the inflammation for as long as possible. To accomplish this, we want the injected corticosteroids to remain in the joint for as long as possible. Ideally, the child is not "active" for the first twenty-four hours after the injection. Some physicians even go so far as to place a temporary cast on the leg if the knee is injected, removing it the next day. Most of us settle for instructing the family to limit unnecessary activities for twenty-four hours.

It is also necessary to remember that the corticosteroids to be injected are typically mixed with lidocaine (the medicine used when the dentist numbs your teeth or when you need stitches in the emergency room). This has the advantage of immediately making the joint numb. *Be sure to tell the physician if you are allergic to lidocaine.* Since the joint will be numb for several hours after the injection, everyone should be careful. Just as you could bite your lip and not know it after seeing the dentist, a child could injure the injected joint and not know it. This is one of the reasons why athletes who get their joints injected and then go back in the game end up in so much trouble.

BIOLOGICS

The biologics are a new class of medications that have allowed us to provide dramatic relief to children with severe arthritis. They are designed to target a specific molecule that plays an important role in the inflammatory process. Each of the biologics has strengths and weaknesses that I discuss below. Because the biologics relieve arthritis by directly affecting the immune response, they are immunosuppressive. As a result, the biologics carry the same risks of infection and possibly late development of cancer that are discussed in the section on immunosuppressive medications above. The stronger the biologic or the higher the dose given, the greater is the risk of infection.

Parents often worry that because the biologics are new medications, we do not know what will happen to someone who takes them for ten years or more. Of course, until a medication has been in use for ten years, it will be impossible to know for sure what effects it will have. However, you would not go out and buy a ten-year-old model television or computer or other technologically sophisticated device. You'd want the latest.

All of the medications that have been licensed for use in the United States have undergone several years of testing in animals and patients before they were licensed. Before you insist that you have to know what the effects of ten years of the medication might be before you allow your child to take it, remember that pediatric rheumatologists know quite well what ten years of uncontrolled arthritis will do to your child. There are remote risks of undiscovered long-term medication side effects, but there are many uncontrollable risks in everyday life. We recommend these medicines because we know for sure that ten years of uncontrolled arthritis will cause significant disability.

Etanercept (Enbrel)

Etanercept was the first widely available biologic. It has made a dramatic difference in the care of children with JA. Many pediatric rheumatologists feel it is the most significant advance in many years. It is effective for most children with polyarticular onset arthritis, spondyloarthropathies, and psoriasis-associated arthritis and some children with systemic onset arthritis. It may prove to be effective for many other forms of childhood rheumatic disease, but this has not been fully investigated. Although etanercept is also effective for children with severe pauciarticular onset arthritis, it is rarely necessary for that disease.

Etanercept was initially studied in children with severe disease who were not responding adequately to methotrexate. All of the data that have been published indicate that methotrexate plus etanercept is better than methotrexate alone. There is little published data regarding the use of etanercept without methotrexate in childhood. However, I have used etanercept without methotrexate in many children who did not tolerate methotrexate or whose parents did not wish them to take methotrexate. The two drugs do not need to be given together. Etanercept works quite well alone.

Etanercept works by interfering with the function of a molecule called tumor necrosis factor alpha (TNF-α). This is a very important messenger molecule that is released into the circulation by an activated cell and causes the cells that receive the message to become activated. When large amounts of TNF-α are in the circulation, people tend to feel very ill. The etanercept molecule consists of two artificial receptors for TNF-α attached to a larger molecule (Fc receptor) that allows the etanercept to be cleared from the body. The effects are often very impressive. Parents frequently report striking improvement within hours of the first dose. For most children, the improvement continues for as long as the child remains on etanercept. Early studies suggest that by blocking TNF-α activity, etanercept not only prevents symptoms of the disease, but also allows healing of the bone and joint damage to begin.

The major disadvantages of etanercept are that it is costly (though not in comparison to the cost of untreated disease) and must be given by subcutaneous injection twice weekly. That means that parents or the child will need to learn how to give the shots. Alternatively, the shots can be given in the physician's office, by a visiting nurse, or another individual. However, since subcutaneous injections are easy to do, most parents learn to do them without difficulty.

Common side effects of etanercept include runny nose, soreness or skin reactions at the injection site, and headaches. Few parents or children feel these are significant when measured against the dramatic relief of arthritis symptoms. Periodic monitoring of blood tests is required, as with every medication, but significant problems are few.

There are several important considerations regarding uncommon side effects for children on etanercept. The most important is the increased risk of infection. As discussed previously, every drug that reduces the body's inflammatory response, thereby reducing the arthritis, also reduces the inflammatory response to infections. This increases the risk that an infection could escape the body's control and become life-threatening. Fortunately, such episodes are extremely rare.

Because of the risk of severe infections, if a child receiving etanercept looks sick, he or she should see the physician sooner, not later. Further, I recommend not giving the injections to children with fever unless the fever is part of the disease they are being treated for (and then only with care). Skin and lung infections may be the most important to watch for. Infection is a risk with all of the immunosuppressive medications used for children with severe arthritis.

Another concern is that all of the drugs that affect the immune system are associated with altered immune regulation that may lead to the development or worsening of other diseases. Some children receiving etanercept have developed minor serologic abnormalities related to lupus, and this needs to be monitored. However, medically significant problems appear to be extremely rare. Etanercept can prevent serious damage from arthritis. For the majority of children, allowing the arthritis to continue is far more worrisome and dangerous than the remote risk of a serious side effect from etanercept.

Parents often ask how long their child will need to continue on etanercept. This is a very difficult question to answer. Although etanercept often does an excellent job of controlling disease, it does not cure disease. It's like the child who looks at the sleeping lion at the zoo and asks why the big cat is in a cage. Etanercept cages the arthritis. Take the cage away and no one can be sure what will happen. I have had two experiences with children who were "miraculously cured" by etanercept, so much so that the family thought there was no reason to continue the shots or return for their appointments. After six or eight weeks off medication, the disease came back much worse than before.

At the present time, a child who is doing well on etanercept should continue on the medication. Several of my families have tried to space out the dosage interval or gradually reduce the dosage, but the arthritis has flared. The proper means of discontinuing etanercept remains to be determined. In the few children for whom etanercept has not been beneficial, there have been no problems with discontinuing it.

All parents worry about giving their children a medication without a clear indication of how and when they will be able to stop the medication. However, seeing a child with significant arthritis suddenly and dramatically improve provides an immediate reminder of how much trouble the child was having. *It is true that parents and physicians should be worried about giving a child a medication without a clear indication of how and when to stop. But they should be far more worried about allowing a child to have active uncontrolled arthritis and all its complications without a clear indication of how and when the arthritis will stop.*

Infliximab (Remicade)

Infliximab is another very useful biologic for the treatment of children with arthritis. It is an antibody that is directed against TNF-α. Infliximab directly reacts with TNF-α molecules in the body and carries them away. Not only does it attack TNF-α in the circulation, but it can also attack TNF-α molecules on the surface of cells destroying both the TNF-α and the cells. It seems to be a very potent treatment for severe arthritis. It is effective for most children with polyarticular onset arthritis, spondyloarthropathies, and psoriasis-associated arthritis and some children with systemic onset arthritis. It may prove to be effective for many other forms of childhood arthritis.

In the published information on infliximab, it is used in conjunction with methotrexate. This is because the antibody molecule that is the active part of infliximab sometimes stimulates an immune response where the body produces human antichimeric antibodies (HACAs). These HACAs will attack the infliximab molecule and block its effect. There is reason to believe that methotrexate reduces the incidence of allergic reactions and other complications that may interfere with how infliximab works. It is also believed that taking methotrexate slows the formation of HACAs. If a child cannot tolerate methotrexate and requires infliximab, it may be useful to treat him or her with one of the other immunosuppressive drugs.

The major difficulties associated with infliximab relate to its administration. Infliximab is given as a periodic intravenous infusion. It can be given in a physician's office, in a hospital infusion unit, or by a visiting nurse. The dosage regimen is variable. After the initial doses that are given more frequently, infliximab may be given monthly or every other month. The optimal dosage regimen and frequency are not the same for every patient. Allergic reactions seem to be more common with infliximab than other biologics, and some patients need to be medicated for these. As a result, the first dose of infliximab is normally given under a doctor's supervision. Even after the first dose, any side effects during administration should be promptly reported to the physician for evaluation.

Infection is a concern with infliximab, just as it is with other immunosuppressive and biologic agents. Tuberculosis is a particular concern and children should be screened for tuberculosis and tuberculosis exposure before infliximab is begun. The use of very high doses of infliximab is clearly associated with a marked increase in the risk of infection.

If a child is running a fever or there are other reasons to suspect that there might be an infection, the dose of infliximab should not be given. Significant side effects of infliximab except for mild allergic reactions and infections are very rare. All of the concerns related to altering the immune system with immunosuppressive medications should be considered. As with etanercept above, the ultimate duration of infliximab therapy is unclear.

Adalimumab (Humira)

This is the newest of the biologics. It is an antibody to TNF-α that can be given as a subcutaneous injection either every week or every other week. Preliminary indications are that it is as effective as infliximab, with greater convenience. However, more experience is necessary before any definite comparisons can be made between adalimumab and etanercept or infliximab. Some of my patients who were not getting an adequate response to etanercept have improved once they switched to adalimumab. Because adalimumab is a "fully humanized" antibody (see the Glossary), there should be fewer side effects and less development of HACAs than with infliximab. As our experience grows, the strengths and benefits of adalimumab will become more obvious. It has been very helpful for some children with uveitis.

Kineret (Anakinra)

Kineret is a novel biologic agent that works by blocking a messenger called IL-1, preventing its attachment to the IL-1 receptor. The experience with kineret in children is limited. Unlike infliximab, adalimumab, and etanercept, which are given less often, kineret needs to be administered as a daily subcutaneous injection. It may be associated with abnormalities on the routine blood tests and local pain at the injection site. It also has a slow onset of action. The combination of a slow onset of action and a daily need for injections is often unsatisfactory for young children. They don't feel better fast enough to be willing to tolerate the everyday shots.

Although kineret is effective, the ultimate place for this agent in the treatment of childhood arthritis is uncertain. In animal models, blocking IL-1 substantially reduced joint damage due to arthritis. However, this effect is seen only over a period of time. Like the other biologics, kineret is primarily used in association with methotrexate. However, it has also been shown to have beneficial effects when used without methotrexate.

Kineret has all of the side effects associated with other immunosuppressive drugs. Unfortunately, the combination of kineret with etanercept resulted in an increased incidence of infections. Until there is further information, the appropriate place for using kineret in children with arthritis is uncertain.

MISCELLANEOUS AGENTS

Thalidomide (Thalomid)

Thalidomide is a medication that was initially used as a sedative. It was rapidly withdrawn from the market because it causes significant birth defects if taken by pregnant women. It was subsequently discovered to have very potent anti-inflammatory effects. Although parents and physicians initially are concerned on learning that thalidomide is known to cause birth defects, *none of the immunosuppressive drugs is safe to give to pregnant women.* Fortunately, in pediatric rheumatology, pregnancy is rarely an immediate concern. There is no evidence that thalidomide has any lingering effects more than a month after it is discontinued. Thalidomide is very effective for some children with systemic onset, psoriasis-associated, and polyarticular onset arthritis who have not responded to other medications.

Thalidomide may cause abnormalities in the routine blood tests, including decreased white blood cell count and elevated liver enzymes. Routine monitoring is required. Thalidomide is associated with nerve irritation that can produce pain and tingling. This should be monitored for. Continued treatment with thalidomide could result in permanent nerve damage. However, in the dosage recommended for children with arthritis this has not been a significant problem to date.

The use of thalidomide currently requires extensive monitoring to assure that the patient is not at risk for becoming pregnant. Although it seems improbable for small children, one can never be too careful. At the present time in the United States, only physicians who have registered with the company that provides the drug can prescribe thalidomide.

This drug may become more important in the future because it down-regulates the genes that are responsible for synthesis of many inflammatory molecules. (In other words, it tells the genes in the body to make less of them.) In the United States, biologics are being used to attack these molecules, but the biologics are very expensive. When I teach in foreign countries, often the doctors are all interested in hearing about the new biologic agents, but no one can afford them. Thalidomide may be similarly effective and is much less expensive.

Intravenous gamma globulin (IVIgG)

Intravenous gamma globulin (IVIgG) received a lot of attention in the early 1990s. It is still used for many diseases by some physicians, but the cost is extremely high and its use has largely been supplanted by the biologics. IVIgG always appeared to be helpful, but in controlled studies the benefits were always marginal. Some physicians still believe this is an excellent medication for systemic onset arthritis and dermatomyositis. It is very effective for children with Kawasaki disease (see Chapter 17). The difference is that Kawasaki disease is an acute illness. Once you have treated a child for Kawasaki disease with IVIgG, in most cases the illness is cured.

The use of IVIgG seems to suffer from a phenomenon called tachyphylaxis. What that means is that the effect of treatment decreases with each successive dose. Children treated with IVIgG often seemed much improved initially, but they would require more and more IVIgG over time (usually, more frequent treatment) with less and less effect. As a result, the benefits of IVIgG for chronic conditions such as arthritis and dermatomyositis are less clear. It is a useful therapy for children with immune deficiency diseases who do not make enough of their own IgG, because in those cases it is simply a replacement therapy.

Many parents and physicians initially chose IVIgG because they felt this was a safer therapy. With extensive experience, it has become clear that significant negative side effects may occur. Like infliximab, this therapy must be given as periodic intravenous infusions and may be associated with allergic reactions. In general, this therapy should be restricted to specific situations such as Kawasaki disease and some hematologic disorders.

Gold sodium thioglucose and gold sodium thiomalate (Myochrysine, Solganol, "gold shots")

Gold shots were the standard of therapy for difficult arthritis in adults and children when I began my career. For many children, they were dramatically effective, bringing a slow but steady resolution of the arthritis. The major difficulty with gold shots is that they require painful intramuscular injections. The injections are given weekly until the arthritis is well under control and then slowly spaced out over longer intervals.

Since gold shots could have significant impact on the blood-forming cells, most physicians do routine blood work before every dose. Frequent testing and doctor visits are a major inconvenience. However, gold shots were effective for many children with arthritis. Side effects beyond the inconvenience of frequent physician visits were most often limited to minor changes in the blood tests. Severe side effects do occur, but they are infrequent.

Over the past twenty years, most physicians have replaced the use of gold shots with methotrexate and now the new biologics. Methotrexate is usually given in oral form and is far more convenient. It is unclear where gold shots belong in the current approach to therapy. There are many children whose arthritis disappeared when they were treated with gold shots. However, some children ultimately relapsed after the gold shots were discontinued. The biologics, such as etanercept, clearly provide a quicker and greater level of relief with less apparent toxicity. I almost never use gold shots now, but there may still be a place for them.

Auranofin (Ridaura)

Auranofin is an oral version of gold salts given as daily pills. It was developed in an effort to overcome the inconvenience associated with weekly gold shots. Unfortunately, auranofin does not seem to be as effective as gold shots. It has just as many side effects. It is rarely if ever used in childhood.

D-penicillamine

D-penicillamine is a chelating agent (see the Glossary) that was widely used for the treatment of children with JA and morphea and scleroderma. It is clearly a disease-modifying agent but has a very slow onset of action and a high frequency of toxic reactions. Routine blood test abnormalities, skin rashes, kidney irritation, and neurologic abnormalities all occur. As a result of the slow onset of improvement and the high frequency of side effects, D-penicillamine was rapidly replaced by methotrexate for the treatment of children with arthritis. D-penicillamine may still have a role for children who have not responded to other medications, but it is rare to see it used for arthritis in childhood.

D-penicillamine has long been the standard recommended therapy for children with morphea and scleroderma (progressive systemic sclerosis). Although some physicians report good effects, most physicians with extensive experience find D-penicillamine to have a high frequency of toxicity and only minimal efficacy. The right therapy for scleroderma remains controversial, but I prefer methotrexate. For most children with scleroderma or morphea, methotrexate has greater efficacy and less toxicity than D-penicillamine. Nevertheless, there are well-respected physicians who continue to use D-penicillamine for scleroderma.

Plasmapharesis (apharesis). Plasmapharesis is not a medication. It is a technique by which the patient's blood is removed from the body so the plasma (see the Glossary) can be removed and replaced, while the blood cells are returned to the patient. If there is a toxic element in the plasma, plasmapharesis will remove it.

At one point, plasmapharesis was considered a possible therapy for a wide variety of diseases. However, it was found to lack lasting beneficial effects. Today, plasmapharesis is not routinely used for the therapy of children with any rheumatic disease. However, it is occasionally beneficial for crisis management in children with systemic lupus erythematosus or antiphospholipid antibody syndrome. Controlled studies do not convincingly show any sustained benefit from plasmapharesis after the acute crisis. Over time, the toxic effects mount, while the therapeutic efficacy decreases.

COMBINATIONS OF MEDICINE

It is a great frustration for parents to have a child with active arthritis who is receiving multiple medications and does not seem to be getting better. When the physician recommends a new medication, parents inevitably ask, "Which one is this replacing?" Sometimes we are adding a new drug without discontinuing one of the others. This frustrates many parents. It is important to understand that the immune system is the body's defense against infection. Throughout history infection has been a major cause of death in childhood. Thus, children who had strong immune systems were much more likely to survive.

> Imagine if you were given the job of reducing traffic in Manhattan—there are just too many cars! At first, you might simply close one of the many bridges into the city. That would be effective when you first did it, but quickly you would notice that there are a lot of bridges into Manhattan. Some people may have stopped going into the city, but others changed to a different bridge.
>
> The next step would be to stop traffic on all the bridges. That would have a very good effect at first, but then you would realize that there are four tunnels. Pretty quickly, the tunnel traffic would go way up and traffic in the city would begin to climb again. If you start stopping tunnel traffic, you would discover that people would start using the ferries more.
>
> Just to make matters worse, if you could completely stop the traffic into Manhattan, the people living in the city would starve. Thus, there is no simple answer. You would need to adjust and test varying combinations of bridge and tunnel restrictions to find one that accomplished your goal of reducing traffic sufficiently without causing harm to the people in the city.

As a physician prescribing medicine for a child with arthritis, I need to find the right combination with the best effect for the child and the fewest side effects. Often this means attacking the problem from several different directions. I try to stop one bridge and one tunnel to get the right balance of letting necessary traffic in and reducing cars. There is no perfect solution for traffic or arthritis.

A nurse with whom I have worked for more than ten years summarized it best: "When I first saw you prescribing so many different medicines for children, I was scared. Now we've worked together for over ten years and I see how well the children have done. We didn't get such good results before. Now I understand that aggressive therapy works."

ROUTINE SUPPLEMENTS

Parents are always anxious to make sure they are doing everything possible for their children. In the United States it is rare to find anyone whose diet is truly deficient. However, some kids are fussy about meat, vegetables, and so on. The best way to deal with this is to make sure your child takes a single multivitamin each day. This should be a vitamin that is appropriate for your child's age. Check with your physician if you are unsure.

Many children with chronic active disease are anemic. As a result of the chronic blood loss, some of them will become iron-deficient. In other children, the problem is that they don't utilize the iron in their bodies well. If your child has arthritis, make sure you give him or her a vitamin with iron. However, remember iron is toxic if the levels are too high. Don't give iron pills unless directed to do so by the physician. If you've been giving them for a long time, remind the physician to check the levels. Excessive iron causes damage to many organs.

Calcium supplementation is also very popular at the present time. Calcium is included in our daily diet, but not all of us get enough every day. Most routine multivitamins don't contain a large amount of calcium. However, there is a reason for this. Calcium tends to cause upset stomachs and constipation. (People won't buy vitamins that cause these problems.) If your child is not getting a balanced diet, speak to your doctor about a calcium supplement. However, be aware that calcium does cause constipation and upset stomachs in some people. Like iron, calcium is necessary, but too much can be harmful. Don't overdo it. Let your doctor know what you are giving your child.

Most of the other vitamins and minerals are adequately replaced by a single multivitamin daily. There is always a lot of talk about extra this or extra that. No one is quite sure when extra is good or not. However, it is clear that *too much vitamin A and too much vitamin D are harmful.* Do not supplement these beyond your doctor's recommendation. In most cases, a daily multivitamin is more than enough.

> The best intentions don't always work out as you would expect. One of my teenage patients came from a family with a strong family history of kidney stones. He had never had any problems, but some of the adults in his family had developed kidney stones in their forties. When my patient became ill, his mother wanted to do everything possible. She gave him extra calcium and extra vitamin C. As a result, she also gave him kidney stones.

IMMUNIZATIONS

The following are several important questions that I am repeatedly asked about immunizations.

- Do they cause juvenile arthritis or other rheumatic diseases?
- Are they safe for children with rheumatic diseases?
- Should my child be vaccinated?
- *And the question too many people forget to ask: What about vaccinating my other children?*

The most important thing to understand about immunizations is that they have saved millions of lives. Routine vaccination against smallpox eliminated a terrible and often fatal disease from the world (current bioterror issues are not relevant to this discussion; I discuss smallpox vaccination for children with rheumatic diseases below). Although it may take a full generation, routine immunization against hepatitis B will also save hundreds of thousands of lives. You will find it nearly impossible to locate a young American doctor with experience treating polio, measles, mumps, rubella, or their complications because routine vaccination has made these diseases very rare. This is a wonderful thing. At present, every American child is routinely vaccinated against polio, tetanus, measles, mumps, rubella, pertusis (whooping cough), and hepatitis B.

To meet the current recommendations of the American Academy of Pediatrics, children receive at least fifteen vaccinations during the first three years of life. Pauciarticular onset juvenile arthritis frequently starts in young children in this age group, so chances are that children often develop the disease within a few months of a vaccination. Since the injections cause a fever and pain, it is natural for parents of a child with arthritis to suspect that the injection may have played a role.

A proper study would require evaluating the frequency of juvenile arthritis in a large group of children who did not get properly vaccinated. However, it would be unethical to do this. What I can tell you is that I have been practicing for more than twenty-five years and have practiced in areas where routine vaccinations were not always done (because people did not come to the doctor). There does not appear to be any increase in the incidence of juvenile arthritis among properly vaccinated children. *We know there are small risks associated with routine vaccination, but the risks of the diseases we are being protected against are far more severe.*

However, while I believe it is important that all normal children receive vaccinations, *the situation for children who have arthritis is more complicated.* Here there is a diversity of opinion among doctors. In addition, the answer depends on what medications your child is taking. What I am stating here are only my own views.

Most often your child will have received polio, tetanus, measles, mumps, and rubella immunizations before developing arthritis. This will make life easier for everyone. Although several doses of vaccine are recommended, children get some protection from even a single dose. A child who has never been vaccinated against these diseases is a special case that will require careful consideration between the parents and physician.

If a child has received the three routine vaccinations scheduled up to six months of age and the first measles, mumps, rubella vaccination, then the child should not receive any further vaccines while the arthritis is active. For children who are off medications or taking only a routine NSAID and if the arthritis has been fully controlled for six months, then one can carefully consider giving vaccinations.

Rubella is the only vaccine that routinely causes transient arthritis as a side effect. I would check to see whether a child has a reasonable titer of immunity (this is a routine blood test) and not revaccinate with rubella if the child is immune. I would avoid live vaccines (e.g., the chickenpox vaccine [herpes zoster], and the smallpox vaccine) in any child who has active disease or is receiving immunosuppressive drugs. These recommendations are detailed in the box on the following page.

A major issue that is often overlooked by physicians and families is the possible spread of live virus vaccines among close contacts. If your child is receiving medications that impede the ability to fight infection (including but not limited to corticosteroids, methotrexate, and biologics), not only should they *not* receive live vaccines but neither should their brothers and sisters. The altered virus contained in these vaccines can spread from one child to another and cause severe problems in an immunologically compromised child. You must also be careful about letting your child come in close contact with other children who have been recently vaccinated.

Notes on other vaccines

Flu shots. Hotly debated by physicians. There is no right answer.

Pneumovax. It is now recommended by the American Academy of Pediatrics that young children receive the pneumovax vaccination early in life. It prevents many types of serious pneumonia and other infections caused by the same family of bacteria. Most older children have not gotten it. It should be given to children if you think you are going to put them on immunosuppressive medications, but it must be given before you start the immunosuppressive medication for it to be most effective. There is evidence that it still has some benefit even if the children are on immunosuppressive medicine. This is safe because it is not a live vaccine.

Recommendations for vaccinations in children with rheumatic disease

Child with arthritis off all medications and well for six months or more
All vaccines recommended may be given, but avoid rubella if the child has a positive titer, indicating immunity to rubella.

Child with arthritis on NSAIDs, but well for six months
Most routine vaccinations okay but avoid rubella if the child has a positive titer
No live vaccines (e.g., chicken pox [herpes zoster] and smallpox). There is risk of disease and Reye's syndrome.

Child with arthritis on immunosuppressive medications: Corticosteroids, biologics (e.g., etanercept, infliximab, anakinra, and adalimumab), and cytotoxics (e.g., methotrexate, mycophenolate mofetil, cyclophosphamide, and azathioprine)
No vaccinations to the child
No live vaccinations to siblings or household contacts.

Child with active arthritis within the past six months (no matter what the medications)
No vaccinations (not all doctors agree).

Meningitis (meningococcal vaccine). The meningococcal vacine is frequently recommended for college freshman. It is not essential and the risk of meningococcal meningitis is very low. I would not dissuade parents who want their child to have it.

Smallpox (vaccinia). Smallpox was and still is a terrible condition that is often fatal. Worldwide vaccination programs have led to the elimination of this disease except as a biowarfare threat. *This is a live virus and has a significant risk of causing trouble to anyone who is immunosuppressed.* It is also a member of the herpes family of viruses that has been linked to Reye's syndrome.

Should the disease become a real threat, it will be necessary to immunize as many people as possible. For children on NSAIDs only, the risk would be acceptable under those circumstances. For children on immunosuppressive drugs, it would be necessary to stop those drugs at least fourteen days before vaccination and maintain the child off the drugs for a month after the vaccination (if the CDC makes official recommendations for this situation, we should all follow them. But so far they have not.) The risks of doing this will have to be considered for each child's situation.

23

Alternative Medicine

Vitamins and Supplements

Whenever I finish explaining a new medication and a parent asks me, "Is there another choice?" I know that something is worrying him or her. One of the biggest problems in medicine is fear of side effects. It's a lot like flying. When you get on the airplane and the flight attendant talks about the life jacket under the seat in front of you, you cannot help but think, "If there's a real chance we're going to land in the water, I'm getting off this plane." Surely, the flight attendant feels the same way. However, the government requires that passengers be informed about the life jacket and other safety precautions. Similarly, physicians are required to tell you about possible side effects of medications. If they thought there would be any serious ones, they would not give you the medicine. However, the physicians and the flight attendant are required to give you this information because no one knows for sure when something might go wrong.

You cannot get to a far away place without the risks of driving, flying, taking a train, or taking a boat. You cannot treat illness without the risk of side effects. *Whether you take the prescribed medications, buy over-the-counter medications, ignore your problem and figure it will go away, or buy health food "cures," there are risks associated with every choice. The only difference is whether or not those risks are clearly explained to you.* The physician is required to do that, but you have to read the warnings for yourself on over-the-counter medications.

A quick search of the Internet for the words "arthritis+alternative+cure" turned up over 120,000 Web pages. Searching for "arthritis+diet" turned up over 500,000 Web pages. Some recommend you avoid red meat, some recommend rub-on creams, some recommend "dietary" supplements.

Can all of these people really be wrong? Surely, some of these sites have useful information.

There are many things to remember when you consider using supplements and alternative medicines. First and foremost is that *none of these diets or creams or "supplements" is subject to any regulation regarding truth of their claims, the purity of the product, or even that what it says on the label is what is in the product.* Many supplements have been found to contain little if any of the ingredients highlighted on the label, but some have been found to be contaminated with heavy metals and other substances that are known to be bad for you. The harmful contaminants were not listed on the labels. (If you are curious, I found over 4,000 web pages discussing harmful contaminants in supplements. See supplement+harmful+contaminant.)

READ THE LABEL CAREFULLY AND DON'T BELIEVE EVERYTHING YOU READ

There is no such thing as a medication or food to relieve bone or joint pains that has positive effects that has no risk of side effects. It is with dismay that I see parents bring in all sorts of things found in health food stores, noted on the Internet, advertised on television, or seen in the newspapers. They want me to say that it's all right to give it to their child. Most would not be fooled for a moment if the item promised stock market riches or a new way to keep your car from needing gasoline.

There are lots of unscrupulous individuals who will sell you anything to get your money. Health aids are a billion-dollar-a-year business. Most are harmless except for the expense and may have a positive "placebo effect." However, many are potentially harmful, especially for people who really do have a problem. Moreover, their use may delay proper diagnosis and treatment. There are no rules restricting what salespeople can say in stores or can be claimed on the Internet. The small print always says, "This item is sold as a food supplement not a medication and these claims have not been evaluated or validated by the FDA." FDA-approved drugs are made in factories that are carefully inspected. The medications are checked to be sure that they are really what they say the are and to be sure they contain no contaminants that could be harmful.

Prescription medications are provided by licensed physicians who have been trained in their use and who do not have a financial incentive for you to take the drug. What do you know about where that health food or miracle cure was made, what's really in it, the training of the people recommending it, or their financial incentive to sell it? You would be shocked to read the reports about many of these products that have been investigated.

Many people assume that physicians are automatically against anything they did not prescribe. If you read through all the literature on alternative care, you'll even find statements such as, "Doctors are not going to give you this because it will cure you. Then you will not have to go back and they will not make any money." Nothing could be further from the truth. It is against the law for doctors to have a financial interest in the drugs they prescribe. If peanut butter from the supermarket would cure arthritis, I'd be thrilled to send my patients straight to the checkout counter.

In the sections that follow, I discuss vitamin and mineral supplementation, alternative diets, dietary supplements, and herbal cures. You will find I favor some types of supplementation and oppose others. Several key points need to be considered.

- Although manufacturing, advertising, and distribution of medications are tightly regulated by the FDA, there is no regulation of recommendations for diets or dietary supplements.
- The manufacturers of supplements can claim whatever they wish without doing testing of any kind.
- There is no independent testing to determine whether what the label says the supplement contains is in fact in it.
- Nor is there independent testing to make sure that the supplement does not contain harmful things.

When you meet someone who is sure that a special diet or supplement made his or her arthritis better, remember they may or may not have the same disease you or your child has. Second, large-scale studies of adults with arthritis have clearly documented a substantial "sugar pill" (placebo) effect. In studies of new medications, patients are divided into two groups. One group gets the new medication; the other gets an identical-appearing sugar pill. In virtually every such study, one-third of the patients receiving the sugar pill report dramatic improvement. They are not lying. They feel better. Whether this was due to spontaneous improvement, psychological effects, or other factors varied from patient to patient. But the sugar pills did not make them better.

No matter what anyone tells you, there is no such thing as an active ingredient without possible side effects. *Anything that has real effects has the potential of side effects.* Physicians are prevented from owning pharmacies or selling you medications in their offices. This is to prevent them from having a financial gain in prescribing a medication. In contrast, the people selling vitamins and supplements are salespeople who have been trained to sell you their products. Many are on direct commission. That means the more you spend, the more they are paid. Recently, some physicians started selling vitamins and supplements in their offices (and making a profit on them). This was declared unethical by several medical societies and may soon be illegal.

VITAMINS

Every child with chronic disease should be on a daily vitamin that contains the appropriate amounts of vitamins A, B (all types), C, D, E, and K, folic acid, iron, and calcium. Children with iron deficiency may need additional iron supplementation. Children should also be getting adequate daily calcium. However, the iron-containing medications may cause upset stomach. Overdosage of iron can be fatal, so keep the pills in a safe place and give extra iron (more than a regular multivitamin contains) only on a doctor's advice.

Calcium in excess causes upset stomach and constipation. In severe excess, calcium can also contribute to kidney stones (especially if combined with a lot of vitamin C, which acidifies the urine). Beyond the recommended basic daily requirement, extra vitamins must be given with caution. Most vitamins have a tremendous safety range. However, vitamins A and D are stored in the body and may reach toxic levels. Too much vitamin A or D can cause severe illness and even death.

When you buy your vitamins I strongly recommend you stick with an established brand from a major national manufacturer. Not all vitamin pills are the same. Some pills will claim a large amount of an ingredient, but it may not be in a form your body can use. Spinach is a famous example of this problem. It is full of iron, but not in a form that is very usable when you eat it. In addition, you have no way of knowing what the filler in the vitamin is or what it may be contaminated with.

In the 1980s many people developed eosinophilic fasciitis after taking a B vitamin supplement. It's never been conclusively proven, but it is thought that the main ingredient was improperly manufactured. Unfortunately, a number of vitamin makers bought the main ingredient from the same company. If your local coffee shop or newsstand is selling vitamins at the checkout counter, it's because they make a profit on them. If you never heard of a brand, I suggest you avoid it.

SUPPLEMENTS

Supplements need to be divided between plant extracts and a large variety of chemicals. *You have to remember that "all-natural" does not mean safe. The hemlock that poisoned Socrates was an "all-natural" product.* Sometimes parents or patients ask whether they can take the medicine in a more natural form. It is useful to consider the history of aspirin. The original form was derived from willow tree bark, clearly an all-natural product. When chemists looked at it carefully, they discovered the active ingredient was salicin. However, while salicin was much more effective than the original bark extract, it caused severe upset stomach. Aspirin is chemically modified salicin that is much easier on the stomach than the all-natural form of the drug.

> If you are standing in the aisle of your local pharmacy or health food/nutrition store and trying to decide which of all the products to buy, remember this. There is a large counter containing many different remedies for coughs and colds. But if you have a documented streptococcal sore throat, every doctor recommends penicillin (unless you are allergic). *Why is only one drug recommended for streptococcal sore throat? Because it has been proven that penicillin works. Why are there so many different remedies for coughs and colds? Because none of them has ever really been proven to work well.* If one had, we would all buy that one and the other brands would be gone. *How many different products do you see in the health food or nutrition store claiming that they will cure arthritis?*

Glucosamine

One supplement that has been shown to be of benefit for people with **osteoarthritis** is glucosamine. Glucosamine is a raw ingredient used by the body in manufacturing cartilage. Several studies have shown that adults with osteoarthritis who were taking glucosamine felt better than those taking sugar pills. However, osteoarthritis is due to breakdown of cartilage with age. This is not the cause of the problems in children with arthritis. Still, side effects of glucosamine are usually mild. In contrast, chondroitin sulfate, which is often marketed with glucosamine, has failed to show benefit in studies and been shown to cause an increased frequency of stomach upset.

Fatty acid supplementation (Omega 3 and similar products)

Omega-3 fatty acids have been recommended for people with arthritis since the 1980s. The omega-3 fatty acids are oils found in large amounts in cold-water fish. There was tremendous excitement when these compounds were initially described as helpful, and extensive studies were done. These fatty acids alter the synthesis of inflammatory mediators in the body. However, to demonstrate the claimed effect it's necessary to take ten or more capsules every day.

When careful studies of patients taking omega-3 fatty acids were done, the researchers were able to show that many of the adults with rheumatoid arthritis were much better in six to eight weeks. However, by twelve weeks the body readjusted itself and began to make increased amounts of the inflammatory mediators again. All the benefits found in the early phase of the studies disappeared, and there were no long-term benefits. The major side effects of omega-3 fatty acids are increased bruising and prolonged bleeding. It's also very expensive if you take the amount necessary to show a short-term effect.

Flaxseed oil is another source of essential fatty acids that is frequently recommended for the treatment of arthritis. There is no long list of negative side effects, but there is no convincing evidence it helps, either. Other sources have suggested that evening primrose, black currant, and borage oil may be beneficial by increasing omega-6 fatty acids. However, all of these products have failed to demonstrate a positive effect when compared with identical-appearing fake capsules. In addition, they can cause side effects, especially if they are contaminated.

In the never-ending search for a better solution, a wide variety of additional agents are being screened and tested for use in patients with arthritis. What you must remember is that *anything with real effects can have possible side effects*. Many additional dietary supplements will appear with claims that they help arthritis sufferers. We hope that one of them will ultimately turn out to be beneficial. However, just as you would never accept a doctor's prescription for your child for a new drug that had not been approved by the FDA and on which no safety testing had been reported, just because a friend told you it might help, you should not be trying new dietary supplements any more willingly. A number have been taken off the market after being proven unsafe. If something is proven safe and effective, everyone will know very quickly and I'll be recommending it.

DIETS

I am a strong proponent of a healthy, balanced diet. Many different sources recommend that people with arthritis should avoid all sorts of foods. There are the no nightshade diets, the no red meat diets, the avoid fungus diets, the low gluten diets, the vegetarian diets, and many more. *Going on a special diet makes us feel as if we have taken some control over our destiny.* Taking that important step to regain control makes all of us feel better.

I never argue with a family that tells me they have adopted a special diet and the child feels better (as long as it is a healthy diet). However, large-scale testing has not shown any of these diets to be particularly beneficial for children with arthritis. The only exception is children with celiac disease. These children may develop arthritis as one manifestation of their disease and will do better on a low-gluten diet. If you are unsure, double-check that your child has been checked for this; the initial screening is a simple blood test. Most will not have celiac disease, but we need to find the few that do.

From time to time I see children who have been placed on strict elimination diets because the family believes the arthritis is due to a food allergy. Although families sometimes convince themselves of short-term benefits, I've never seen a child get better over the long term. These diets put your child through useless deprivation and damage their growth and their self-image. The only food intolerance truly associated with arthritis is celiac disease, which is easily tested for.

ALTERNATIVE MEDICAL SYSTEMS

We all know stories of people who got better after they prayed to a certain saint, went to Lourdes, had acupuncture done, or took up Zen, among other therapies. Taking care of children for many years has made it clear to me that I cannot always explain why their symptoms get better or worse on a given day. The diseases do wax and wane over time. Someone is going to get lucky and get better right after doing something unlikely to really help. There is no reason in the world why you or I should argue with them that it is a coincidence. They will know they got better and they will try to convince you to do the same thing. Be very careful.

If anything worked consistently, we'd all be recommending it. I'd be just as happy to send you to a certain acupuncturist, to a church, or to the supermarket for peanut butter. But, rest assured, I have lots of families who took their children to Lourdes, the Dead Sea, or the acupuncturist, or tried all the other things you hear about. If one of them worked more often than random chance, I'd be telling you about it.

In this era of global travel and communication, there is no hidden cure being used in some remote part of the world that we do not know about. I frequently teach in Asia and Africa. The question there is always whether I can help them get more American medicines. No one has ever come up to me and said, "Here, take this stuff home, it will cure everyone." In Vietnam, you will see vendors selling snake wine for rheumatism. The dead snake is still in the bottle. I wonder why the labels are in English and the prices are in dollars. Nothing on the bottles is written in Vietnamese.

CONCLUSIONS

Everyone wants to feel he or she is doing everything possible for children with arthritis. However, before you buy a dietary supplement, ask yourself the following questions.

- Would you accept a prescription for the same thing from your doctor?
- Have you ever heard of the manufacturer?
- Is any proof supplied for the claims made?
- Is there any certificate of approval of the plant where it was manufactured? Where is it?
- Who is recommending this and what is their training?
- Are they going to make a profit if you buy this?
- If you are going to make your child take this, would you take it yourself?

- What do you know about possible side effects or possible interference with the medicines your child is supposed to be taking?
- Have you discussed this with your child's doctor?

If you're afraid to discuss supplements you want to give your child with the doctor, either do not give the supplements or find a doctor you are not afraid to talk to. I discuss these things with my patients all the time. If it's essentially harmless, I'll tell you. I stop families from doing things or giving children things only if I believe they are unsafe.

24

Understanding Laboratory and Diagnostic Tests

X RAYS

Each type of diagnostic test has its proper place in evaluating children with muscle, bone, or joint pain. If a bone is painful, it is appropriate to begin the evaluation (after a complete history is taken and a thorough physical examination is done) with an X-ray radiograph to eliminate the possibility of fracture or structural abnormality. X rays are also useful to determine whether bones are out of alignment or abnormally curved. An X ray may be the only study necessary to establish the diagnosis of a broken bone, slipped capital femoral epiphysis, scoliosis, or many other orthopedic conditions (see Chapter 3). However, for children with juvenile arthritis, lupus, or many other rheumatic conditions, the X ray may be useful only to exclude orthopedic problems.

X rays are almost always necessary when there is any history of trauma before the onset of pain or when there has been a sudden change in the child's condition. However, the bones are not fully calcified in young children, and the use of X rays to evaluate arthritis is of little value except in the most severe cases. Once the initial X rays have been done, follow up X rays are necessary only if a fracture is suspected or if there is a structural abnormality that must be monitored. For children with rheumatic disease, periodic X rays provide little information that cannot be gained from careful examination of the joints and their range of motion. However, X rays are important if there is a sudden change or if the problem is not resolving in the expected manner.

CAT SCANS

Instead of the X rays striking film after passing through the body, as in a regular X ray radiograph, **CAT (computer axial tomography) scan** X rays are recorded by a computer that creates a three-dimensional picture. These pictures may reveal far greater detail than regular X rays and provide a lot of additional information. *Many families are confused about the relative roles of CAT scans and MRI.* This is easy to understand if you recognize that although the two machines look similar, they operate in a very different manner. The CAT scan passes X rays through the body. Anything that absorbs X rays, such as bone, blocks their passage and shows up white on the film. Various tissues absorb X rays to differing degrees and can be seen on the CAT scan.

MRI

Magnetic resonance imaging (MRI) works on the principle of nuclear magnetic resonance. All you need to know is that this allows the machine to locate water molecules in the body (although it can be set to find other molecules). The machines are calibrated so that they can detect differences in the concentration of water molecules in different tissues, and, using sophisticated computer programs, this allows them to construct a picture of the tissues. The MRI is excellent for making a picture of the soft tissues of the body that are filled with water molecules (remember, we are all made up of about 70% water). However, bone tissue contains very little water and does not show up well on MRI. The bone marrow contains water and shows up well, and the cartilage covering the ends of the bones shows up well, but not the bones themselves. As a result of these differences, a CAT scan will give a much better picture of a structural abnormality of bone, but an MRI will show a torn ligament or damaged cartilage that cannot be seen well on the CAT scan.

BONE SCANS

There are a number of other diagnostic tests that may be useful in dealing with bone and joint problems. One of the most common is the **bone scan**. Bone scanning is based on the uptake of the radioactive isotope technetium 99 (Tc-99) by active bone cells. Normal bone cells are not very active, but if there is an injury, arthritis, infection, or tumor, the bone cells become active in trying to repair the damage. When they become active, they take up more calcium and related substances. When Tc-99 is injected, active bone cells take it up. Because it is radioactive a picture of where it went in the body can be made using a gamma counter. When a bone scan is done, the patient is given an injection of Tc-99. Later the patient lies on a special table while a gamma counter passes over him or her and makes a picture of where the Tc-99 went. Areas with increased Tc-99 are areas of irritated bone.

This test can find areas that are too small to be obvious on regular X rays or CAT scans. It can also find areas where the bone cells have been irritated but obvious changes have not taken place. As a result, this test is very good for finding things such as osteomyelitis (bone infections) and osteoid osteomas (small, benign bone tumors) before they are evident on X ray. Although the actual lesion may not be large, the irritated bone will show up quite brightly. One advantage of a bone scan is that it allows the physician to evaluate the entire body for areas of bone irritation. Thus, it can help to find unsuspected problems.

GALLIUM SCANNING

Gallium scanning is another method of looking for areas of inflammation by injecting a radioactive substance (Ga-67). Areas of inflammation in soft tissues such as liver, spleen, lung, muscle, and other tissues take up the radioactive gallium to a greater degree than normal tissues. Increased uptake of gallium can be used to find infections, tumors, and other problems. The machinery used is the same as the machinery used in the bone scan. Again, this has the advantage of allowing the evaluation of the entire body.

Although bone scans and gallium scans are done using the same machinery, they cannot be done simultaneously. Bone scans are completed the same day, and the Tc-99 is rapidly removed from the body. The gallium scan procedure is done over a period of three days. This is because it takes the Ga-67 longer to reach the tissues. In addition, the Ga-67 takes a long time to leave the body. As a result, *if both tests are necessary, it is important to do the bone scan first.* The gallium scan can then be started the next day. It is necessary to wait more than a week after a gallium scan has been done (for the Ga-67 to clear the system) before a bone scan can be done.

Risks of radiology tests

Every parent is concerned about the risks of exposure to X rays or radioactive isotopes. It would be foolish to expose anyone unnecessarily to these sources of radiation. All people who work in these areas wear badges and protective aprons if they are going to be directly exposed. At the same time, the risk to children who have these tests is generally negligible. The two things to remember are, first, the risk of undetected disease is far greater than the risk of damage from the test; and second, even crossing the street or riding in the car to the supermarket involves a certain level of risk. It is important to do what needs to be done.

DIAGNOSTIC ULTRASOUND (SONOGRAPHY)

Ultrasound is a relatively new technology that may allow us to study muscles, bones, and joints at far less cost and without the risks associated with radiation. At the present time, the use of ultrasound to evaluate joint swelling and tendon inflammation is rapidly advancing. These tests may be available to your doctor and may be quite helpful in evaluating problems in the muscles and joints. Ultrasound can also be used to guide the doctors when they need to inject joints that they cannot see, such as the hips.

SYNOVIAL FLUID ASPIRATION

Synovial fluid aspiration is often done in the physician's office. However, sometimes it is done in the radiology department because physicians want to use X-ray guidance (or ultrasound, as described above) to make sure the needle is in the right place. Synovial fluid aspiration consists of taking some of the fluid out of an inflamed joint. This is normally done for the purpose of analyzing the fluid to look for evidence of infection, bleeding, or tumors. In children, the test is done most often to exclude the possibility of infection. Even children who are known to have arthritis can develop an infection in the joint. If there is any question, the physicians will want to remove fluid from the joint and send it for appropriate testing. This testing should include a Gram stain, culture, cell count, protein, and sugar analyses. These tests are described in greater detail in the section on synovial fluid analysis later in this chapter.

Parents often wonder why the physicians do not simply take all the fluid out while they have a needle in the swollen joint. Unfortunately, the fluid will rapidly reappear. Medications are needed to stop the process. (Imagine that your kitchen faucet is stuck open and the sink is overflowing. If I come in with a bucket and empty the sink, the problem will stop for a short period. However, if I don't turn off the water or unplug the blockage, the sink will just fill right back up and start to overflow again.)

PULMONARY FUNCTION TESTING

Pulmonary function testing (PFT) is a special set of tests to measure the child's ability to breathe. This consists of two parts. The first part measures the ability of the lungs to move air in and out. The second part measures the ability of the lungs to move oxygen from the air inhaled into the lungs to the blood passing through the lungs. Both parts must work properly for a child to breathe easily.

The first thing that happens when a child is sent for pulmonary function testing is that he or she is set up to breathe into a big machine. Then the child is encouraged to breath normally at first. After that the technician will have him or her breathe in and out as hard as possible, then as fast as possible. This may be repeated after a medication called a bronchodilator is given. The bronchodilator is used to reverse changes due to constriction of the airways by asthma or a similar illness. So if the tests improve after the child uses a bronchodilator, it suggests that part of the problem is asthma or a similar disease.

Rapidly breathing in and out allows the doctors to see how well the lungs are moving. There are two types of problems. Obstructive lung disease describes when something is getting in the way of the air flow. This is rare in children with rheumatic disease. Restrictive lung disease describes when the lungs themselves are not moving well. This can be due to weakness, but more often it means the lungs themselves are stiff. Most often, this happens when the lungs are involved by scleroderma, but it can happen with other rheumatic diseases.

The final part of PFTs is a test called a diffusing capacity (DLCO). In this test, the child inhales a special sample containing a small amount of an easily measured gas. The child is instructed to hold his breath for ten seconds and then exhale. When the child exhales the breath is analyzed to see how much of the special gas was kept in the lungs and how much came back out again. This tells the doctors whether or not it was easy for the inhaled gas to cross into the bloodstream. If there are problems, it means that it is hard for oxygen to get into the blood even though it is being moved in and out of the lungs properly. If the child is not getting enough oxygen, he or she will feel out of breath all the time.

OTHER TESTS

There are a number of other diagnostic tests that are specific to different diseases. Rather than discuss each of them here, I have included them in the sections related to those diseases where they are relevant. If you have concerns about a test not discussed here, ask your physician for more information.

LABORATORY TESTS

Before I begin to discuss the details of various laboratory tests, it is important to understand that the results must be viewed as part of the total picture of the patient. *A set of laboratory tests is no replacement for a good history and physical examination. Abnormal laboratory tests can be a mistake, and a child can have all normal laboratory tests and still be seriously affected by arthritis.*

Children who complain of bone and joint pains but have "normal laboratory tests" often confuse parents and physicians. Many of the rheumatic diseases are associated with abnormal laboratory tests, but there are rheumatic and musculoskeletal diseases in which all the tests are normal. *Normal laboratory tests do not mean that a child cannot have arthritis or another rheumatic disease. It is especially important to realize that* **juvenile arthritis is almost never associated with a positive test for rheumatoid factor**. Conversely, many children are found to have mild laboratory abnormalities but do not have rheumatic disease.

It is also important to remember that laboratory tests are not always accurate. In this day of cost saving, centralization, and rapid turnover, everyone should be very careful in interpreting laboratory values. Sometimes children are referred to me with abnormal laboratory tests that are normal when the test is repeated. Other times children have been told there was nothing wrong because the test was normal, but a repeat test in my office is abnormal.

> A few years ago a child came to me who was complaining of hip pain on both sides. A physician had ordered an arthritis panel and the report came back that the child was both antinuclear antibody (ANA)- and rheumatoid factor (RF)-positive. Since these tests "confirmed" the diagnosis of arthritis, the child was begun on medications. The child was sent to me to be evaluated for treatment with stronger medication for her arthritis because she had failed to get better with six months of treatment. X rays revealed the child had bilateral slipped capital femoral epiphyses (an orthopedic condition requiring surgery; see Chapter 3). The original physician did not do X rays or further testing once he had the positive ANA and RF, because those results had "confirmed" the diagnosis. Those tests were negative when repeated. The original laboratory's results were incorrect.

Over the years I have had numerous children referred because of laboratory tests that were incorrect. In addition, many children whom I care for (who repeatedly test positive for their disease) are occasionally reported to have negative tests. They are, of course, positive again when I next repeat the test. Incorrect results may be a consequence of a machine not operating properly, the blood being mishandled en route to the laboratory, the wrong person's name on the sample, the wrong results being entered in the computer by a keyboard operator, and many other causes. *Always recheck a result that does not make sense, or a key result that would change the course of treatment, if it does not fit the clinical picture.*

CBC and MCV

A **complete blood count (CBC)** is one of the most routine blood tests; yet it can provide a lot of useful information. The first thing reported is the hemoglobin and hematocrit. These are measures of the amount of red blood cells in the blood. If the child has a low hemoglobin level, it means he or she is anemic. The anemia may be from many different causes but should prompt further investigation. Many children with severe arthritis are anemic. However, a child may have normal results and still have arthritis or another condition. Anemia may be evidence of more severe disease, inadequate diet, bleeding (including bleeding from an irritated stomach lining), increased destruction of red cells, or decreased production of blood cells. Each of these reasons for anemia has many possible causes. The hematocrit measures the same thing as the hemoglobin, although it is reported in different units. Most laboratories then report a group of tests called RBC, RDW, MCV, MCH, and MCHC. These tests tell you whether the red blood cells are normal in size and help differentiate causes of anemia. In general, only the **mean corpuscular volume (MCV)** is important in bone and joint conditions. This is just a fancy way of describing the size of the red blood cells.

When the MCV is very low (the red blood cells are too small), usually this occurs because there is not enough hemoglobin (the oxygen-binding protein) in the cells. This is most often the result of iron deficiency but can also be caused by genetic diseases in which hemoglobin is not properly made (see thalassemia below). In rheumatic diseases, the MCV is often low. In part this is because children with chronic disease often absorb iron poorly, and in part it may be due to irritation of the stomach lining by medications, which leads to chronic loss of small amounts of blood. Often anemia and a low MCV are due to a variety of factors acting together. A high MCV may indicate an increased number of young cells called reticulocytes. However, it can also be caused by folate deficiency (folate is a vitamin). Sulfasalazine and methotrexate are two drugs used by rheumatologists that antagonize folate. Thus, a high MCV can be an early sign of problems from these medicines, but children on methotrexate should be receiving supplemental folate to prevent this problem. If necessary, folate may also be given to children on sulfasalazine.

A normal MCV with a low hemoglobin level may be a "normochromic normocytic anemia," which is the first phase of iron-deficiency anemia. It may also be a manifestation of hemolytic anemia. In hemolytic anemia, the body is rapidly destroying the red blood cells because of a metabolic or autoimmune problem. In an effort to compensate, the bone marrow starts releasing large numbers of young cells called reticulocytes. These young cells are very large so their MCV is high. However, the automated machine that performs the CBC typically produces an average reading. Thus, young cells that are large and old cells that are small may average out to a normal number despite low hemoglobin. (Some newer machines used to do CBCs will detect this situation.) However, this situation can be detected easily by ordering a reticulocyte count to identify the young cells. Often children with hemolytic anemia do need more iron. Hemolytic anemia may be an isolated problem, but it may also be caused by certain medicines and a number of rheumatic conditions, including systemic lupus erythematosus. Hemolytic anemia due to drugs occurs with increased frequency in children who lack an enzyme found in normal red blood cells called G6PD. This condition is called **G6PD deficiency** and is more common in children of African heritage. Any child with hemolytic anemia should be carefully investigated.

Genetic diseases in which hemoglobin is not properly made may cause bone pain because the bone marrow expands to make more red cells. Diseases with abnormal hemoglobin that produce bone pain include sickle cell disease and the carrier state for sickle cell disease. **Thalassemia** is another disease associated with abnormal hemoglobin production and very low MCV values that may cause bone pain. Mild thalassemia, or "thalassemia minor" (the carrier state), often has a low MCV but has no symptoms. Thalassemia major is a severe disease associated with marked anemia. Because the bone marrow is overactive in children with thalassemia major, these children may have bone pain and bones that appear very abnormal on X ray. However, these children are usually diagnosed early in life and under the care of a hematologist. Abnormal hemoglobin production is best analyzed by a test called a hemoglobin electrophoresis.

TIBC and Fe

When a child is anemic, it is important to determine whether he or she is getting enough **iron (Fe)** in the diet and absorbing it. If not, the iron will be low, while the **total iron bind capacity (TIBC)** will be high. If these values are normal and the child is anemic, it suggests that there is a problem in making hemoglobin that is not related to iron deficiency.

WBC count

White blood cells are a critical component of the body's defense against infection. A low **white blood cell (WBC) count** is called leukopenia. If the white count goes too low, the child is vulnerable to infections. If the count goes too high, it suggests that that child is under physiologic stress. Infection is one of the possible causes of this type of stress. However, certain medications will make the count go up as well. Very high WBC counts can occur in diseases such as juvenile arthritis (especially systemic onset juvenile arthritis), severe infections, and leukemia (a cancer of the white blood cells).

Very low WBC counts can be the result of leukemia (if the cancerous white blood cells are not being released into the circulation). More often a low WBC count is the result of medications or certain viral infections. Many of the medications used in treating children with rheumatic diseases cause low WBC counts in some children. Whenever a child's count is too low, careful attention should be given to all of the medicines the child is taking. This should not be limited to the medicines for rheumatic disease. It may be the result of another medicine or two medicines interacting. If your child is having a problem, make sure your doctor knows about *all the medicines and supplements* your child is taking.

Certain diseases, such as systemic lupus erythematosus, may be associated with more rapid destruction of the white blood cells and result in a low WBC count. Certain severe infections may also do this. Leukemia and some forms of cancer may make the WBC count too low or too high. A rare cause of very low WBC counts is a condition called **aplastic anemia,** in which the bone marrow elements that make the white blood cells, and others, fail.

When the laboratory reports the WBC count, it also reports the percentage of each different type of cells: neutrophils, lymphocytes, monocytes, basophils, and eosinophils. Normally, the neutrophils make up the greatest percentage. In young children (under the age of five), lymphocytes are often increased. Eosinophils are often increased in people with allergies. They may also be increased in children with parasitic infections. Certain uncommon rheumatic diseases (such as eosinophilic vasculitis, some cases of scleroderma, and Churg Strauss syndrome) are also associated with a significantly increased number of eosinophils. Significantly increased numbers of monocytes or basophils are very rare.

Platelet count

Platelets are the sticky pieces in the blood that initiate the formation of a blood clot when someone is cut. They are rapidly made in the bone marrow and the number may fluctuate quickly. The platelet count is often very high in people who are under stress or chronically ill. Kawasaki disease and iron-deficiency anemia are often associated with platelet counts over 600,000. Low platelet counts may result from certain medications that lead to decreased production. In addition, the platelet count may go down because of increased destruction in children with idiopathic thrombocytopenic purpura (ITP), systemic lupus erythematosus, Felty's syndrome, macrophage activation syndrome complicating systemic onset JRA, thrombotic thrombocytopenic purpura (TTP), or an infection. It may also be low because of decreased production in someone with leukemia, lymphoma, or aplastic anemia. At times there may be several different problems contributing to the low platelet count. If the platelet count is low without obvious explanation, the hematologist may recommend a bone marrow aspiration. This will allow examination of the cells that make platelets (megakaryocytes). If these cells are active, then the low level of platelets must be the result of increased destruction. If they are inactive, there is decreased production of platelets. In addition, a bone marrow aspiration may provide clues to the cause of decreased production.

ESR

Erythrocyte is just another word for red cell. There are several variations of the test for **erythrocyte sedimentation rate (ESR)**, but all of them reflect how the red cells interact with each other in the blood and how fast they settle to the bottom of a test tube. Children with severe illness often have a high ESR and this may prompt referral to a rheumatologist. *Often parents know their referring physician became worried when he or she saw the high "sed rate,"* and they will ask me what that means. It is important to understand that the sedimentation rate is based on an observation and was not designed as a test. When blood collected from a patient is left to stand in the test tube, it will separate just like the oil and vinegar in salad dressing. The red cells in the blood will settle to the bottom of the tube, leaving clear fluid on top. The measurement of how far the red cells settle toward the bottom in one hour (in a specially designed tube) is the erythrocyte sedimentation rate.

Doctors observed a long time ago that the red cells generally fell to the bottom much faster in sick patients than in healthy ones. Thus, the ESR is a screen for how sick someone may be. But, of course, there are exceptions. Some people are sick and the ESR is not abnormal, and some people with abnormal ESRs do not have an obvious explanation. The normal ESR value varies with the age and sex of the patient and from laboratory to laboratory, so it is important to know the normal value for where your test was done.

If the blood is left to sit for a long time or is not properly processed, the test is unreliable. This is a problem with many large centralized laboratories outside hospitals. The following warning is included with the results of every ESR specimen sent to a well-known national laboratory: "ESR specimens are stable for 4–6 hours at room temperature (12 hours if refrigerated). ESR results trend lower with increased specimen age." Unfortunately, neither you nor your physician knows how long the time was between when the blood was drawn and when the test was performed. Nor do you know whether the blood was refrigerated. Even if you have your specimen drawn by the laboratory's own facility, the answers to these questions are unavailable. This is why I look at trends and never believe an isolated ESR value.

How fast the red blood cells settle to the bottom of the test tube is determined by how they interact with each other. If they stay far apart, they fall relatively slowly. If they are pulled close to each other, they will fall faster. Studies have indicated that red cells fall faster in some people because of electrostatic interaction between the cells. This interaction is due to small molecules stuck to the surface of the cells that cause the cells to move closer together. Most of these small molecules are acute phase reactants. Acute phase reactants are proteins and similar materials that the body makes when it is under physiological stress. The greater the stress, the more the acute phase reactants, the faster the cells fall, and thus the higher the erythrocyte sedimentation rate goes. *The problem is that physiological stress is a very broad concept and elevated erythrocyte sedimentation rates can result from many different conditions.*

It is very hard to be comfortable when a child has an elevated ESR without an obvious explanation. Most often it simply goes up when a child has a cold or other infection and comes back down when the infection is gone. The ESR is also elevated in many children with rheumatic diseases and many other illnesses. At the same time, children with pauciarticular JA or spondyloarthropathies may be having all sorts of problems and their ESR may be normal (see Chapters 7 and 9). Whenever I am sent a child with an elevated sedimentation rate, I begin by taking a careful history and doing a careful physical exam to look for the reason the ESR is elevated. After that, I do further blood tests to look for other evidence of elevated acute phase reactant levels. It is important to investigate further until the explanation is found. However, in rare cases, children have abnormal ESRs for which no explanation is apparent.

CRP

C reactive protein (CRP) is an acute phase reactant that is made in the liver. Levels of CRP go up rapidly and come down rapidly, as well. Because the ESR measures a variety of acute phase reactants, the ESR and CRP generally move together. Some physicians prefer one test to the other, and many use both. It is thought that the CRP may go up faster and come down sooner than the ESR. It is a common myth that CRP elevation indicates infection over another cause of inflammation, but many children who have rheumatic diseases have high CRP levels without infections. The CRP is reported to be more stable after the blood is drawn and may have greater use for this reason.

Chemistry panel, metabolic panel, or a serum multichannel automated chemistry (SMAC)

The chemistry panel consists of a variety of tests that document primarily the function of the liver and kidneys. In some hospitals, the test includes electrolytes and a lipid profile, but there is some variation between laboratories in the list of tests included.

Serum glucose refers to the amount of sugar in the blood. The level may be elevated or decreased in diabetics but is usually normal in children with orthopedic and rheumatic diseases. It may go up in children being treated with steroids. If the blood has been allowed to sit for too long before being processed, the value will go down. The **blood urea nitrogen (BUN)** level is a measure of kidney function. It is elevated in children with impaired kidney function. It often goes toward the top of normal to slightly over in children receiving nonsteroidal anti-inflammatory drugs (NSAIDs) because these drugs decrease the rate at which the kidneys cleanse the blood (the glomerular filtration rate, or GFR). These slight elevations are normal and should not be a cause of concern. The **creatinine (Cr)** level is also a measure of kidney function, but it is not affected by mild changes in the GFR the way the BUN is. Because children normally have lower creatinine levels than adults, the BUN/creatinine ratio may become very elevated. This is not something to be concerned about if the underlying values are normal. *One concern is that many laboratories do not report age-adjusted normal values. A creatinine of 1.2 mg/dl is normal for an older adult, but very abnormal for a child under the age of ten years.* If the laboratory is not using age-adjusted normal values, the value of 1.2 mg/dl will not be indicated as abnormal in the child's results.

Sodium, potassium, chloride, and carbon dioxide are electrolytes. Their levels may indicate abnormal kidney function or, under certain circumstances, other metabolic abnormalities. Their levels should be normal in children with orthopedic and rheumatic conditions unless there is significant internal organ involvement. *It is important to recognize that the electrolytes, like the glucose and the ESR, are very sensitive to proper handling.* If the specimen is mishandled (too warm, too cold, or sits out too long), these values may become very unreliable due to the metabolic activities of the cells in the blood.

Low **sodium levels (Na)** may be the result of fluid retention, brain injury, or medications. Children with very low sodium levels may have problems including weakness and muscle cramps, but values above 130 are rarely troublesome. High levels of sodium suggest dehydration or kidney disease. Like the sodium level, the potassium level (K) is normally regulated by the kidneys. Low levels of potassium also cause weakness and muscle cramps. High levels may interfere with heart rhythm, and very high levels are dangerous. Don't give extra electrolytes to someone unless you know their kidneys are working properly or you have been directed to do so by your doctor. Low sodium levels with high potassium levels can occur in diabetics and in people who have poorly functioning adrenal glands.

Serum **calcium (Ca)** measures the level of calcium in the blood. It may be abnormal in children with disease of the parathyroid gland, which secretes a hormone to regulate calcium levels. It may also be abnormal in children with kidney disease, vitamin D intoxication, or other metabolic abnormalities. These problems may result in bone and joint abnormalities or pain if they persist for an extended period. Low calcium may be associated with severe muscle cramps. **Vitamin D-dependent rickets** may cause problems in children who do not get enough of the vitamin and is associated with a low calcium level and joint pains. However, rickets is extremely rare in the United States because most dairy products contain supplemental vitamin D. Rickets is typically diagnosed by a characteristic abnormal appearance of the bones on X rays.

Most often the serum **chloride (Cl)** level is normal. A very low chloride level can occur in someone who is sick and vomiting a lot. *If you are dealing with a teenager who chronically has low chloride levels, you need to consider the possibility of bulimia (throwing up after eating to avoid gaining weight). Teenagers won't always admit to this unless confronted with the evidence. If an increased amylase level accompanies the low chloride, it strongly suggests the possibility of bulimia. The amylase comes from irritation of the salivary glands by the persistent vomiting.*

Carbon dioxide (CO_2) levels in the blood go up and down as part of the mechanism that controls acid-base balance. If the CO_2 level is significantly off, a thorough metabolic workup should be done by the physician. However, the CO_2 level is another of the tests that may become abnormal because the blood specimen was allowed to sit for too long before it was processed.

Phosphorous (P) is another electrolyte that is often measured. Phosphorous is closely related to calcium metabolism. Children with kidney problems or calcium metabolism problems may have too high or too low a phosphorous level. Otherwise, the phosphorous level is rarely abnormal. *Note that children who are using too much antacid may develop low phosphorous levels (hypophosphatemia).* The antacids contain chemicals that bind the phosphorous in the intestines and prevent it from being absorbed.

Albumin is a serum protein manufactured by the liver that serves as both a building block and a carrier molecule. If the level is low, it may be the result of decreased production or increased loss. Decreased production may be the result of liver disease or poor nutritional intake. Increased loss may result from loss through the gastrointestinal system or loss through the kidney. In either case, it needs to be investigated. Systemic lupus erythematosus and amyloidosis are among many diseases that may cause increased loss of albumin through the kidney. This is easily detected by urine tests for protein.

Whenever the serum albumin level is low, the body must compensate by increasing other elements in the blood to maintain an appropriate osmotic balance. Most often the body increases the level of cholesterol in the blood to accomplish this. High cholesterol and low albumin are commonly found in children with kidney disease. Changes in diet are not likely to have any effect on these problems if the kidney or liver diseases that cause the problem are not corrected. If the body is not able to maintain an appropriate osmotic balance, water tends to leak out of the blood vessels, producing swelling. Painful swollen feet in children may be a sign of kidney malfunction and low albumin levels. *Sometimes the first clue is that socks are leaving deep marks on the feet or calves.*

In addition to measuring the albumin level, the comprehensive metabolic panel also includes the total protein, the total globulin, and the albumin-globulin ratio. These are obtained by measuring the total protein and the albumin. The globulin is then determined by subtracting the albumin from the total protein, and the albumin-globulin ratio is determined simply by dividing the albumin level by the globulin level. Globulins are larger proteins in the blood that include a number of acute phase reactants as well as immunoglobulin molecules. The level of acute phase reactants goes up in people who are ill, and so the globulin level goes up in people who are ill. At the same time, the albumin level often goes down when people are sick. The combination of factors often leads to a decreased albumin-globulin ratio. Low globulin levels also may be an indication of low immunoglobulin levels. Low levels of immunoglobulin may be associated with a variety of problems, discussed below.

Bilirubin is commonly included in the comprehensive metabolic panel. Most often it is reported as "total" and "direct" bilirubin. The liver produces bilirubin from breakdown products in the blood. Direct bilirubin has been completely processed by the liver, while "indirect" bilirubin has not. Liver disease is the most common cause of significantly elevated bilirubin levels. If the bilirubin level is too high the child will look jaundiced, or yellow. In children with rheumatic or musculoskeletal disease, the most common cause of a significantly increased bilirubin level is hemolysis (the breakdown of red cells). This can occur after bleeding internally or if there is increased breakdown of red cells by antibodies. This complication, autoimmune hemolytic anemia, is often seen in children with SLE. Because red cells also contain SGOT (see below) physicians may initially be confused into thinking that children with elevated bilirubin and SGOT levels have a problem with the liver, when in fact the liver is fine, but too many red cells are being broken down.

SGOT/ALT is an enzyme contained in muscle cells, liver cells, and red blood cells. Damage to any of these can result in increased amounts of SGOT being present in the blood. If the SGOT is elevated without obvious explanation, it is important to be sure that muscle enzyme testing (CPK and aldolase) is done to look for muscle diseases, as well as a reticulocyte count to look for hemolytic anemia. Normal CBC and chemistry panels do not include the proper tests to look for these problems, and an elevated SGOT may be the only hint. But in a child with hemolysis due to excessive red cell destruction, the bilirubin level will also go up. This does not happen with muscle disease. If the elevated SGOT is the result of problems with the liver, there should be a significant elevation of the SGPT, as well (see below).

SGPT/AST is another enzyme that is primarily found in the liver. Thus, if the SGOT level is elevated but the SGPT is not, it suggests that the source of the SGOT is outside the liver. Mild elevations of SGPT level can occur from disease outside the liver if the SGOT level is also elevated. There are many different liver diseases that may result in an elevation of the SGPT level. The SGPT level may also rise if the liver is being irritated by medications. Methotrexate is known to irritate the liver in some children, but the NSAIDs and many other drugs may also cause liver irritation in some children. This is why it is important to monitor these tests routinely in children on medication.

It should always be remembered that some rheumatic diseases may cause damage to the liver, and some liver diseases may cause bone and joint discomfort. This is especially true in patients with infectious hepatitis. All children with significantly elevated liver enzyme levels need careful evaluation.

The level of lactic acid dehydrogenase, **LDH**, another enzyme measured in the blood, goes up with damage to red cells, the liver, or other types of cells. When there is increased cell turnover, the LDH level can be very high. Many physicians believe that an LDH level over 1,000 units means that the child must have a tumor, but children with rheumatic diseases, such as systemic onset JRA, and other systemically ill children may have very high LDH levels (well over 1,000 units). However, if a child is thought to have pauciarticular JRA and the LDH is very high, something is wrong. These children should be carefully evaluated for leukemia or bone tumors.

Just like children with elevated SGOT or SGPT levels, children with an elevated LDH level must be investigated carefully to determine the cause. It may be in any of many different organ systems. Damage to many tissues—including the brain, heart, lungs, liver, blood cells, muscle, or spleen—all may result in elevated LDH levels.

Alkaline phosphotase is an enzyme that is associated with bone growth. Because children have actively growing bones, the normal alkaline phosphotase value for children is much higher than the normal value for adults. If the laboratory is not reporting age-adjusted values, a normal value in a child may be reported as abnormal. Alkaline phosphotase is also found in the gallbladder. In an adult, an elevated alkaline phosphotase may indicate gallbladder disease, but this is a rare problem in children. (Note: Children with sickle cell disease can get gallbladder problems.) Occasionally, children have values of alkaline phosphotase many times the expected normal value without any apparent illness. The significance of this finding is unknown.

The level of **uric acid** is another laboratory value frequently reported in the comprehensive metabolic panel. Uric acid is a breakdown product of DNA. Thus, increased uric acid means that either there is increased breakdown of cells or the kidneys are not properly clearing the uric acid, or both. Children sick with hemolytic uremic syndrome have high uric acid levels. So do children with leukemia. Sometimes children with elevated uric acid levels and joint pain are referred for possible gout. These children should be carefully evaluated for other problems. Gout is essentially unheard-of in childhood except in the setting of kidney disease or cancer chemotherapy, where the drugs are causing many tumor cells to die very quickly and the kidneys cannot handle the load. For all intents and purposes, *children do not get gout.*

Muscle enzymes: creatinine phosphokinase and aldolase

Creatinine phosphokinase (CPK) is an enzyme produced by a variety of cells in the body. It can be released from both skeletal and heart muscle and from the brain. Although it may be elevated in adults with myocardial infarctions, the most frequent cause of elevations in childhood is muscle inflammation. This may occur in children with dermatomyositis, scleroderma, or mixed connective tissue disease. Sometimes the CPK is elevated with extensive exercise. I have had a number of children referred to me over the years because of elevated CPK levels after working out with weights or practicing for the football team. They often had CPK levels many times the upper limit of normal. After two weeks of rest the results were back to normal limits.

The level of CPK is also elevated after some viral infections. One winter there was a viral epidemic (influenza?) in which many children began to complain of pain in their calves. Their CPK levels were in the thousands, and many physicians became concerned. All of these children had normal tests a few weeks later when their viral infection had resolved. There are children with elevated CPK levels that persist despite rest and for which no explanation can be found. This situation is discussed in Chapter 6 on dermatomyositis.

Aldolase is another muscle enzyme that may be elevated in children with muscle damage. In general, the aldolase is less sensitive to muscle inflammation than the CPK, but there are children with dermatomyositis who have elevated aldolase levels and a normal CPK. Aldolase can also be increased in children with liver inflammation secondary to infectious mononucleosis or viral hepatitis.

One of the biggest problems with our current system of ordering laboratory tests is that many useful tests have been eliminated from the standard panels. As a result, the tests may all be normal because the right test to diagnose the disease was not included. LDH and CPK are well-known examples of this. Children with dermatomyositis act tired all the time and want to be carried because their muscles are painful and weak. Early in the course of the disease, the LDH, CPK, and aldolase levels may be elevated before there are any other indications of muscle disease. However, the LDH and CPK are no longer included in the normal metabolic panel. Thus, it is not uncommon for me to see a child because the parents keep insisting there is something wrong, but the pediatrician cannot find anything and "the lab tests are all normal." Sometimes the answer is obvious when the proper tests are done.

Quantitative immunoglobulins (IgG, IgA, and IgM)

Immunoglobulins are the antibodies made to fight infections. These are measured in the blood by the total protein but can be more precisely measured by specific tests. In a normal immune response, the body recognizes and processes a foreign antigen and begins making antibodies against it by making IgM. As the immune response matures the body begins to make IgG. IgA is also made in the secondary stage. There are additional antibody classes—IgE and IgD—that play a role in specific diseases.

If you cannot make any antibodies, you have **agammaglobulinemia**. Children with agammaglobulinemia usually die of infections unless they receive a bone marrow transplant. IgG is the main class of immunoglobulin used by the body to fight infection. Without treatment, total deficiency results in death from infection. Partial IgG deficiency can take many forms. There are several subclasses of IgG. If only one is missing, the child may have frequent infections, but otherwise do well. Children may also have a generalized low level of IgG. Children with these generalized low levels may have trouble handling viral infections and have an increased frequency of joint pains and limping episodes when they have viral infections. Defining these low levels is difficult. Large studies have shown that the normal levels of immunoglobulins in young children are highly variable. I have seen a number of young children (four to six years of age) with low levels that are still normal who limp whenever they get viral infections. Thorough investigation has not found any additional abnormalities. As the children get older and their immune system matures, this stops happening.

IgA deficiency is an important special case of immunoglobulin deficiency. IgA is the body's defense against external bacteria at mucosal surfaces. Thus, IgA is found in the gut, in the saliva, and in the upper airways. Children with IgA deficiency have an increased incidence of colds and ear infections but in general do well. However, IgA deficiency is much more common in children with rheumatic disease than it would be if the two conditions were unrelated. It is important to recognize children with IgA deficiency not only because they have an increased incidence of infections and rheumatic diseases, but also because they can have major problems with transfusion reactions. There are many stories of these children getting into trouble when they need a transfusion because all of the tests for red blood cell compatibility are done correctly, but the children are having a "transfusion reaction" due to the IgA in the donor's blood.

IgE is primarily associated with allergic reactions. High levels of IgE usually indicate a very allergic individual. They can also be found in children with eosinophilic vasculitis (see Chapter 15). IgD levels are almost never measured. There is a very rare syndrome called hyper-IgD syndrome that causes children to have recurrent fevers and abdominal pain.

Specialized tests

In trying to understand all of the specialized laboratory tests performed by physicians, it is necessary to understand how these tests come about. Imagine that I have asked you to develop a quick and rapid test to detect fire engines. Since we need fire engines to conduct the test, I have sent you to the scene of several fires to start your work. Pretty quickly you come back and report that you have a very useful test to detect a fire engine. It is almost invariably a big red truck at the scene of a fire. You and I go to a few fires and the test looks extremely useful.

Then we stand on the corner of the highway and pull over all of the big red trucks that go by. Few, if any, are fire engines. What went wrong? All tests have important characteristics called sensitivity and specificity. Sensitivity means no false negatives (everybody with the disease is found by the test). Specificity means no false positives (everybody who has a positive test has the disease). No test has perfect sensitivity and specificity. Further, the results depend on where the test is done. At the scene of a fire, the red truck test is useful, but not on the highway. A positive test should always be considered in light of the setting (i.e., why it was done).

Antinuclear antibody (ANA) testing used to be very significant in diagnosing children with rheumatic disease. When the test was originally set up, a positive test in a child who did not have rheumatic disease was rare. The main problem with the test was that the results were difficult to compare between different laboratories. Each lab used its own materials for running the test and did its own calibrations. In the early 1980s it was decided that a standardized test would be better. This requires that every laboratory use the same substrate.

A uniform cultured human cell line, called Hep2, was agreed on for the standard. But there are so many variables in performing ANA testing that it is still not safe to compare results between different laboratories. Furthermore, this cell line gives low titer (see below) positive results much more frequently than the old method did. As a result, positive tests that do not mean the child has a rheumatic disease have become very common. In one reported study, one-third of children who were admitted to the hospital as part of having their tonsils out had low titer positive tests for ANA when their blood was checked. None of these children had rheumatic disease. Higher titer positive tests are more meaningful. However, having only a low titer ANA does not guarantee your child does not have disease. As a result the situation has become very confused.

Many parents want to know what an ANA test is. The test was developed in the 1950s, but it began with an observation in 1948. On a cold winter day a physician named Hargraves placed a test tube containing bone marrow blood cells from a patient with lupus in his coat pocket. He had to carry it back to his laboratory in another building. When he examined the marrow under a microscope in his office, he found cells that had engulfed (eaten) the nuclei of other cells. This had never been reported before. It was discovered that this was a common finding in patients with lupus, but only if the specimen was kept warm for 10 to 15 minutes after it was taken from the patient. This is called the LE (lupus erythematosus) cell phenomenon. As doctors looked for an easier way to do the test, they discovered that the LE cell phenomenon occurred because there were antibodies on the surface of the cell that was engulfed.

In the ANA test, serum from the patient is placed on top of layers of Hep2 cells on a microscope slide. The serum is then washed off and a special antibody that sticks to the patient's serum is applied and then the slide is rinsed. If the patient does not have ANA, the serum rinses right off the Hep2 cells and so does the special antibody. However, if the patient's serum sticks to the Hep2 cells, the special antibody will stick to it. This special antibody is labeled so that it glows under fluorescent light. If the patient has ANA present, the patient's serum has stuck to the nucleus of the Hep2 cell. Using a fluorescent light a green glow can be seen coming from the special antibody that has stuck to the patient's sera where it stuck to the nucleus of the cell. (Think of a sandwich. The first layer is the nucleus of the cell. If the serum contains ANA, there is a second layer of the patient's serum sticking to the nucleus of the cell. The third layer is the special antibody. It will not stick if there is no second layer. But if it does stick, it is easy to see.) At first this was checked by mean of a microscope, but now machines do it automatically.

The titer of the ANA refers to how much the patient's sera can be diluted and still give a positive reading. Sera are initially screened after being diluted forty times (1:40). If the screen is positive, then further tests are done at 1:80, 1:160, 1:320, and so on, until there is no detectable fluorescence. The last dilution at which the fluorescence can be seen is the ANA titer.

Positive tests for ANA are found in a wide variety of conditions. They are certainly found in children with SLE, but they are also found in children with a wide variety of other rheumatic diseases. They may briefly appear after a wide variety of infections (especially viral infections where the virus has damaged the nuclei of the cells it infected). Positive tests for ANA have been seen in many children with no identifiable disease and in some children with many different diseases. The presence of a positive ANA should prompt consideration of a rheumatic disease, but it may be a false lead.

A positive test for ANA is also important in children with arthritis. *In children with any of the various forms of juvenile arthritis, the complication of eye disease occurs more frequently in children who have a positive test for ANA than in children who have a negative test* (see Chapters 7 and 8). Despite extensive investigation, the explanation for this association is unknown.

If you wonder what it is that the antibodies that make up the ANA are sticking to, you are in good company. This has been examined extensively. There is no single answer, but we have learned a lot from this test. When people were looking at the results, they noticed that there were several different patterns of fluorescence (ANA pattern). The most common ANA pattern is called homogeneous. Some children have a speckled ANA, and some children have a shaggy or **rim pattern ANA. Homogenous pattern ANA** occurs in many different people and is not disease-specific. **Speckled pattern** is also common at low titer, but at higher titer may be associated with mixed connective tissue disease or scleroderma. *Rim pattern is almost always a sign of active lupus.*

Determination of whether the different patterns of ANA were associated with antibodies to different parts of the nucleus was very difficult in the 1970s. Researchers did not have all the advanced techniques that are available now. At that time scientists tried dipping the cells in different chemicals and to see whether it changed the ANA test. In doing this it was discovered that one group of patients went from positive to negative, and whatever the antibodies were reacting to could be "extracted" by the chemical solution. This led to the term **"extractable nuclear antigen" (ENA)**.

Many years of research have resulted in our understanding that ENA consists of a number of different pieces: Ro, La, Sm, and RNP (Ro comes from Robert, the name of the patient in whom the antibody was first found; La from Lane; Sm from Smith; and RNP stands for ribonucleoprotein). Different patterns of how antibodies reacted to these pieces tend to correlate with different patterns of disease. The interpretation of these various patterns is found in Chapters 11 and 12.

Another early finding was that some of the antibodies detected by the ANA test were directed against DNA and that people with high titers of anti-DNA antibodies were often sicker. At first the tests for antibodies to DNA were fairly crude, but they have improved a lot over time. These tests used to be separated into tests for single-stranded DNA (ssDNA) and tests for double-stranded DNA (dsDNA). Tests for ssDNA have mostly disappeared, as they were very nonspecific and occurred in a wide variety of situations. Most anti-DNA tests today measure dsDNA. High titers of anti-dsDNA are much more specific for lupus than a positive ANA. However, there are children with anti-DNA antibodies who have other diseases. Sometimes a child is very sick with a viral infection and anti-DNA antibodies appear as part of the immune response to the virus. These usually go away within a few months. When you are looking at anti-DNA antibody tests, the lab may have run a *Crithidia lucilliae* assay. Many sources of DNA contain DNA in chains. These chains may have damaged ends. The damaged ends often caused positive tests that were not truly meaningful. Crithidia is a microorganism that has circular DNA. There are no loose ends. Thus the Crithidia test avoids this problem (it's done just as I described for the ANA above). A positive test for anti-DNA antibodies using Crithidia is more meaningful. However, even this test is occasionally positive in children who don't have SLE.

Antineutrophil cytoplasmic antibodies (ANCAs) are relatively newly described. Unlike antinuclear antibodies that react with materials in the nucleus of the cell, these antibodies are reacting with elements in the cytoplasm of neutrophils (one type of white blood cell). The cytoplasm is the body of the cell surrounding the nucleus. There are two major variations. cANCA reacts with proteinase 3, a substance found in granules that are spread diffusely throughout the cytoplasm of neutrophils. pANCA reacts with myeloperoxidase. This is also a component of neutrophils granules, but because of its electrostatic charge, when the cell is fixed for staining myeloperoxidase tends to move toward the nucleus. The resultant staining pattern is perinuclear (around the nucleus). With continued investigation it has become clear that pANCA may also represent antibodies to lactoferrin (a common protein) and other substances in the blood.

How and why pANCA and cANCA occur is unclear. Their importance lies in their association with Wegener's granulomatosis, pauci-immune glomerulonephritis, Churg-Strauss syndrome, other systemic vasculitis syndromes, and inflammatory bowel disease. These antibodies are measured by rheumatologists evaluating children with unusual symptoms or symptoms that suggest one of these diseases. If the antibodies are present, then more extensive testing is indicated. For example, if a child with arthritis is complaining of stomach pains, it may be due to medications. Endoscopy will quickly tell whether it is due to stomach irritation or inflammatory bowel disease (IBD). However, endoscopy is an invasive test that requires being anesthetized. If the symptoms are nonspecific, I will start by changing the medications. If the same child has pANCA, I will be quicker to investigate the possibility of IBD by endoscopy. Unfortunately, the association of the antibodies with these diseases is incomplete. Some patients with the diseases do not have the antibodies, and some people with the antibodies do not have these diseases. As with so many other tests in rheumatic disease, we recognize the association but do not yet fully understand the how and why.

Anti-saccharomyces cerevisiae antibodies. *Saccharomyces cerevisiae* is a fungus that commonly occurs in the large intestine. Antibodies to this fungus **(anti-saccharomyces cerevisiae antibodies, or ASCA)** occur more often in children with IBD than in normal people. These antibodies are not routinely measured by rheumatologists but are increasingly being used by gastroenterologists in the evaluation of children who may have IBD. Studies have shown ASCA to be common in children with Crohn's disease, which is one type of IBD.

Serum complement levels. Complement levels are tests done in children with possible lupus. Although the complement system consists of many separate components, only C3 and C4 are routinely measured. **C3** is typically depressed in children with active lupus and may be a warning of more active disease to come. However, the predictive value of a change in C3 level is the subject of much debate. There are few diseases other than lupus that cause a low C3.

C4 is also frequently low in children with lupus. However, the significance of a low C4 is less clear. This is discussed in much more detail in Chapter 11. Many laboratories will also report a **CH50**, but this is not a complement component. CH50 is a test that measures the function of the entire complement system. If any one of the components of the system is low then the CH50 will be low.

C1q and **C2** are two other complement components that can be measured, but these are not tested routinely. Genetic deficiency of C1q is associated with an increased risk of developing lupus. The risk of developing lupus is also increased in children who are deficient in C2 or C4. Deficiency of C4 does not cause any obvious illness, but deficiency of either C2 or C3 is associated with increased infections. Children with complete genetic deficiency of C3 often die of infections. Children genetically deficient in C2 have an increased incidence of infections and of rheumatic diseases but may live a normal life if they are recognized and given antibiotic prophylaxis. Most physicians think that C2 deficiency is extremely rare, but I have several children with C2 deficiency in my practice. You have to look for it to find it.

Anticentromere and anti-Scl-70 antibodies are antibodies that are associated with forms of scleroderma. Anticentromere antibodies are often present in children with CREST syndrome, and anti-Scl -70 antibodies may be present in children with systemic scleroderma. These antibodies are very significant if they are present. Most children who test positive for the antibodies will ultimately turn out to have the disease. However, I have seen false positive results and low titer positive results that have turned out not to mean anything.

Like all diagnostic tests, tests for anticentromere and Anti-Scl-70 antibodies are useful when they are done in people who you suspect have the disease, but you must be very careful in interpreting them if they do not fit the clinical picture. Not every laboratory does these tests well. Before you get concerned about a positive test that does not make sense, make sure the test has been repeated in one of the nationally recognized laboratories (see the section on resources toward the end of this book). Unfortunately, the absence of these antibodies does not guarantee that you do not have one of these diseases. They are found in less than half of affected patients and less often in children than in adults.

Anti-Jo-1 antibody is one of a variety of antibodies that have been described in adults with muscle disease. Some doctors still look for this antibody in children with muscle disease, but it is very uncommon in childhood. Adults with this antibody tend to have a more difficult disease course. There is a growing belief that patients who test positive for this antibody have a completely different disease from other patients with myositis.

Factor VIII, or Von Willebrand's factor, is one of the blood clotting factors. If you do not have any factor VIII, you have **hemophilia** (a serious bleeding disorder). In children with other types of inflammatory disease, the factor VIII level will rise and fall as an acute phase reactant. Some physicians like to follow this level in children with muscle disease or other diseases in which the blood vessels tend to be involved. A rising level suggests more disease activity, while a falling level suggests things are better.

Antigliadin antibodies, antitissue transglutaminase, and antiendomyseal antibodies. Testing for antigliadin antibodies, antitissue transglutaminase, and antiendomyseal antiboeis is done in the detection of children with celiac disease (gluten-sensitive enteropathy). This is an uncommon disease in which patients are sensitive to a protein in wheat called gluten. Whenever they eat too much of this protein, they get abdominal pain and diarrhea. Interestingly, people with this disease develop arthritis and other autoimmune diseases more often than would be expected. To test for this disease, physicians order tests of antigliadin antibodies and antitissue transglutaminase. Antigliadin antibodies can be of the IgG type or the IgA type. IgG-type antigliadin antibodies are very common and probably not meaningful. IgA-type antigliadin antibodies should raise suspicion of celiac disease. Antitissue transglutaminase and antiendomyseal antibodies are much more specific for celiac disease (i.e., a child with these antibodies is much more likely to have the disease). Unfortunately, everyone who tests positive does not necessarily have the disease, and a negative test does not guarantee you could not. However, these tests are helpful in deciding which children with abdominal complaints should be evaluated further. The diagnosis of celiac disease depends on a biopsy of the small bowel that demonstrates the classic findings under the microscope.

Rheumatoid factor. *The most important thing to know about **rheumatoid factor (RF)** is that children with arthritis are most often negative. The test is positive only in one small subgroup of children and should not be used to make the diagnosis of juvenile arthritis.*

Measuring the RF is an old test that, like ANA, was discovered rather than designed. The original version was the Rose-Waaler test, described in 1948. In this test, it was found that the rheumatoid arthritis patient's sera caused sheep blood cells coated with IgG to clump together. The test has been refined and explored over the years. It measures the presence of IgM antibodies directed against IgG in the blood. This test is very useful in diagnosing an adult with rheumatoid arthritis and must be positive for the patient to be "sero-positive." However, most children with JA are negative. Why these antibodies are present in adults with rheumatoid arthritis remains unclear. It is thought to mean that the IgG in these patients is altered in some way. RF is found in some normal people, people with a variety of rheumatic diseases, and in people with various infections, especially subacute bacterial endocarditis (SBE).

Positive tests for RF in children with bone or joint pain occur in a few specific situations. Adult-onset RA by definition occurs after sixteen years of age. However, since the disease does not always proceed as described in the literature, it occasionally starts earlier. So there are children with true adult-type RA that starts in the early teenage years. This is not common. Children with certain infections, including SBE, also may have a positive RF test, as can children with other rheumatic diseases. A child with joint pains, a positive RF, and a positive ANA should be carefully evaluated for the possibility of scleroderma or mixed connective tissue disease. These conditions are often associated with a positive ANA and a positive RF.

You may hear about "hidden" rheumatoid factor. This is a very confusing subject. Typical RF is IgM directed against IgG. Because IgM has a unique structure that is very large, it is easy to detect these antibodies. Using special techniques, one can measure IgG and IgA antibodies against IgG, which are smaller and not detected by the normal RF test. These "hidden" rheumatoid factors are found in some children with juvenile arthritis. However, these tests are not commonly done, and their proper interpretation remains unclear.

Lyme titer. Lyme disease testing is a key element of the evaluation of any child with arthritis in areas where the disease is endemic. There are many different laboratories doing Lyme testing, and a variety of techniques are used. It is very important that you understand the difference between a screening test and a meaningful positive test. If you have a very good test for a disease that is expensive to perform, you do not want to do it on every child that might have the disease. This is especially true if there is an easier test that will identify children who do not need the costly test. This is the situation for Lyme. The easy test is an ELISA (enzyme linked immunosorbent assay) that identifies antibodies in the blood against spirochetal antigens. *Borrelia burgdorferi* is the agent that causes Lyme disease. It is a spirochete and has spirochetal antigens. However, there are many spirochetes, all of which have spirochetal antigens. Some of these spirochetes are normally found in saliva. *If a child has Lyme disease he or she will have a positive ELISA for antibodies to spirochetes, but so will many children who have been exposed to spirochetes other than Lyme.* All children with a positive ELISA should then be tested on a Western blot. The Western blot determines exactly which spirochetal antigens the antibodies in the child's blood are reacting with. Since it separately tests many different spirochetal antigens, the Western blot can distinguish between antibodies found only in people with Lyme disease and antibodies found in people exposed to other spirochetes. *Thus, a positive Lyme*

ELISA identifies only the people who need to be tested further. A positive Western blot indicates definite exposure to Borrelia burgdorferi, *the spirochete that causes Lyme disease.* The Western blot isn't done on everyone because it is a much more expensive test.

There are several points to remember. A child with a positive Western blot has definitely been exposed to *Borrelia burgdorferi* and needs to be treated for Lyme disease. However, that does not prove that Lyme is the cause of the child's symptoms. Lyme disease and exposure to *Borrelia burgdorferi* are very common in many parts of the United States. Thus, people with other problems may also have a positive test for Lyme, even though Lyme may have had nothing to do with their symptoms. In one study, people who lived in an endemic area for Lyme, who felt well and were shopping in a local shopping center, were asked to give blood specimens for testing. Over 10 percent were positive for Lyme disease. If more than 10 percent of the random population tests positive for Lyme, that means over 10 percent of the people with other problems will test positive for Lyme even though Lyme is not the cause of their problem. *If a child tests positive for Lyme, he or she certainly should be treated. But if the symptoms continue, retreatment may not be the right answer. There may well be another problem.* Conversely, some people worry about having Lyme disease, but test negative. This is unlikely unless the laboratory makes a mistake. It is always a good idea to repeat the test if you are concerned. Treatment and repeated treatment in the absence of a positive test may lead to a delay in the diagnosis of the real problem.

I have seen and treated many children with real Lyme disease. However, the child that stands out was sent to me from an area where many children get Lyme. His test was negative, but he had a very painful hip. Over a period of six months he was treated with antibiotics repeatedly for Lyme disease, without improvement. Then he was referred to me for treatment of difficult Lyme disease. I did further testing and found he had a tumor irritating his hip. Only when we took out the tumor did he get better. The problem was never Lyme disease.

Thyroid function tests are often done in children with joint problems because both excessive thyroid hormone (**hyperthyroidism**) and too little thyroid hormone (**hypothyroidism**) are often associated with diffuse aches and pains. Both hyperthyroidism and hypothyroidism also may be associated with fatigue and muscle weakness. In addition, autoimmune diseases such as SLE may be associated with antibodies that interfere with thyroid function.

The main thyroid function tests are **T3 (triiodothyronine), T4 (thyroxine), and TSH (thyroid-stimulating hormone)**. T3 and T4 are hormones produced by the thyroid gland that regulate the body's metabolism. TSH is secreted by the pituitary gland and influences the function of the thyroid. In children with rheumatic disease, we occasionally see abnormalities of the TSH without T3 or T4 abnormalities. This can be a warning of problems to come. The best way to think of this is as if you were evaluating a car. If the car is going normal speed and the driver is pushing normally on the gas pedal, everything is fine. However, if the car is going too fast and the driver is not touching the gas pedal (high T3 and T4 but normal TSH), something is wrong. If the car is going normal speed, but the driver has depressed the gas pedal all the way, that also suggests problems (normal T3 and T4 but high TSH). Children with SLE and related conditions often develop autoimmune thyroid disease. Normal T3 and T4 with a high TSH may be the first sign.

Some children with autoimmune diseases have high titers of **antithyroid antibodies** for a long period before they actually have thyroid disease. These may be **antithyroid peroxidase antibodies** or **antithyroglobulin antibodies**. Often children with antithyroid peroxidase antibodies have a family history of Hashimoto's thyroiditis. These children should be monitored carefully for the possibility that they, too, may ultimately develop Hashimoto's thyroiditis. Thyroid antibodies are also seen in some children with SLE and occasionally in children with celiac disease and other autoimmune diseases.

Serum protein electrophoresis (SPEP) is a test that measures the pattern of the proteins in the blood. It is a useful test for multiple myeloma, a cancer of the cells that make antibodies. In multiple myeloma, one particular line of cells is causing the problem, resulting in a "monoclonal spike" (a single sharp peak) that can be easily seen on the SPEP. This virtually never occurs in children. In children with rheumatic diseases, the SPEP usually shows a polyclonal (a broad peak) increase. However, the SPEP may detect IgA deficiency or a low level of other immunoglobulins.

Anticardiolipin and antiphospholipid antibodies were first recognized in lupus patients who had bleeding problems. Doctors noted an association between patients with lupus who bled too much because of what was called "the lupus anticoagulant" and false positive tests for a venereal disease (syphilis). When this was examined, it was found that many lupus patients had an antibody that reacted with the cardiolipin backbone of the spirochete that causes syphilis. Further testing led to the description of anticardiolipin and antiphospholipid antibodies.

Anticardiolipin and antiphospholipid antibodies are not identical, but the same information applies to both. These antibodies were first noted in lupus patients with excessive bleeding, but it was discovered they were also present in lupus patients who had problems from blood clotting (deep vein thrombosis, strokes, etc.). Over time the test began to be done on people who had blood clots or bleeding problems who did not have lupus. It turns out that these antibodies are present in some adults and children with a variety of rheumatic diseases as well as people who do not have any other identified autoimmune disease.

The clotting system works by bringing together several different molecules in a carefully regulated activation sequence. If it is too easy for your blood to clot, you will have excessive clotting. If it is too hard, you will bleed too much. So this is a very delicate balance. The anticardiolipin and antiphospholipid antibodies can interact with these clotting molecules (see Chapter 11). However, these antibodies are not all the same. Some have no effect on clotting. Some get in the way and slow down clotting. Others make the molecules stickier and promote clotting that should not happen. If someone is clotting too much, they need to be on blood thinners. If someone is not clotting, that needs to be corrected as well.

One source of confusion comes from finding these antibodies in someone who is not having problems with clotting. No one is sure what to do. If you look at children who have blood clots without any other explanation, most turn out to have anticardiolipin antibodies. However, it is risky to give anticoagulants to people because they can bleed excessively if they fall, are cut, or are in an accident. It appears that most people with anticardiolipin antibodies are at very little risk. Therefore, if the child has never had trouble with clotting, most doctors either do nothing or just give a baby aspirin daily. However, if a child has had a blood clot, most doctors believe he or she should be treated with anticoagulants.

Anticardiolipin or antiphospholipid antibodies can also affect pregnant women. Women known to have anticardiolipin antibodies should be carefully monitored when they become pregnant. Women who have an excessive number of "spontaneous" abortions often turn out to be anticardiolipin antibody–positive. Of course, all women with excessive spontaneous abortions should be checked.

Clotting studies: PT and PTT. Routine clotting studies consist of two tests: the **prothrombin time (PT)** and the **partial thromboplastin time (PTT)**. The PT measures the ability of blood to clot once it is exposed to thromboplastin (a substance that starts clotting). The values are usually 10 to 14 seconds. The PTT measures the ability of blood to clot when left out of the body without being exposed to anything extra to start clotting. The two tests measure different parts of the clotting system which consists of many different factors.

Anticardiolipin antibodies can prolong clotting, as can many drugs. Some children have prolonged clotting times because they either do not make or do not make enough of the clotting factors. Genetic inability to make a clotting factor is the cause of hemophilia. Low levels of clotting factors may be a genetic defect or the result of liver disease. Vitamin K is important for making the clotting factors, and someone who has prolonged bleeding should be given an injection of vitamin K. It is unsafe to operate on children with a significantly prolonged bleeding time without explanation.

HLA B27 is a genetic marker. Our knowledge about HLA B27 serves to demonstrate both how much and how little we understand about the role of genetics in rheumatic diseases. HLA B27 is inherited, and, like other markers, it is common in some populations and rare in others. HLA B27 seems to have arisen out of Asia. It is common among Northern Europeans (e.g., Scandinavians) but also among the Chinese and some North American Indians.

Eight percent of the Caucasian population is HLA B27–positive, but nearly 100 percent of adults with ankylosing spondylitis are positive. The vast majority of people who are HLA B27–positive do not have arthritis. However, if your child is being evaluated for arthritis, finding that they are HLA B27–positive raises the risk of them having a chronic disease and some day progressing to ankylosing spondylitis.

The easiest way to conceptualize this is to view HLA B27 as a multiplier. Thus, if you have no other genetic predisposition to arthritis, being HLA B27–positive is not significant. However, if you have any genetic predisposition to arthritis, HLA B27 doubles that predisposition. Thus the very worst cases are HLA B27–positive, and children who are HLA B27-positive are at increased risk of problems. However, you may have problems because of your genetic predisposition and still be HLA B27–negative, and you may be HLA B27-positive and have no problems because you do not have any other genetic predisposition. (Note: While this is a helpful way to think about the role of HLA B27, we do not know how HLA B27 actually works.)

HLA B27 is strongly associated with ankylosing spondylitis. It is less strongly associated with Reiter's syndrome, the arthritis of IBD, psoriatic arthritis, and other forms of spondyloarthropathies (see Chapter 9). As with all genetic factors that seem to increase the risk of having arthritis, it is logical to ask why the gene has not disappeared from the population. Although all the details are not conclusively proven, it appears that being HLA B27–positive may protect against developing tuberculosis as well as streptococcal and other serious infections. Thus it is beneficial to keep HLA B27 in the population even though it has a negative effect on individuals who have additional genetic factors that predispose them to having arthritis.

Urinalysis

Examination of a urine specimen **(urinalysis)** is the easiest way to evaluate whether or not the kidneys are inflamed or damaged. When damaged, the kidneys can leak red or white blood cells or protein. A typical urinalysis report will describe the **specific gravity**, which reflects how well the kidney is concentrating the urine. This must be evaluated with reference to whether someone has been drinking a lot or is dehydrated. If a person is dehydrated, the urine should be concentrated and have a high specific gravity. If he or she has too much fluid in the body, the urine should be dilute.

Sugar in the urine is called **glycosuria** and is reported as urine glucose on a scale of zero to 4+. Normal people do not lose any sugar in the urine, but diabetics do. Children being treated with high doses of corticosteroids sometimes begin to lose sugar in their urine. If they do, it is an indication that they are moving toward diabetes and efforts should be made to reduce the corticosteroids. **Ketones** are also reported from 0 to 4+. Normally, there are no ketones in the urine. Ketones are an indication that the body is metabolizing fat instead of carbohydrates. In someone who is sick or has not eaten well for a significant period, this is a normal finding. However, in a diabetic it may be a sign of significant trouble. There may be ketones in the urine because someone has not been eating, but there shouldn't be glucose, too. Anyone with ketones and glucose needs to be evaluated by a physician immediately.

Protein in the urine needs to be monitored carefully. Some people have **orthostatic proteinuria**, which means that their kidneys leak protein when they are standing for a prolonged period. This is a common and unimportant condition. This can be determined by checking a morning specimen. After lying down all night, they should not have protein in their urine. Other people have protein in their urine after a lot of physical activity, especially running. This, too, is not significant. However, if the kidneys are damaged and constantly losing a lot of protein, this can result in **nephrotic syndrome**. This is determined by measuring the twenty-four-hour urine protein excretion (see below) or by comparing the excretion of protein to creatinine in a specimen (the protein-creatinine ratio). Children with lupus may develop nephrotic syndrome as a result of kidney damage. Children with amyloidosis, a rare complication of juvenile arthritis, often have protein in their urine and also may develop nephrotic syndrome.

Mild amounts of protein in the urine may be an indication that drugs or other chemicals are irritating the kidney. If protein appears in the urine after a new drug has been started, it needs to be monitored carefully. One problem is that some of the NSAIDs are excreted in the urine and cause a false positive test for protein on the dipstick. This can be determined by having the laboratory perform a more sophisticated test for protein in the urine.

Urobilinogen indicates the presence of bilirubin in the urine. This occurs only in the setting of liver damage or disease that results in an elevated bilirubin level in the blood (discussed above). This may occur in children with **hemolytic anemia** because all the broken-down blood cells are metabolized into bilirubin. Another cause of a positive test for urobilinogen is the NSAID etodolac (lodine). When etodolac is excreted in the urine, it will react with the test strip and give a false-positive test for urobilinogen.

Occult blood in the urine measures the presence of hemoglobin from broken red blood cells. It suggests that there is bleeding somewhere in the urinary tract. This bleeding may be occurring in the kidney or further down the urinary tract. Most often this is associated with the presence of red blood cells (see next paragraph). However, mild bleeding in which all of the cells are broken before leaving the body may show up only as occult blood. Another cause of a positive test for occult blood is myoglobin. Myoglobin is a muscle breakdown product that is detected by the dipstick test for occult blood. Myoglobin can show up in the urine after muscle damage from crush injuries or even vigorous tackle football games. It may also be seen in newborn babies who had a difficult delivery. It is rarely present in children with dermatomyositis.

Red blood cells in the urine are reported as RBC/hpf. This is a simple count of the number of red blood cells per high-powered field when the urine is examined under the microscope. Zero to five is a normal report. Small amounts of blood can be present after vigorous exercise but should go away quickly. While five to ten RBC/hpf may not be significant, investigation is necessary if it is consistently present. The red blood cells in the urine may come from the kidney, the bladder, or anywhere else in the urinary tract. Many different diseases, renal stones, or drugs may cause red blood cells to be present in the urine. This can also be caused by injuries if a child is struck hard in the stomach or on the back. Some children with juvenile arthritis occasionally have blood in their urine without an obvious cause. Blood may also show up in the urine of girls during the time of menstruation. Sometimes a specimen is contaminated with blood just before a girl realizes her period has started. This is not a cause for concern. The specimen simply needs to be repeated after menstruation is over.

White blood cells in the urine are reported as WBC/hpf. Most often a few white blood cells in the urine result from a specimen collected without proper cleaning. However, large numbers of white blood cells or clumps should be considered an indication of infection, and a urine culture should be performed. White blood cells in the urine may also result from irritation of the kidney.

Casts refer to clumps of red or white blood cells in the urine. They are called "casts" because they are clumps of cells that are held together in the shape of the urine tubules. If red or white blood cell casts are present, it is considered an indication of ongoing significant kidney damage. This is most often seen in SLE but can occur in other diseases that damage the kidneys. Hyaline casts are another type of cast but are not significant.

Bacteria in the urine suggest that either the specimen was not collected in a clean manner or that there is a urinary tract infection. If there is a urinary tract infection, it is usually due to a single type of bacteria, while a poorly collected specimen may contain many different types of bacteria. A leukocyte esterase test may help in detecting a urine infection, as the level of leukocyte esterase goes up when the white cells (leukocytes) are trying to fight an infection. However, this is not always a reliable finding.

Some compounds that are excreted into the urine by the body may condense into **crystals**. Uric acid crystals and calcium appetite crystals are very common. If there are a lot of these crystals, one must consider the possibility of kidney stones. These types of crystals are not normally associated with any of the rheumatic diseases.

Twenty-four-hour urine studies are done to determine exactly how much protein, calcium, and creatinine or how many red blood cells are being lost in the urine. This is the best way to quantify the amount, as the dipstick test is relatively inaccurate and may vary from specimen to specimen during the day. However, the twenty-four hour tests are accurate only if the child collects *all* of the urine. This is best done by collecting the specimen over the weekend. The proper procedure is to have the child get up in the morning and throw away the first urine specimen. Then everything is collected including the first specimen the next morning. If you collect on Sunday, you can take the specimen straight to the laboratory for analysis on Monday. If you collect on Saturday, you'll have to keep the specimen in your refrigerator on Sunday. There are expected values that will alert the doctor if most of the urine was not collected. Don't confuse everyone with an unreliable specimen. Just confess and start over. Newer tests that do not require a twenty-four hour collection are being developed.

Testing cerebrospinal fluid

Cerebrospinal fluid (CSF) covers the brain. It is analyzed by performing a lumbar puncture. A synonymous term for lumbar puncture (LP) is a spinal tap. Although this test always sounds scary to parents and children, it is a relatively easy test in most circumstances. The only time it is unsafe to do a lumbar puncture is if there is increased pressure in the brain. This can be detected by examining the patient's eyes for evidence of increased pressure (the pressure may cause bulging of the optic discs at the back of the eye because they are directly connected to the brain). A CAT scan or MRI of the brain may also detect increased pressure.

The fluid that is withdrawn from the lumbar puncture can be analyzed for evidence of infection, irritation of the brain, bleeding, or other disease. The most important reason for the lumbar puncture is make sure there is no infection. In diseases such as lupus that may affect the brain, the child may start acting strangely. Often there is confusion as to whether the strange behavior is due to the drugs being used to treat the lupus, the child's is being upset about being ill, the illness itself, or an infection. Examining the spinal fluid is the only way to be sure there is not an infection.

The report on the CSF will describe its color, which may be reddish or yellow if there has been bleeding. If the tap is bloody, it may indicate that a blood vessel was nicked during the procedure. This is not a major cause of concern. The doctors can tell whether the blood is from the procedure or comes from bleeding in the brain by looking at the cells. Fresh bleeding does not discolor the CSF after the red cells are spun out, and there will be no damaged or "crenated" red cells in the specimen. If there is a lot of fresh blood in the specimen, the number of white cells must be adjusted to account for the white cells that come from the bleeding.

In the absence of infection or irritation, there should be fewer than ten white cells per cubic centimeter or milliliter in the CSF. Large numbers suggest infection. Another check for infection is the Gram stain. This is a test done in the bacteriology laboratory to look for bacteria in the CSF under the microscope. Sometimes a child will have ten to twenty white cells per milliliter in the CSF. This can be from irritation or infection by a virus. It is less likely this is caused by a bacterial infection, but some of the CSF is always sent to the microbiology laboratory for culture just in case. In addition to the cell count the CSF is analyzed for the amount of sugar and protein present. The amount of sugar will decrease if there are bacteria in the specimen. A low sugar level and high protein suggest infection, but a high protein level with a normal sugar level suggests irritation.

Oligoclonal bands are another finding that suggests irritation of the central nervous system. They are sometimes found in lupus and sometimes in multiple sclerosis, but there may be other causes. If the doctors are worried about infections such as Lyme in the central nervous system, they will measure the concentration of antibodies to Lyme in the CSF and compare it with the concentration in the blood. Higher levels of antibodies in the CSF than in the blood suggest Lyme infection of the central nervous system.

Testing synovial fluid

Synovial fluid is the normal lubricating fluid secreted by the cells that line joints (synovium). If synovial fluid analysis is necessary, a needle is inserted into the joint to withdraw fluid for testing. Synovial fluid testing is very similar to CSF analysis except that the normal values are different. Again the most important reason to do this is to eliminate the possibility of infection. Just as someone with a rheumatic disease that affects the brain could still get an infection, children with known juvenile arthritis can still get infections in their joints.

Whenever a doctor first sees a child with a hot, swollen joint, he or she needs to be sure there is no infection present. An experienced physician may be confident that he or she can distinguish a joint that is not infected, but whenever there is real doubt the joint must be aspirated. All the tests done on the synovial fluid are the same as those done to the CSF. However, in the synovial fluid there may be up to 100,000 cells without infection. Less than 5,000 cells are considered normal. Cells numbering 5,000 to 50,000 are consistent with arthritis but can also be seen with Lyme disease and irritation of the joint. Cells numbering 50,000 to 100,000 may indicate arthritis, Lyme disease, or an infection. Greater than 100,000 cells indicates probable infection.

A Gram stain to look for bacteria is always done no matter what the cell count is, and some of the fluid should be sent for culture by the bacteriology laboratory. If tuberculosis is a possibility, special stains should be done on the fluid (it won't show up on the Gram stain). Special culture techniques are also required if the bacteriology laboratory is going to detect tuberculosis. Protein and sugar are measured just as in the CSF.

Doctors also look for crystals in synovial fluid. In adults, this is useful in detecting gout, in which there are uric acid crystals in the joint, and pseudo-gout, in which there are calcium hydroxyappetite crystals in the joint. However, neither of these diseases occurs in children under normal circumstances. If the synovial fluid is bloody, it may indicate that a vessel was nicked during the procedure. However, there is an infrequent disease called **pigmented villonodular synovitis** that causes bleeding into the joint so that the fluid will be bloody. Usually, this is suspected when there is evidence of old blood in the joint. Old blood in the synovial fluid may also come from an injury.

One important source of error in evaluating synovial fluid may occur when the end of the bone near the joint is infected. In this situation the child may be complaining of knee pain, but the synovial fluid does not reveal evidence of an infection. This is correct in that the joint is not infected, but there is an infection in the end of the adjacent bone. This can be discovered by careful physical examination. A bone scan or MRI will reveal the infection in the bone. During the first few days after they start, infections in bone may not be apparent on X rays.

25

Reconstructive Surgery

Rebecca's parents were very nervous. Rebecca had severe arthritis that had affected her hips. Despite multiple medications from a variety of physicians, things had slowly gotten worse over the last year. Now Rebecca was in my office. Rebecca and her family had hoped that I would have a medication to reverse all of her problems and allow her to walk normally again. Unfortunately, it wasn't so. Rebecca's hip pain was so bad that she rarely ventured out of the house except to go to school. She had begun to use a wheelchair to get from class to class in school. Careful review of her X rays made it clear that medications were not going to make Rebecca's hips better. She needed hip replacements.

The family was very resistant to the suggestion that Rebecca's hips be replaced. I carefully explained she would have much less pain and much better function. When I had Rebecca walk down the hall, she had an abnormal gait because of all the hip pain. The family told me that other children had picked on Rebecca because they thought she walked funny. They were very afraid of what would happen if she had her hips replaced. I called out to my office and had one of my volunteers bring in a pamphlet on total hip replacement. The volunteer, a young lady, walked in, smiled, gave me the pamphlet and walked out again. I asked the family whether they had noticed anything. They replied that I was lucky to have such an attractive volunteer working in my office. They were stunned when I said that the volunteer was one of my patients who had had her hips replaced one year earlier. No one could tell that she had had her hips replaced. The only ones who knew were her friends, who saw how much better and how much happier she was after recovering from the surgery.

The goal of every pediatric rheumatologist is to maintain and restore the fullest possible level of function. In an ideal world, every child would receive proper medical attention early in the disease course and respond dramatically to therapy. Unfortunately, in the real world children do not always receive proper medical attention early in the course of their disease. In addition, some of those who do receive proper medical attention nonetheless fail to respond well.

Many parents are afraid of reconstructive surgery. However, the ability to replace severely damaged joints is one of the most dramatic improvements in the long-term prognosis for children with arthritis. I discuss a number of surgical joint replacements below. With all the modern medications, these are rarely necessary for my patients. Moreover, there are very few institutions that have the experienced surgeons and the necessary facilities to perform joint replacements on children and adolescents with rheumatic diseases. The Hospital for Special Surgery, where I work in New York City, has these specialized facilities, and children who need this surgery are often sent here.

At present we have useful replacements for hips, knees, and shoulders. We can also do useful reconstructive surgery on wrists, elbows, ankles, and feet. These surgeries often dramatically relieve pain and improve function. If a child's activities are being significantly limited by the damage to a joint, it should be replaced if possible.

ANESTHESIA

Whenever surgery is done, it is necessary to anesthetize the patient. This means blocking pain from the area. Most joint replacement surgery used to be done under general anesthesia (the patient was put entirely to sleep and a machine would breathe for him or her). For children with severe arthritis, this was always a major problem. They frequently have neck involvement and it is difficult (and sometimes dangerous) to put the necessary breathing tube in so that they can be put under general anesthesia. In the past if a child had severe neck involvement, it might even be necessary to perform a tracheotomy (make an opening in the neck) so that the child could be properly ventilated.

At the Hospital for Special Surgery, almost all of the joint replacement surgery can be done using regional anesthesia. This means that the child does not have to be ventilated by a machine. (We do make sure he or she is "asleep.") This eliminates the risks of injury to the neck that made it so complicated to do joint replacement surgery for children with severe arthritis in the past.

TOTAL HIP REPLACEMENT

Total hip replacement (THR) surgery is one of the most significant advances in the care of children with severe arthritis. Prior to the widespread availability of THR for children, any child with severe arthritis in the hip was simply placed in a wheelchair when the pain became too great. Few were ever able to resume walking. Now we are able to replace the hips of children with severe pain, and wheelchairs have become far less common.

THR surgery is not performed by pediatric orthopedists. Instead, it is necessary to find an adult orthopedist who does THR surgery and who is experienced in working with children. Those with sufficient experience are primarily found only in large academic centers with extensive experience in pediatric rheumatology. In addition, there are relatively few centers that have the sophisticated resources required to manufacture custom hip replacements for small children. The normal outcome of THR surgery is excellent. I care for a number of children and young adults who have had THR surgery. They could walk right past you on the street unnoticed.

Many parents are concerned about the timing of THR surgery. The appropriate time for surgery is as soon as the child's arthritis begins significantly to limit his or her ability to walk around outside the house. If your child's hip pain is such that you are considering asking for a wheelchair, it is time to be asking for THR surgery instead. For all of us it is far easier to be pushed than to walk. For a child with arthritis, this is many times truer than for a normal child. However, as soon as the child begins to use a wheelchair, he or she begins to lose strength in the legs and begins to develop flexion contractures in the knees. Both of these complications make it much more difficult to recover the ability to walk after surgery. The best outcome is obtained when the use of a wheelchair has been minimized or avoided completely.

Parents sometimes hesitate because they are concerned that the child will stop growing if the hip is replaced. It is important to remember, first, that if the hip is so damaged and painful that the child cannot walk, it is not going to grow. Second, two-thirds of the growth in length of the hip bone (femur) occurs at the end where the knee is. That growth is not affected by THR.

Other parents are concerned because they do not know how long the THR is going to last. It is true that the metal and plastic replacement assembly (prosthesis) may ultimately need to be replaced, but confinement to a wheelchair is not a better option. In experienced hands, hip replacements that become loose or otherwise need revision can be fixed repeatedly. The key is to have an experienced surgeon who is familiar with working with children. I have seen children who were denied hip replacement because "hip replacements are not made small enough." At centers such as the Hospital for Special Surgery, we have a custom fabrication unit that can make whatever size prosthesis we need. We have done surgery on children as young as nine years of age and as small as 60 pounds with excellent long-term results.

ARTHROSCOPIC KNEE SURGERY AND KNEE REPLACEMENT

Total knee replacement (TKR) surgery has been very successful in maintaining the ability of children to carry out their activities of daily living. With improved medications and the ability to suppress arthritis in the knees using intra-articular corticosteroids, TKR due to arthritis has become rare in children. Continuing active synovitis in a knee that has not responded to routine medications or intra-articular corticosteroid injection may be treated with an arthroscopic synovectomy (cleaning out the inflammatory material through a small incision in the skin using a special instrument called an arthroscope). This therapy often provides significant relief but may have to be repeated.

Some children develop avascular necrosis in their knees as the result of corticosteroid usage. This is best treated with TKR. Usually, this does not need to be done in small children and does not result in significant loss of growth. As with hip replacements, knee replacements may need revision over time. However, experienced centers can do this when necessary.

ANKLES

The ankle joint is difficult. As of the time of this writing, it is generally better to fuse the ankle than to replace it. Fused ankles force children to walk without bending their ankles (it's clumsy, but it works). Because the joints of the ankle have been fused, they do not move but they do not hurt, either. The mechanics of the ankle joint are relatively complex and we have not found the mechanical replacements satisfactory.

FOOT SURGERY (TARSAL FUSION)

One of the more difficult problems for children with arthritis is involvement of the joints between the tarsal bones of the feet. These joints are important when you walk over an irregular surface or bend your feet. If they become significantly involved by arthritis, it may result in a lot of pain when walking. A surgical procedure called a triple arthrodesis will fuse these bones together. This results in a stiff foot and will cause difficulty when the child walks over an uneven surface, but it will relieve most of the pain.

WRIST SURGERY

The wrist is often significantly involved in children with psoriatic arthritis and some related spondyloarthropathies. It may also be involved in polyarticular onset juvenile arthritis. There are two major problems. One is a wrist that hurts whenever it is bent. Some children get relief of their symptoms by wearing a splint on the wrist. If there is active arthritis, the splint may even result in the wrist fusing itself.

If the splint does not provide adequate relief, it may be necessary to fuse the wrist surgically. This is not a major surgery. The surgeon will fuse the wrist in a functional position to maintain its strength and functionality. If the wrist is not splinted or fused, there is a risk of progressive subluxation and deformity. When this happens, the wrist is permanently bent (usually downward) and loses function.

From time to time I will see children who are developing marked subluxation of their wrists. This subluxation causes the tendons that extend the fingers to rub on the end of the wrist bone on the little finger side (the ulnar styloid). If this is allowed to continue, the tendons sometimes rupture and the patient loses the ability to open the fingers. An orthopedic surgeon can easily remove the end of this bone (the ulnar styloid), which should improve the situation.

SHOULDER SURGERY

The head of the arm bone (humeral head) is called the glenoid. In some children with severe arthritis this can be damaged and limit the ability to raise the arms over the head and perform other activities. This can interfere with dressing and other activities of daily living. Surgical replacement of the glenoid head is easily done in an advanced center.

26

Family Issues

Most of the parents reading this book will not have a child with a serious chronic condition. They can skip this section. However, *if your child does have a significant disability, or you think your child's medical care is starting to take over your life, please read on.*

In one of my families there were three children; the oldest was a twelve-year-old with severe arthritis. The decision was made that he would have a hip replacement after the end of the school year. Both parents were very concerned and everyone knew that Johnny was expected to be in the hospital for five days after the surgery. All of us would have the same initial response: Ask a sitter or a relative to care for Sally and Timmy (8 and 10 years old) so Mom and Dad can be at Johnny's bedside for the five days. Summer travel plans are off, because Johnny will need a lot of physical therapy to recover and will not be able to travel. *This all sounds reasonable, but it's the wrong answer.*

Instead, Grandma came to take care of Sally and Timmy for the first two days. After it was clear that Johnny was recovering as expected, Dad took off with Sally and Timmy on a trip to one of their favorite places. Mom and Grandma relieved each other in the hospital. At the end of a week everyone was back at home feeling they had gotten lots of attention. Further, it was agreed that if Johnny made good progress in physical therapy, the whole family would go off to an amusement park at the end of the summer. Otherwise, Sally, Timmy, and Mom would go, and Dad would stay home with Johnny. Everyone got attention. Everyone had a shared goal. No one felt deprived or held back.

If you have lived with a child with a chronic condition for any period of time, you know that this places a strain on everyone in the family. *Any chronic childhood illness is not the child's problem; it is the family's problem. No one in the family is spared from the impact of the child's disease. If you try to pretend otherwise, everyone suffers.* Everyone will feel the impact of the attention diverted to take care of the ill child, everyone will feel the impact of the financial burden, everyone will feel the impact of missed vacations. Divorce and psychiatric disease are much more common in families of children with chronic illness than in the normal population.

IS THERE ANY ESCAPE?

There is not going to be a single answer that works for everyone. Families are different. Children are different. The degree to which a child's illness interferes with the family will be different. *Still, there are important points of which everyone should be aware.* First, as parents you have more control over the situation than you think, but you have to take control by confronting the situation. Second, ignoring the problem does not make it go away; it makes it worse. I deal with families every day. The successful ones allow everyone in the family his or her own time and space. If everyone in the family is recognized to have important needs, everyone can work together for the good of the whole family. *Do not neglect your healthy children (or spouse) for the sake of the child who is ill. In the end, everyone will be unhealthy because of the psychological problems this causes.*

None of this advice means you should neglect the child who is ill. None of this advice is easy. Having children is hard work. Having a child with a chronic disease makes it much harder. The key to success is allowing everyone to communicate and express his or her feelings. In many families, Mom is in charge of taking care of the children, including all the doctors' appointments and so forth. *Mom often starts to feel overburdened.* The other children often start to feel neglected because of the time it takes for Mom to deal with the needs of the ill child. Dad often starts to feel neglected as well. This will not work if there is a chronic problem.

The families that cope most successfully do so by having everyone pitch in. Sometimes Dad brings the child to the appointment and Mom stays home with the other children. There have to be special activities for everyone. There will be times when everyone makes a sacrifice for the child with disease. Equally, there should be times when everyone gets to go somewhere special as a reward to make up. Life is not fair, but it can be balanced. If you have several children, make sure each one gets the attention he or she needs. *Don't forget to include yourself on the list of people who need attention and special activities.*

WHOSE FAULT IS IT? THE BLAME GAME

Imagine that you and your spouse are going out to the movies on Saturday night. Your spouse gets home late from visiting with friends and everyone has to rush to get ready. By the time everyone has it all together and you get to the movie theater, they've turned down the lights and are showing the previews. The easy-to-reach seats are full and you have to squeeze past a bunch of people to reach two seats together on the side.

As you squeeze past one gentleman. you hear a plop and your foot gets cold. You just knocked over the large soda that he'd set on the floor. "Oh my goodness! I'm so sorry!" You struggle into your seat feeling guilty and wondering whether you should get up and offer to buy him another soda or to give him the money for it. Now you are mad at yourself for knocking over his soda.

In a few minutes, as you think about it, you are mad at your spouse for making you late getting to the theater. If you'd been on time, you would have arrived while the lights were still on and found better seats. Then you are mad at the man who set his soda down on the floor. He should have known better than to put it there and forget to shift it when he saw you moving into his row. The rows of seats shouldn't be so close together in this theater anyway. Who designed this place? Maybe we should not come back here!

It's the blame game! These are all minor issues. It is unfortunate that all of them are true. Nonetheless, no one of these problems is the explanation for what happened. In reality, no one is to blame and everyone is to blame. Trying to assign blame to any individual party won't solve anything. It's just a normal process of rationalization that we all go through. *If you said out loud any of the things you were thinking to yourself, it would just make the situation worse.* Swallow hard and concentrate on moving on, so everyone can enjoy the movie.

It is not the fault of anyone that your child has an illness. No one should feel he or she is being deprived or punished as a result. Devote time to the child with disease, but make sure you devote time to the other children and your spouse as well. Always look for a way to make things special and balanced for everyone. It's hard work. But it's well worth it. If you feel that your family is off to a bad start, sit down with everyone and talk about it.

Think about what you are going to do so that everyone feels attended to. You may need to call on your friends, relatives, and the local community. Do not be afraid to get help when you need it. There are psychologists, psychiatrists, and social workers who are trained specifically in dealing with the families of children who are chronically ill. I hope you do not need them. But if you do, ask your doctor. He or she knows how to get you help. There are many stories of mothers who selflessly devoted their lives to a child with serious disease. Most of them include divorce, unhappy brothers and sisters who did not do well, and a child with chronic illness burdened by guilt over the disruption of the family. Do not let this be you.

GROWING UP IS HARD TO DO

Another difficult situation for families of children with chronic disease is allowing the young adult to accept increasing responsibility and ultimately total responsibility for his or her care. Some hospitals have special adolescent clinics, while others sponsor specialized transition clinics for older children with chronic disease. In most situations, this type of clinic is unnecessary. If the physicians and family have done a good job of preparing them, as they get older the children will naturally make the transition.

The vast majority of my patients have reached the age where they are able to bring themselves to their appointments. Obtaining a driver's license is the only transitioning experience they need. They understand that just as they can drive themselves to the appointments, they are responsible for being sure that their blood tests are done in a timely fashion, the prescriptions are obtained or renewed, and their medications purchased. It's amazing how much more responsible they suddenly become when they can take themselves places.

There are physicians who feel that all patients need to be transferred to an internal medicine specialist once they reach a certain age. It is certainly true that patients need to be cared for by a physician who treats them in a manner that is appropriate for their age. If a physician is unable to adapt to their changing needs as they grow older, the patient should move on. However, many physicians are quite comfortable caring for patients of diverse ages.

If the physician and patient have been working well together and trust each other, it is not necessarily in the patient's best interest to be forced to move on. I have learned a lot about how to deal with younger patients from my patients who have grown up and feel comfortable talking about how they used to feel. If you treat children as responsible participants in their own care from the beginning, nothing necessarily needs to change when they get older.

Some children with debilitating disease are forced to remain dependent on their parents even when they are clearly no longer children. This is always a difficult situation. Some continue to rely on their parents for all types of support, while others recognize that they qualify for appropriate aid for the disabled (social security disability, etc.) and assume responsibility for their own care. If the individual physician is uncomfortable providing the appropriate resources to deal with these issues, it may be best for the patient to be helped through the process by a multidisciplinary team in a transition clinic. However, this is rarely really necessary. Ask your doctor and your local foundations what resources are available to you and pick the course that best meets the needs of your family. Do not be afraid to ask whether they have social workers available who can help you deal with "the system." These people are there to help you.

DEPRESSION (PATIENT FATIGUE)

Katherine was a young lady who had suffered from chronic recurrences of dermatomyositis since the age of six. Although she was always the official patient of one of the senior physicians, many of us took care of her during our training. By the time she reached her late teens, she had experienced more hospitalizations and setbacks than anyone could count. However, when I last saw her she was doing well. Her medications had been reduced to acceptable levels and she was preparing to go to college. I left and moved on to another institution.

Two years later she came to the hospital between scheduled visits complaining of symptoms similar to those she had had during a very difficult period. When she asked whether the symptoms might mean that her disease was flaring, she was told they could. She drove her car into a freeway pillar at high speed that afternoon. No skid marks. Maybe she just lost control?

I have been discussing how hard it is to be the parent of a child with arthritis. *What I have not talked about yet is how hard it is to be the child with arthritis or another chronic condition.* When children are young, their problems are the responsibility of their parents. The children expect their parents to make them better. For most children with arthritis and the related conditions, this is possible. The vast majority of the children I care for go on to live productive lives. However, the adolescent years of increasing self-awareness and increasing self-responsibility are difficult for everyone. They are even more difficult for children with chronic disease.

During the course of a chronic illness, there will be times when a child or young adult becomes depressed. He or she would be abnormal if this never happened. Parents and physicians need to be paying attention. While a certain amount of depression can happen to anyone, it is well known that some adolescents with chronic disease become suicidal. They feel that they have lost control over their lives and cannot see the light at the end of the tunnel. This may take the form of overt actions or simply failure to take their medications. Everyone should be listening for comments such as, "It doesn't make any difference," "I don't care anymore," "Why do I have to go to the doctor?" *Parents and physicians must keep track of whether the medications are being refilled at appropriate intervals.*

No one should try to tell adolescents with chronic disease that they shouldn't complain. It isn't helpful to tell them things could be worse. *What adolescents need is someone to sit down and discuss their concerns honestly.* It is important to acknowledge their problems while pointing out the positives. It is also important to be proactive. If you are a parent and the doctor just gave you and your child depressing news in the office, talk about it. Don't leave your child to "stew alone." *Don't let him hear you complaining about how hard his illness is for you, either.* If you think he is significantly depressed, ask for help. You might be depressed and need help, too.

There are psychologists and psychiatrists who specialize in dealing with adolescents and children with chronic illness and their families. Some children can be dealt with simply by having an honest conversation with their doctor. Others need an outsider to talk to. Some need medication. *It is important to remember that there is no direct correlation between the doctor's view of how well or badly an adolescent is doing and the adolescent's view.* Parents and physicians must be vigilant.

27

Getting the Best Results for Your Child

After I get a family settled down and the child's care on the right track, someone frequently asks, "Why do I have to come back so often?" I always compare this to making soup. Anyone can take down a cookbook, read the soup recipe, and get two pounds of beef, a large onion, a carrot, noodles, assorted seasonings, a good-sized pot, and a stove. However, there is a lot of room for interpretation when the instructions say, "Cut up the beef and slice the carrot and onion thinly. Add the ingredients to a large pot with water just to cover. Heat over medium heat for two hours, adjust the seasonings and serve."

To someone with a lot of experience making soup, those are adequate instructions. If you make soup every day, you know exactly how to do it to get the result you want. But compare two cooks. One cook reads the book, finds the ingredients called for, puts them in a pot of water, sets it on medium heat, and walks away for two hours. The cook who makes soup all the time has picked exactly the beef, onion, and carrot he or she wants and knows how to prepare them for the soup. After the pot is on the stove, the experienced cook checks the soup every ten to fifteen minutes, adjusts the heat, tastes the seasonings, and makes all the other small adjustments that come from experience. Which cook do you think is likely to make the better soup? Similarly, your child's health requires continual monitoring, reevaluation, and adjustments for the best outcome.

This is the most important chapter of this book. Everyone wants the best results for his or her child, but not everyone understands that you have to go out and get them. Reading this book means you are off to a good start. You are looking at this book because you want more information. If you were planning a vacation to Hawaii, it would not be a good idea simply to call the first travel agency you found in the phone book or walk into the first one you saw on the street. Most of us would begin by asking our friends if they or some one they knew had been there. Were they pleased with the trip? What airline did they go on? Where did they stay? What did they see? Who made the arrangements? Similarly, you should invest as much time as possible in picking the specialist to care for your child's disease.

THERE ARE THREE MAJOR DETERMINANTS OF THE OUTCOME OF ANY PROJECT

- Your level of effort and knowledge
- The effort and knowledge of the people who work with you
- Luck

No one can control luck, so it is very important to maximize your efforts and your choice of people with whom to work. First and foremost, you need a primary physician you trust. If you simply picked your doctor from a book or you go to a group where you get a different doctor every time, make sure someone is listening to your concerns. If you think something is wrong with your child, make sure the doctor listens and examines your child carefully.

Remember, growing pains do not occur during the daytime. I've seen far too many children with significant problems dismissed repeatedly as growing pains. Few pediatricians have any training in muscle, bone, and joint diseases. Many think they have never seen a case of arthritis in childhood. Do not be afraid to press your concerns or to seek another opinion. Sometimes you have to insist. This book will help you determine whether there is really something wrong, but it is not a replacement for a good doctor.

CHOOSING A SPECIALIST

Once your primary physician agrees that you need to see a specialist, ask him or her why you are being referred to the one chosen. You should be looking for the best doctor for your child. It may be the one in your plan, the one in the same building, the one in the same group, or the one in the same hospital. Or it may not.

Ask questions! Ask the primary physician whether he or she would take his or her child to the doctor who was recommended for your child's complaints. Ask the specialist about your child, and ask the doctor about himself or herself. If the doctor is uncomfortable answering you or the answers make you uncomfortable, this might not be the right doctor for you. No one doctor is the right one for everyone.

Children with muscle, bone, joint, or arthritis pain often are sent to an orthopedist for a possible injury. If there is no history of an injury, be suspicious. Some orthopedists have little or no experience with childhood arthritis. I often see children with arthritis who were originally told they must have a hairline fracture that did not show up on the X ray. If the problem promptly resolves itself, there is no cause for concern. However, *if the problem keeps coming back, or there are repeated problems in many joints, a more detailed investigation is needed.* The appropriate sections of this book will help you to know when you need to go further.

Finding a specialist on your own is not difficult. In every large urban center, there are organizations such as the Arthritis Foundation, the Lupus Foundation, and the American Academy of Pediatrics (see the Appendix). These organizations can direct you to the certified doctors in your area, but they may not be willing to choose among them. See which doctors are associated with the better hospitals in your area. In major cities, there are often newspapers or magazine articles reporting who are the top doctors. You can even find books listing the top doctors in America. The doctors on these lists are not all the same, but they should be well trained and well regarded in their specialty.

Unless you live in a very small town far away from any large academic center, you want a physician who fulfills the following criteria:

- Is board certified in the specialty
- Preferably is certified in the pediatric specialty (many specialists trained in internal medicine only rarely see children)
- Answers your questions in a way you can understand
- Takes time to explain what is happening
- Treats you and your child in a way that makes both of you comfortable

WHAT IF THE DOCTOR RECOMMENDED ISN'T IN MY INSURANCE PLAN?

You must consider how much your child's well-being means to you and find the best care you can. Muscle, bone, and joint diseases are one area of medicine where the right or wrong decision now can make a difference for the rest of your child's life.

AGGRESSIVE VERSUS CONSERVATIVE APPROACHES

There are physicians who are very active in their fields, who attend the annual scientific meetings of their medical specialties each year, teach at universities, and publish their own work describing advances in the field. Other doctors take care of children the same way they were taught to during their training many years ago. Fortunately, medicine has been making rapid advances over the past five years and there are many new and exciting therapies. You want a physician who is going to make sure your child gets the best possible care. They may not be teaching or publishing, but they should be up-to-date.

There are "aggressive" and "conservative" physicians. *What you want as a parent is a physician who is conservative when appropriate and aggressive when appropriate,* not one who is always aggressive or always conservative. Some muscle, bone, and joint diseases tend to resolve over time. These are best treated conservatively. Some get steadily worse: the longer you wait before you stop them, the more damage accumulates. You need a physician who can tell which is which and respond appropriately. The only way to know what your physician is thinking is to ask. Do not be afraid to ask questions!

Second opinions

One of the most difficult issues for parents is when their child does not seem to be getting better. First, be sure you are doing what the doctor recommended. If you are, let the doctor know your concerns and discuss them with him or her. Parents are always worried about getting a second opinion. A good doctor knows that the child's health is the most important thing. If a family wants a second opinion, a good doctor will not act insulted. Instead, he will encourage the family. However, you should make sure you go to a well-qualified physician for the second opinion.

Ask your doctor. If he or she is confident, you will be sent to someone he or she believes is a valuable source of further information. If your physician is not confident, that may be all the more reason to go. Your relationship with your doctor is a major factor in determining your child's outcome. Make sure you have a good one.

CONFLICTING ADVICE

Conflicting advice is one of the hazards of getting a second opinion. What should you do when you get conflicting advice from two different doctors? Sometimes some of the advice is just plain wrong. However, far more often it reflects different points of view.

> Imagine if you wanted a really good chocolate cake. If you asked all your neighbors to recommend a bakery, they might all agree. More likely, they would recommend several different bakeries. If they all agree, it's easy. But suppose you went to the different bakeries and asked each baker how he made his chocolate cake. They probably would not agree on all the ingredients. However, it's unlikely that any of them would stay in business very long if their cakes did not come out well. Similarly, discuss the difference of opinion with the physician you trust. Often there are varied approaches. Is your doctor flexible? Can he or she explain the choices? *But remember, while either of two different ways to bake a cake may work, a combination of the two often will not.*

Frequently, when I am evaluating children for a second opinion, the parents are quite confused if I give advice different from that of the original physician. Rheumatology is not a textbook science. If there were one correct answer, everyone in the field would agree and life would be simple. Parents feel confronted by the need "to make the right choice" for their child. Yet every physician brings a different level of training and experience to the examining room. As a physician, I can only make sure I explain the plan well, discuss the options, and explain why I prefer the option I recommend.

In some situations, I recommend a course of treatment that is not in the books. If all the answers were in the books, experience wouldn't count. Since I see children from all over the world with difficult conditions, it is my job to be offering the benefit of my experience and testing new ideas. These children were sent to me because the answers in the books didn't work. New therapies that work ultimately make it into the books, but there are often delays of several years between when a new therapy is tested and found to work and when it is described in the books.

Some physicians feel that it is up to the parents to decide which treatment plan to follow. They lay out all the options and say, "You choose." If the physicians with all of their training cannot agree, how can the parents choose? *Physicians must not take away the parents' ability to choose for their child but certainly should accept the responsibility of recommending what he or she thinks is the best course.* Parents, in turn, must decide what makes sense to them and which physician they are most comfortable working with.

There is no easy answer for parents who get conflicting advice. You need to know the doctors' backgrounds and level of training. Is one specialist widely respected in his or her field? Is the specialist someone who is teaching new physicians in the field? Ask these questions. Sometimes the advice that is most difficult to accept is what you really need to hear.

If you ask enough doctors, sooner or later you'll probably find one who says what you want to hear. Is that the best therapy? In the end, it is important to remember that you need to trust your doctor and have faith in his or her recommendations. If you do not, you need a different doctor. Unless you are working with a doctor who is not a specialist in the field, in most situations the quality of your working relationship with your doctor will have a greater impact on the outcome than most other factors.

Often a family will come to me and tell me that they have heard about a different medicine from a friend, neighbor, and so on. I will discuss that medicine with them and tell them why I think it is or is not a good idea. Often it is simply one of many choices. If they are anxious to try it, I'm flexible enough to go along, as long as I believe it is safe to do so. If I do not believe it's a good idea, it's my job to explain why. *If you have questions, get answers. Do not sit still and do nothing.*

FOLLOWING ADVICE AND KEEPING APPOINTMENTS

Mrs. Smith could never understand why Jennie didn't do well. Jennie always seemed to be having some type of joint complaints, but every time Mrs. Smith took her to see a doctor, they wanted to do all sorts of blood tests and make Jennie take medicine. Frequently, she'd fill the prescription because Jennie was complaining a lot. But when Jennie

> wasn't better in two weeks or complained of a stomachache, Mrs. Smith would just stop giving her the medicine and cancel the follow-up appointment. After all, there was no sense in going back to have the doctor see how Jennie was doing on the new medicine; she wasn't taking it. After a few months or a year, Jennie's complaints would increase and Mrs. Smith would go back to the doctor and try another medicine for a few weeks, but none of them ever controlled Jennie's arthritis. Mrs. Smith even tried a couple of different doctors. *You'd think this story couldn't be true, but I've seen and heard it over and over again.*

It may seem obvious, but following your doctor's advice and keeping your appointments are the most important things you can do. All of us are a little bit lazy. All of us want to believe the problem will just go away if we ignore it. But if you smelled smoke in your house, would you just ignore it?

All too often I see children who were supposed to be back in two weeks who come back in six months. They still have the problem. Often the parents will say that the child took a few of the pills, and then had a stomachache, so they stopped. Instead of calling the doctor to discuss the problem, they did nothing until everything got worse again. The more damage you let accumulate, the harder it is to fix. If you do not like the advice, call and discuss it with your doctor or find another doctor. Prescriptions left in pockets or purses and pills sitting in bottles in the medicine cabinet will not fix the problem. You must take responsibility for getting your child proper care.

Every parent is concerned about giving his or her child medication. Every parent is worried about side effects. This is a valid concern. Medicines do have possible side effects. You need to be sure that you are following up with your doctor and that he is monitoring your child appropriately (see Chapter 22). However, imagine how silly it would look to let your house burn down because you are afraid of water damage from the fire hose. The vast majority of children who have done poorly in my experience did so because their parents were afraid of the medications and wouldn't give them. If the doctor thought the medicine was a greater risk than the disease, she would not recommend the medicine. You must follow through if you want to get good results.

PROPER MONITORING

This is a key aspect of your child's care. If your child is on medication, he or she needs to be monitored for possible side effects. Careful monitoring is how physicians minimize problems. The reason for periodic blood tests is to detect problems before they become obvious. Skipping your appointment because your child looks fine to you robs your child of the chance to have a problem detected before it becomes serious. Of course, most children don't experience side effects, but no one knows who will and who will not. By the time your child does not look fine, the problem may have progressed to a serious stage that is not easily reversed.

It's easy to skip the periodic monitoring appointments when your child is off medication. However, the same principle applies. We can never be sure a rheumatic disease is gone forever. If you did not notice your child's problems right away at the beginning, will you immediately notice them coming back? Your specialist is trained to detect the earliest signs of disease activity. Do you want to take advantage of his or her skills or rely on yours? The best results come from both you and your physician, each doing his or her part. You should take your child to his routine follow-up appointments. You should also bring your child to the doctor in between scheduled appointments if you suspect something is going wrong.

DEALING WITH INSURANCE COMPANIES

Dealing with insurance companies is one of the most frustrating aspects of medical care. They have no problem insisting that you make your payments each month. But somehow they often have problems paying you for your claims. Make sure your claim forms are properly completed and promptly sent in. Your insurance company will reject your claim for any mistake. Do not be afraid to call and ask where your money is. Keep a log of your phone calls. Write down the name and telephone extension of each person you talk to. Do not be afraid to ask for a supervisor. Do not take "No" for an answer. Good records are vital.

Following up with insurance companies is a good example of the squeaky wheel getting the grease. Parents who keep after the insurance companies most often get paid. Parents who accept denials or small payments get what they accept. If you need a procedure or medication authorized by the insurance company, keep after them. I often have to get on the phone and sometimes I have to speak to the medical director of the plan. *However, you have to keep pushing the insurance company to move your appeal up the ladder.* Your doctor cannot simply call them. They call the doctor when you've pushed them far enough.

Do not assume that the person on the other end of the phone has any real knowledge of your case. I've had "medical directors" of insurance companies tell me they did not know children could get arthritis. You are not dealing with a group of people who understand your needs and are concerned about your child's health. I've had representatives deny medications because they could not spell them. When I spelled it for the person on the phone she said, "Oh, that's in my computer. It's okay." They simply did not understand how the medication was pronounced and spelled.

When you are dealing with your insurance company, you are dealing with an organization that is trying to make a profit, that means reducing expenses. In many states, there are independent review panels. Often when insurance companies realize it is going to cost more to fight you than to give in, they will give in. You have to make them realize that you are going to fight for what you deserve.

DEALING WITH FRIENDS AND NEIGHBORS

To someone who does not have a child with a chronic problem, this section might sound unnecessary. However, all of us know how hard it is to deal with the questions and the stares when you are out in public with a child who looks or acts "different." My number one goal as a physician is to make it so that no one will be able to tell your child has a problem, but we don't always succeed completely. The hardest part of this is that many people who stare or ask impolite questions are simply well meaning and curious. *They don't realize that they are the ten thousandth person to ask you that same question!* As always, there is no easy way out. However, this is one of those situations where practice makes perfect.

Rule 1. The public does not have a right to your medical information. We have strict confidentiality laws in this country about what your doctors, nurses, and other health care providers can say about your family to the public. You shouldn't be worrying that you have to tell everyone who asks you all your medical information. In fact you have no obligation to answer them at all. However, staring back is likely to create an uncomfortable situation for everyone.

I recommend that you make up an answer that is as short and simple as you can. When you are answering questions from strangers, it does not need to be true. I prefer simple, silly answers so that they realize you are politely telling them to "bug off."

> STRANGER: "Where did that red mark on your child's face come from?"
> PARENT: "That's where the Martian's rocket sled brushed against her as they were rushing to take off." Then turn around and go on with your business.

See how long that conversation lasts! *Your answer can be whatever you want. Practice it day in and day out so that you can say it without thinking and without being bothered.*

This same rule applies when your child is talking to adults and to other children. As your child gets old enough to talk to you about being asked questions, teach him or her what you have learned. First, make sure he or she understands that the illness is not his or her fault. Make sure he or she understands that the illness is not something "bad" about him or her. Then, help your child practice a silly answer to give strangers. Encourage him or her to do this until your child is comfortable with it. Explain that the sillier the answer, the clearer it is that the problem is none of that person's business.

Rule 2. You do have to provide some information to your employer, your baby sitter, your child's teachers, and other professionals with whom you interact. If it's someone who has some "need to know," you will have to give a better answer. However, you still don't have to give the whole long story. I'm a strong believer in educating parents about the different types of arthritis and the different risk factors. But when you are talking to your employer, all you need to say is, "My child has arthritis." If your employer claims to have never heard of that, suggest buying this book! *Remember, educating the public is one of my main goals in writing this book. You don't need to sit there and explain it all. Let people buy this book and read it if they want more information.*

Rule 3. Everyone needs someone to talk to. Don't brush off everyone in your life with the easy answers. It's up to you to decide whom you can truly confide in and take comfort from. If you find someone who is a good listener and supportive, you can confide whatever you think is important. You should explain this to your child as well. However, children are likely to get hurt because of this by someone at some point. It's a normal part of growing up. Try to help your child with deciding whom to talk to, and support him or her if problems arise.

DEALING WITH SCHOOLS

Many children with relatively minor problems escape having significant problems at school. But if your child has a chronic condition that is obvious to everyone or even a mild condition that prevents full participation in physical education, the school will need to know. Some schools are extremely obliging and a quick note saying the student should be allowed to "self-limit" in physical education is sufficient. Other schools follow stricter guidelines.

There are a number of important things to know when dealing with your child's school. The most important is that the Americans with Disabilities Act put all the power on your side. If a few notes and an occasional phone call are all that is needed, it's great. However, if the school is being difficult, you may need an individual education plan (IEP), as described later in this section.

For most children with mild to moderate disease, everything can be handled easily. Often children need some leeway in physical education and perhaps a second set of books so they do not have to carry a heavy load of books back and forth to school. A quick note from the doctor's office is often sufficient. If there are going to be a lot of missed classes, if your child needs extra time to get from class to class or extra time on exams because of difficulty writing, you'll probably need an IEP. In most districts, this is not a major problem. However, IEPs take time and effort and often cost the school district money. If the school administration discourages you from asking for an IEP because "you do not want to label your child," make sure you are getting what you need. If you are, great! Otherwise, push for the IEP.

What is an IEP? This is a formal meeting at which you present your position regarding the needs of your child. You are entitled to have a parent advocate present with you at the meeting. The teachers, the administration, and the counselors will also be there to help devise a good plan for your child. The school district is supposed to supply whatever is necessary to facilitate your child's education. Some parents go too far, but some school districts resist senselessly. You should certainly get your child's basic needs met. Do not be afraid of this process. It's designed with your child's best interests in mind. Moreover, the rules are slanted in your favor. But some school districts "forget" to tell you what you and your child are entitled to. Wise parents have spoken with their physician and their local specialty society before the meeting. If necessary, there are even lawyers who specialize in representing parents at IEP meetings. Fortunately, they are rarely necessary.

LOCAL HELP ORGANIZATIONS

There are local help organizations for parents of children with a wide variety of conditions. See the Appendix for a listing. These organizations can be very helpful in directing you to other parents who have had similar experiences. They can provide useful information regarding the nature of your child's condition, experienced doctors, and other resources. They can also help you to find experts for dealing with the many problems of insurance, school, and so on. Many of the national help organizations now have Web sites, as well.

THE ULTIMATE RESPONSIBILITY FOR YOUR CHILD'S OUTCOME RESTS WITH YOU

We are all little kids at heart. We would like someone to come along and play parent and take responsibility for all of our problems. Unfortunately, that is not going to happen. As I said at the beginning of this chapter, the outcome of every project is a combination of hard work, picking the right team, and good luck. You must do the hard work. You must pick the right team. This means you must carefully choose the doctors who take care of your child. Once you have chosen them, you must follow their advice. If you do not understand or do not like the advice, ask questions. Get answers. If you are not satisfied, get a second opinion. Then ask more questions.

You must decide how far you are willing to go to get the answers. I have children who fly in to see me from countries halfway around the world because their parents want the best. On the same day, I may see a mother who tells me that it took her an hour to drive into Manhattan from the suburbs and that "it's too much trouble."

There are parents who for years have continued seeing doctors who were not taking good care of their children. There are other parents who simply went on seeking second opinions until they found someone willing to say what they wanted to hear—even though it was wrong. *Even after you have found a doctor that makes you comfortable, you have not transferred the responsibility for your child's outcome to the doctor. You must make sure your child takes the medicine, does the exercises, keeps the appointments, gets the blood tests, and gets the treatments needed.* It's not easy to find the time. It's not easy to pay for. It's not easy to take on the responsibility. It's not fun. It's not fair. But if you want the best outcome, it's not optional.

It is extremely difficult to have a child with any kind of chronic illness. It is an extremely heavy burden for many parents to bear. You have to educate yourself and navigate the fine line that allows you to get the best outcome for your child. Never be afraid to ask questions. Never be afraid to find another doctor if your doctor seems afraid or too busy to answer. Raising children is hard work. Raising children with an illness is harder. Remember, there are many people and resources out there that will be happy to work with you. You have to find them. You have to ask for help. They won't come looking for you.

28

What Else Can I Do?

This is a question every parent wants to be able to answer. I hope you are already doing everything you can for your child. What else can you do? *You can help others!* There are many volunteer organizations around the world that work with children and families with rheumatic diseases. Many of them are listed in the section on resources that follows. If you have time, energy, or resources left over after dealing with your child's problems, you can help. Every volunteer organization needs more help in whatever way is possible.

I'm not going to tell you which organization to donate to or how. That is an individual decision. You should ask your physician which organizations are the most helpful for his or her program. You may want to donate to research, teaching, or patient care. You may wish to restrict your funds or make them available for any purpose.

As you think about how to help, let me make a few simple points.

- Children with arthritis don't get the attention they should in physician education, research spending, or the public eye. Can you help?

- Many organizations are focused on "finding the cure." Wouldn't it be nice if we could say we funded the research that solved the problem? Indeed, it would! *However, the biggest problem is the lack of public awareness. Most children I see who do poorly do so because it took too long for everyone to realize they had a rheumatic disease. Then it took too long for their parents to find a physician who was educated in diagnosing and treating these diseases.* There is a great need for money to be spent on educating physicians about childhood arthritis.

- You can direct your efforts to improving research, improving education, improving access to care, or any combination of these efforts. These problems exist in every country of the world. Proper treatment by an educated physician will solve the problems of more than 98 percent of the children with musculoskeletal diseases. But there aren't enough educated physicians in the world.
- Just as I've encouraged you to go out and get the necessary care for your child, we all need to go out and get the necessary resources for the care of all the world's children. Of course, there are problems other than musculoskeletal disease, but this is the area of my interest. It's not appropriately recognized and it is clearly underserved.
- Have you written your congressman lately? Do they know children get arthritis?

All of us can do more. Someone reading this book may have a million dollars to donate. More likely, you are like the rest of us. You don't have a million dollars to donate. Do you have the time to talk to parents of another child with arthritis who are confused and uncertain where to turn? Do you have the time to help in another way?

I do not know how we will cure the rheumatic diseases or who will discover the key. I do know that I can help by increasing public and physician recognition of children with arthritis and encouraging the prompt referral of these children to an appropriate specialist. I do not know what you personally can do to help. But I do know that if you take a few minutes to think about it, you will be able to think of something you can do. Do it!

Appendix: Resources

There are thousands of organizations, Internet sites, books, and similar resources for families of children with musculoskeletal diseases and other problems. There is no way I could list all of them here. I have listed the major organizations and others with which I have worked. I'm sure this list is incomplete. Many of these organizations have a Web page that may direct you to many others. I have also listed some Internet-based groups that provide support for children with chronic illness and their parents. But be careful: some of the information on the Internet is excellent, but much of it is not reliable.

My own Web page is the pediatric rheumatology home page: http://www.goldscout.com.

There is more information in this book than I can put there, but I regularly update that site with the latest information.

Organizations Dedicated to Helping Children with Musculoskeletal Diseases

Organizations Without a Specific Disease Focus

National Institute of Arthritis and Musculoskeletal and Skin Diseases
(301) 495-4484 or (877) 22-NIAMS (toll free)
Information Clearinghouse
National Institutes of Health
1 AMS Circle
Bethesda, MD 20892-3675
http://www.niams.nih.gov

The Food and Drug Administration (FDA)
(888) INFO-FDA (1-888-463-6332)
U.S. Food and Drug Administration
5600 Fishers Lane
Rockville, MD 20857-0001
http://www.fda.gov

The American Academy of Pediatrics
(847) 434-4000
National Headquarters:
The American Academy of Pediatrics
141 Northwest Point Boulevard
Elk Grove Village, IL 60007-1098
http://www.aap.org

The American College of Rheumatology
(404) 633-3777
1800 Century Place, Suite 250
Atlanta, GA 30345
http://www.rheumatology.org/index.asp

The American Academy of Orthopedic Surgeons
(847) 823-7186 or (800) 346-AAOS (toll free)
6300 North River Road
Rosemont, IL 60018-4262
http://orthoinfo.aaos.org

Organizations Dedicated Primarily to Arthritic Conditions:
juvenile rheumatoid arthritis, spondyloarthropathy, ankylosing spondylitis, psoriatic arthritis (information on other conditions may be found at some)

The Arthritis Foundation
(800) 283-7800
Arthritis Foundation
P.O. Box 7669
Atlanta, GA 30357-0669
http://www.arthritis.org

The American Juvenile Arthritis Organization (AJAO)
http://www.arthritis.org/events/ajao_programs_services.asp
is now part of the Arthritis Foundation and may be accessed via its contact numbers.

The Arthritis Society of Canada
(416) 979-7228
The Arthritis Society (National Office)
393 University Avenue, Suite 1700
Toronto, Ontario M5G 1E6
Canada
http://www.arthritis.ca

Arthritis Insight
http://www.arthritisinsight.com
This is a Web-based, question-and-answer site with information for children and adults.
The children's info is at http://jraworld.arthritisinsight.com.

Creaky Joints
http://www.creakyjoints.com
This is a site for children, teenagers, and young adults to share ideas, complaints, and the knowledge that they aren't the only ones in the world with arthritis.

The Spondylitis Association of America
(800) 777-8189
14827 Ventura Blvd., #222
Sherman Oaks, CA 91403
http://www.spondylitis.org
This group works with persons with ankylosing spondylitis and with spondyloarthropathies.

National Psoriasis Foundation
(503) 244-7404 or (800) 723-9166 (toll free)
6600 SW 92nd Ave., Suite 300
Portland, OR 97223-7195
http://www.psoriasis.org

Organizations Dedicated Primarily to Vasculitic Diseases:

systemic lupus erythematosus, scleroderma, Kawasaki disease, dermatomyositis

The Lupus Foundation of America, Inc.
(301) 670-9292
1300 Piccard Drive, Suite 200
Rockville, MD 20850-4303
http://www.lupus.org

Juvenile Scleroderma Network, Inc.
(310) 519-9511 (phone or fax)
24-hour helpline: (888) 881-2848
1204 West 13th Street
San Pedro, CA 90731
http://www.jsdn.org

The Scleroderma Foundation
(978) 463-5843 or (800) 722-HOPE (4673) (toll free)
12 Kent Way, Suite 101
Byfield, MA 01922
http://www.scleroderma.org

Raynaud's Association
(914) 682-8341; fax (914) 946-4685
94 Mercer Avenue
Hartsdale, NY 10530
http://www.raynauds.org

Kawasaki Disease Foundation
(978) 887-9357
6 Beechwood Circle
Boxford, MA 01921
http://www.kdfoundation.org

The American Behcet's Disease Association
(800)-7behcets
P.O. Box 19952
Amarillo, TX 79114
http://www.behcets.com/home.ivnu

Sjogren's Syndrome Association
(800) 475-6473
8120 Woodmont Ave., Suite 530
Bethesda, MD 20814
http://www.sjogrens.org/

The Myositis Association
(202) 887-0082
1233 20th St. NW, Suite 402
Washington, DC 20036
http://www.myositis.org

Organizations Dedicated to Other Diseases:
fibromyalgia, chronic fatigue syndrome, etc.

The American Association for Chronic Fatigue Syndrome
(206) 781-3544
515 Minor Ave., Suite 18
Seattle, WA 98104
http://www.aacfs.org/html/contact.htm

The Chronic Fatigue and Immune Dysfunction Syndrome Association
(800) 442-3437
The CFIDS Association of America, Inc.
P.O. Box 220398
Charlotte, NC 28222-0398
http://www.cfdis.org/contact/contact-us.asp

The American Fibromyalgia Syndrome Association
(520) 733-1570
AFSA, Inc.
6380 East Tanque Verde, Suite D
Tucson, AZ 85715
http://www.afsafund.org

The National Fibromyalgia Association
(714) 921-0150
2238 N. Glassell Street, Suite D
Orange, CA 92865
http://fmaware.org/index.html

The Pediatric Network
http://www.pediatricnetwork.org/index.htm
This site is intended for children with fibromyalgia, chronic fatigue syndrome, and related conditions and their families.

Specialized Laboratories for Rheumatic Disease Testing
(not a complete list)

Rheumatology Diagnostics Laboratory
(310) 253-5466 or (800) 338-1918 (toll free)
RDL, Inc.
10755 Venice Boulevard
Los Angeles, CA 90034
http://www.rdlinc.com/

Specialty Laboratories
(800) 421-7110
2211 Michigan Avenue
Santa Monica, CA 90404-3900
http://www.specialtylabs.com/contact_us.asp

Prometheus Laboratories, Inc.
(888) 423-5227
5739 Pacific Center Boulevard
San Diego, CA 92121-4203
http://www.prometheuslabs.com/

Mayo Medical Laboratories
Multiple sites and phone numbers.
See the Web page for details for your area.
http://www.mayoreferenceservices.org/mml/index.asp

Miscellaneous Resources

Individual Education Plans (504). There are many organizations discussing IEPs found on the Web but I don't have any recommendation for a particular one.

"A Guide to the Individualized Education Program by the Office of Special Education and Rehabilitation Services U.S. Department of Education." July 2000. http://www.ed.gov/offices/OSERS/OSEP/Products/IEP_Guide

Parent Advocacy Coalition for Educational Rights
(952) 838-9000
8161 Normandale Boulevard
Minneapolis, MN 55437
http://www.pacer.org

Other School-Related Issues

"Bandaids and Blackboards"
Joan Fleitas, Ed.D., R.N, Associate Professor of Nursing
Fairfield University
Fairfield, Connecticut 06430
http://www.faculty.fairfield.edu/fleitas/contents.html
This site is dedicated to helping children with chronic disease and their parents deal with school-related issues.

Information for Patients on Various Medical Procedures

The virtual hospital total hip replacement page:
http://www.vh.org/adult/patient/orthopaedics/hipreplace/index.html

The virtual hospital total knee replacement page:
http://www.vh.org/adult/patient/orthopaedics/kneereplacement/index.html

The virtual hospital has a variety of other useful pages found at
http://www.vh.org

Textbooks for Physicians

Cassidy, J., and R. Petty. *Textbook of Pediatric Rheumatology*, 4th ed. Philadelphia: W.B. Saunders, 2001. This is the standard textbook. All of the rheumatic diseases discussed here are covered, with many references.

Isenberg, David A., Patricia Woo, and P.J. Maddison, eds. *Oxford Textbook of Rheumatology*, 2nd ed. Oxford Medical Publications. New York: Oxford University Press, 1998.

Anderson, Steven J., and J. Andy Sullivan, eds. *Care of the Young Athlete*. Rosemont, IL: American Academy of Pediatrics and American Academy of Orthopedic Surgeons, 2000.

Greene, Walter B., M.D., ed. *Essentials of Musculoskeletal Care*, 2nd ed. Rosemont, IL: American Academy of Pediatrics and American Academy of Orthopedic Surgeons, 2001.

Other Books for Parents

Aldape, Virginia Tortorica, and Lillian S. Kossacoff. *Nicole's Story: A Book About a Girl with Juvenile Rheumatoid Arthritis*. Minneapolis, MN: Lerner Publications, 1996.

Horstman, Judith, William J. Arnold, Brian Berman, J. Roger Hollister, and Matthew H. Liang eds. *The Arthritis Foundation's Guide to Alternative Therapies*. Atlanta: Arthritis Foundation and Longstreet Press, 1999.

Lockshin, Michael. *Guarded Prognosis: A Doctor and His Patients Talk About Chronic Disease and How to Cope with It*. New York: Hill & Wang, 1998.

Wallace, Daniel J., and Janice Brock Wallace. *All About Fibromyalgia.* New York: Oxford University Press, 2002.

Wallace, Daniel J. *The Lupus Book: A Guide for Patients and Their Families.* New York: Oxford University Press, 2000.

Lane, Nancy E., ed. *The Osteoporosis Book.* New York: Oxford University Press, 1998.

Glossary

amyloidosis: A rare condition of abnormal protein deposition that may damage the kidneys or other organs. Although often described in the old literature, it rarely affects children with arthritis in the modern era

aortitis: Inflammation of the aorta. The aorta is the main blood vessel carrying blood out from the heart to the rest of the body. Although it can be inflamed in many places, most often it is inflamed right at the junction with the heart. This produces inflammation of the valves, which may leak as a result.

arthralgia: Pain around the joint without swelling, redness, or limitation of motion as required for the definition of arthritis.

arthritis: Pain, swelling, redness, or limitation of a joint (any two). There are two types of arthritis. Osteoarthritis is a mechanical problem that results from injury or gradual wear and tear. Inflammatory arthritis is the result of an abnormal response by the tissues that make up the joint, as if there was an infection present. Most cases of inflammatory arthritis in childhood are "idiopathic," meaning we do not know its cause. This is the most common type of arthritis in children.

biologics: Injectable medications that include in their makeup either antibodies directed against human molecules or receptors for human molecules. These antibodies or receptors are usually produced by living cells in culture.

bisphosphonates: A group of drugs that serve to prevent the removal of calcium from the bones. The result over time is that patients with osteoporosis who are treated with bisphosphonates have fewer fractures than those who are not treated. However, the drugs are not safe in pregnancy and are cleared only slowly from the body. Thus, the safety of their use in someone who might become pregnant is uncertain.

bone scan: A specialized test using a radioactive tracer that is taken up by bone cells. Since irritated bone cells are more active, increased accumulation of the tracer is characteristic of infections, fractures, and arthritis or bone tumors (see Chapter 24).

CAT scan: A computer-assisted tomogram. This is an X ray–based technique that allows physicians to see bony structures in much greater detail. Because it uses X rays, it is better for seeing bones than the MRI (see Chapter 24).

celiac disease: This is an inherited condition in which the child is intolerant of the gluten found in wheat, barley, rye, etc. It is the result of an inherited defect where the immune system attacks the structure of the small intestine whenever gluten-containing foods are eaten. This syndrome has a wide variety of possible symptoms, including muscle, bone, joint, and arthritis pain (see www.niddk.nih.gov/health/digest/pubs/celiac).

chelating agent: A chemical that reacts with another chemical, binding to it and inactivating it. An arthritis medicine that works as a chelating agent binds to an inflammatory molecule and prevents it from causing inflammation.

chimera: A monster in Greek mythology composed of different animals. Many of the new biologics are antibodies against messenger molecules that are normally present in the body. Once an antibody that recognizes the messenger molecule is made in an animal, scientists try to make a version that can be given to patients. If part of the original animal antibody remains, the biologic is chimeric (part man: part animal). If a person being treated with the biologic in turn makes an antibody against the animal portion of it, this is termed a human anti-chimeric antibody (HACA). These are important because they reduce the effect of the biologic being used as treatment.

controlled clinical trial: A study in which two groups of patients with disease of similar severity are given different treatments. Ideally, these trials are "double blind, placebo controlled," meaning that neither the doctor or patient knows which treatment is being given to which patient.

cyclooxygenase inhibitor: Typical nonsteroidal anti-inflammatory drugs that block the action of cyclooxygenase. Cyclooxygenase is the enzyme that converts prostaglandins into inflammatory mediators that cause pain, redness, and swelling.

epiphysis: The end of a long bone, making up the joint, that is separated from the middle of the bone (the shaft) by the growth plate. When the growth plate closes, the epiphysis is united with the main bone. Damage to the epiphysis slows growth and limits mobility.

"fully humanized antibody": If an antibody has been "humanized," it means it has been carefully modified to look to the human immune system as if it was made in the human body. This is in contrast to chimeric antibodies (see **chimera** above for more information).

glenoid: The top, rounded part of the bone where the upper arm joins the body at the shoulder.

growth plate: The growth plate is the junction between the middle of the bone (the shaft) and the end of the bone. Adults do not have a growth plate because they have finished growing. However, in children, the growth plate appears on X rays as an irregular dark line across the bone. The major bones of the body have growth plates near both ends.

heliotropic: Literally, "sun loving." It refers to a rash in children with dermatomyositis that occurs in areas that are exposed to the sun, typically on the face and the eyelids.

hirsutism: Increased growth of hair on the body.

immunomodulator: A drug or chemical that alters the activity of the immune system to make it either stronger or weaker.

MRI: Magnetic resonance imaging is a specialized study that uses nuclear magnetic resonance to map the positions of water molecules in the body, allowing a very accurate picture of the soft tissues, constructed with the aid of a computer (see Chapter 24).

myoglobin: A muscle breakdown product. Under normal circumstances, it is rapidly cleared from the body. In someone with extensive muscle damage from myositis or a crush injury, increased levels of myoglobin may show up in the blood or urine.

necrotizing enterocolitis: A severe inflammation of the lining of the intestines; requires immediate medical attention

nemaline myopathy: An uncommon, inherited muscle disease that causes progressive weakness. It is diagnosed by a muscle biopsy that shows a specific pattern of abnormal muscle cell structure.

night splints: Splints used to hold the legs (or arms) out as straight as possible in order to prevent worsening of flexion contractures at the knee (or wrist). They are typically fashioned by making a cast as if the child had fractured the bone. This is allowed to dry, then cut lengthwise so it can be taken on and off. Called night splints or night resting splints because they are used when the child is in bed, they are uncomfortable, but important. They do not make the flexion contractures get better, but they prevent them from getting worse.

nocturia: The need to urinate during the night.

NSAIDs: Nonsteroidal anti-inflammatory drugs, such as ibuprofen (see Chapter 22).

onycholysis: Lifting off of the end of the finger nail due to inflammation. Often associated with psoriasis, it can occur as the result of allergies, infections, drug effects, and other conditions.

osteoarthritis: Arthritis that comes with age. It is due not to the body mistakenly thinking there is an infection, but to gradual wear and tear on the joints from years of use. Some people get it at an early age because they abused their joints or because their joints are not made up of the best material. Children do not get osteoarthritis.

osteopenia: The condition of having bones with insufficient calcium deposits.

osteoporosis: The condition of having a much more significant degree of bone weakness than in osteopenia. It results from either too little calcium being deposited in the bones or too much calcium being taken out of the bones.

penetrance: A term used by physicians when discussing genetic conditions. When genes were discovered that indicated whether or not a child had a disease, in some cases children were found who had inherited the gene for the disease although they did not have the symptoms. This is called incomplete penetrance.

pericardial effusion: A collection of fluid in the pericardium (the sack which contains the heart). Small ones are not important, but large ones may interfere with heart function.

pigmented villonodular synovitis: A rare orthopedic condition in which abnormal synovial tissue bleeds repeatedly, diagnosed on the basis of an MRI and confirmed by a synovial biopsy.

placebo effect: The positive effect gained by thinking one is doing something helpful (even if one is not). The classic example is the improvement in complaints noted by people taking pills that contain nothing but sugar. Interestingly, in many large studies it has been shown that almost one-third of people with bone and joint complaints will improve when given placebo. There is also the **nocebo effect**, which is when people taking pills that contain nothing but sugar complain of being made worse or developing side effects.

plasma: When it first comes out of the body, blood contains red blood cells, white blood cells, platelets, and many different chemicals. If the blood is prevented from clotting and the cells are removed by centrifugation, the clear fluid left is termed "plasma." If the blood is allowed to clot, then the clear fluid left is termed "serum"; see below.

prostaglandins: A group of chemicals synthesized by the body from fatty acids. Many play a role in inflammation, while others are hormones and chemicals that regulate other processes.

proteinuria: The loss of protein into the urine. Very small amounts can occur in many situations, but larger amounts may be a symptom of illness affecting the kidneys and lead to damage.

pseudoporphyria: Porphyria is a serious disease that causes sun sensitivity, abdominal pain and madness (King George III is supposed to have had it). Pseudoporphyria refers to the development of an unusual rash when people taking certain drugs are exposed to the sun. NSAIDs cause this in a small percentage of children who take them (see chapter 22).

reticulocyte: In the body, the average red blood cell lasts 120 days. Thus, new red blood cells are constantly being made and old ones destroyed. When they are very young, red cells are larger and have a darker color when stained. These young red cells are called reticulocytes. Normally, they make up 8 percent of the red blood cells. If more reticulocytes are present, there is an abnormal loss of red cells due to bleeding or destruction that is more rapid than normal.

sausage digit: A finger or toe in which the entire digit is swollen, not just the part around the joints. This is a frequent early finding in children with psoriatic arthritis, but it is usually mistaken for an injury that fails to resolve. When it doesn't get better with time or antibiotics, the child may be sent to a surgeon for a possible tumor. This should be avoided. It is a common finding in children with arthritis, which needs to be treated with anti-inflammatory drugs (see Chapter 9).

sclerodactyly: Tightening of the skin over the fingers.

serial casting: Used to reduce flexion contractures. Because muscle spasm plays an important role in causing the contractures, it is important to relax the muscles as much as possible and then extend the joint. With serial casting the muscles are relaxed and then the leg (or arm, less frequently) is placed in a cast for 24–48 hours. This allows the muscles to relax. When the cast is cut off it is often possible to extend the leg further. When this is done repeatedly to reduce a flexion contracture it is called serial casting.

seronegative, seropositive: Used with many different blood tests, this term refers to whether the test is positive or negative. An adult patient with rheumatoid arthritis who tested negative for rheumatoid factor would be "seronegative." If the patient tested positive, he or she would be "seropositive."

serum: What is left when blood is removed from the body and allowed to clot and the clot is removed. It differs from plasma because some of the chemicals present in plasma are used up when the clot forms and are not present in serum.

sickle-cell disease: A disease in which the hemoglobin molecule is defective (HbS) and tends to deform (sickle) under certain conditions. People with one gene may have bone pain and joint damage under certain circumstances. People with two genes often have serious problems.

somatization: The expression of something in the body. Thus, a somatization disorder is a disorder in which a problem (which may not be a physical one) is incorporated into the body and expressed as a physical problem. It is important to understand that this is not a conscious decision.

spirochete: A type of long, slender bacteria. There are a large number of spirochetes found in various parts of the body that do no harm. However, the organism causing Lyme disease (*Borrelia burgdorferi*) and the organism causing syphilis (*Treponema pallidum*) are both spirochetes.

telangiectasia: A small area of abnormal blood vessel growth that results in a red spot that may be visible on the skin. (Imagine a small normal blood vessel as a length of yarn and a telangiectasia as a knot.)

thalassemia: A type of disease in which there is a genetic abnormality of hemoglobin production. Because there are two different genes for different parts of the hemoglobin molecule and everyone has two of each gene (thus, four involved genes), there are varying degrees of seriousness. In some cases, persons with one good gene and one abnormal gene have low levels of hemoglobin and no other problems (thalassemia minor). People with two defective genes or the wrong defective genes have much worse problems (thalassemia major). Because blood cells are made in the bone marrow, conditions that cause increased blood cell production may cause pain in the bones or cause the bones to have abnormal structure.

thyroiditis: Inflammation of the thyroid gland. This may be due to a variety of problems including the production of autoantibodies in some rheumatic diseases. Depending on the cause and stage of the inflammation, the thyroid gland may produce too much or too little thyroid hormone. Either can produce symptoms that include muscle, bone, or joint pain.

tryptophan (L-tryptophan): An essential amino acid promoted to improve health for a variety of reasons. Unfortunately, improperly made L-tryptophan was widely sold and caused a large number of people to become ill with a syndrome that resembled eosinophilic myalgia (see Chapter 23).

urethritis: Inflammation of the very end of the urinary tract (the urethra). Because the inflammation is at the very end, it is often associated with pain on urination.

Waldenstrom's macroglobulinemia: A rare form of chronic cancer of the plasma cells. It is associated with Sjogren's syndrome in adults, but rarely, if at all, in children.

Index

NOTE: Readers looking for medications and treatments for conditions are advised to look under the name of the condition. Page references in **bold** refer to primary treatment of topics. Page references in *italics* refer to text boxes and illustrations.